Patient voices in Britain, 1840–1948

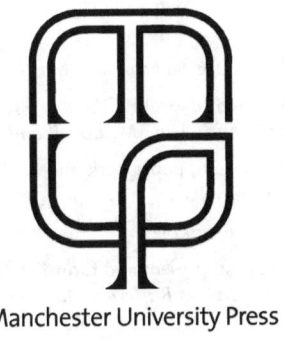

Manchester University Press

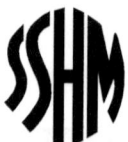

## SOCIAL HISTORIES OF MEDICINE

Series editors: David Cantor, Elaine Leong and Keir Waddington

*Social Histories of Medicine* is concerned with all aspects of health, illness and medicine, from prehistory to the present, in every part of the world. The series covers the circumstances that promote health or illness, the ways in which people experience and explain such conditions, and what, practically, they do about them. Practitioners of all approaches to health and healing come within its scope, as do their ideas, beliefs, and practices, and the social, economic and cultural contexts in which they operate. Methodologically, the series welcomes relevant studies in social, economic, cultural, and intellectual history, as well as approaches derived from other disciplines in the arts, sciences, social sciences and humanities. The series is a collaboration between Manchester University Press and the Society for the Social History of Medicine.

*Previously published*

Migrant architects of the NHS *Julian M. Simpson*

Mediterranean quarantines, 1750–1914 *Edited by John Chircop and Francisco Javier Martínez*

Sickness, medical welfare and the English poor, 1750–1834 *Steven King*

Medical societies and scientific culture in nineteenth-century Belgium *Joris Vandendriessche*

Vaccinating Britain *Gareth Millward*

Madness on trial *James E. Moran*

Early Modern Ireland and the world of medicine *Edited by John Cunningham*

Feeling the strain *Jill Kirby*

Rhinoplasty and the nose in early modern British medicine and culture *Emily Cock*

Communicating the history of medicine *Edited by Solveig Jülich and Sven Widmalm*

Progress and pathology *Edited by Melissa Dickson, Emilie Taylor-Brown and Sally Shuttleworth*

Balancing the self *Edited by Mark Jackson and Martin D. Moore*

Global health and the new world order *Edited by Jean-Paul Gaudillière, Claire Beaudevin, Christoph Gradmann, Anne M. Lovell and Laurent Pordié*

Accounting for health: Calculation, paperwork and medicine, 1500–2000 *Edited by Axel C. Hüntelmann and Oliver Falk*

Women's medicine *Caroline Rusterholz*

Germs and governance: The past, present and future of hospital infection, prevention and control *Edited by Anne Marie Rafferty, Marguerite Dupree and Fay Bound Alberti*

Leprosy and identity in the Middle Ages: From England to the Mediterranean *Edited by Elma Brenner and François-Olivier Touati*

# Patient voices in Britain, 1840–1948

Edited by Anne Hanley and Jessica Meyer

MANCHESTER UNIVERSITY PRESS

Copyright © Manchester University Press 2021

While copyright in the volume as a whole is vested in Manchester University Press, copyright in individual chapters belongs to their respective authors.

Electronic versions of Chapters 1 and 2 are also available under a Creative Commons (CC-BY-NC-ND) licence, thanks to the support of the Wellcome Trust, which permits non-commercial use, distribution and reproduction provided the editors, chapter authors and Manchester University Press are fully cited and no modifications or adaptations are made. Details of the licence can be viewed at https://creativecommons.org/licenses/by-nc-nd/4.0/

Published by Manchester University Press
Oxford Road, Manchester M13 9PL

www.manchesteruniversitypress.co.uk

British Library Cataloguing-in-Publication Data
A catalogue record for this book is available from the British Library

ISBN  978 1 5261 5488 0  hardback
ISBN  978 1 5261 8240 1  paperback

First published 2021

The publisher has no responsibility for the persistence or accuracy of URLs for any external or third-party internet websites referred to in this book, and does not guarantee that any content on such websites is, or will remain, accurate or appropriate.

Typeset
by New Best-set Typesetters Ltd

*To the patients and caregivers finding their voices in the time of COVID-19. And to Amelia and Arthur, who were voiceless but loved.*

# Contents

| | |
|---|---:|
| List of figures | page ix |
| List of tables | xi |
| List of contributors | xii |
| Acknowledgements | xiv |
| Introduction: searching for the patient – Anne Hanley and Jessica Meyer | 1 |

### Part I: Locating the patient: new approaches

| | |
|---|---:|
| 1 The non-patient's view – Michael Worboys | 33 |
| 2 Family not to be informed? The ethical use of historical medical documentation – Jessica Meyer and Alexia Moncrieff | 61 |

### Part II: Voices from the institution

| | |
|---|---:|
| 3 Lunatics' rights activism in Britain and the German Empire, 1870–1920: a European perspective – Burkhart Brückner | 91 |
| 4 Narrating and navigating patient experiences of farm work in English psychiatric institutions, 1845–1914 – Sarah Holland | 125 |
| 5 The patient's view as history from below: evidence from the Victorian poor, 1834–71 – Paul Carter and Steve King | 154 |

### Part III: User-driven medicine

6 Respiratory technologies and the co-production of breathing in the twentieth century – Coreen McGuire, Jaipreet Virdi and Jenny Hutton — 183
7 The patient's new clothes: British soldiers as complementary practitioners in the First World War – Georgia McWhinney — 223

### Part IV: Negotiating stigma and shame

8 'Dear Dr Kirkpatrick': recovering Irish experiences of VD, 1924–47 – Lloyd (Meadhbh) Houston — 255
9 'I caught it and yours truly was very sorry for himself': mapping the emotional worlds of British VD patients – Anne Hanley — 299

Index — 338

# Figures

1.1 Graphic representing the 'symptom iceberg'. A slide from a presentation by Dr Pete Smith OBE on 'The Self Care Challenge for Primary Care', reproduced with his kind permission. *page* 35
1.2 Advertisement from the *Yorkshire Post* (13 February 1943). 51
2.1 Cyril Charles Schramm Casualty Form – Active Service. 74
3.1 Portrait Louisa Lowe (1820–1901). Reproduced from Louisa Lowe, *The Bastilles of England; or, The Lunacy Laws at Work* (London: Crookenden, 1883), frontispiece. 96
3.2 Presumably Adolf Glöklen (1861–c.1935), demonstrating his healing device for breathing therapy. Reproduced from Adolf Glöklen, *Therapeutische Tief-Atmungs-Gymnastik* (Heidelberg: Jünger, 1912), 22. 103
6.1 The Drinker Respirator and Drinker-Collins Respirator (1939). From L.J. Witts, G.R. Girdlestone, R.G. Henderson, P.M. Tookey Kerridge, G.W. Pickering, C.L.G. Pratt, E. Schuster, A. Topping and N.F. Smith, '"Breathing Machines" and Their Use in Treatment: Report of the Respirators (Poliomyelitis) Committee', *Medical Research Council Special Report Series, No. 237*

(London: His Majesty's Stationery Office, 1939), Plate 1. Contains public sector information licensed under the Open Government Licence v3.0. 196

6.2 The Bragg-Paul Pulsator and Burstall Jacket Respirator (1939). From L.J. Witts, G.R. Girdlestone, R.G. Henderson, P.M. Tookey Kerridge, G.W. Pickering, C.L.G. Pratt, E. Schuster, A. Topping and N.F. Smith, '"Breathing Machines" and Their Use in Treatment: Report of the Respirators (Poliomyelitis) Committee', *Medical Research Council Special Report Series, No. 237* (London: His Majesty's Stationery Office, 1939), Plate 3. Contains public sector information licensed under the Open Government Licence v3.0. 198

8.1 Graph showing letters sent to Dr T.P.C. Kirkpatrick per year for the period 1924–47. 261

# Tables

1.1 Actions taken by survey participants for each symptom experienced in the preceding two weeks — 35
8.1 Breakdown of Dr T.P.C. Kirkpatrick's correspondents by class — 263
8.2 Breakdown of letters to Dr T.P.C. Kirkpatrick by subject — 263
8.3 VD clinic attendance figures for Dr Steevens' Hospital, 1919–24 — 264
8.4 Breakdown of letters to Dr T.P.C. Kirkpatrick by size of settlement — 284

# Contributors

BURKHART BRÜCKNER is Professor of Social Psychology and Health Promotion at University Hochschule Niederrhein, Mönchengladbach, Germany.

PAUL CARTER is the Principal Records Specialist at The National Archives, UK.

ANNE HANLEY is Lecturer in History of Science and Medicine at Birkbeck, University of London, UK.

SARAH HOLLAND is Assistant Professor of History at the University of Nottingham, UK.

LLOYD (MEADHBH) HOUSTON is Stipendiary Lecturer and Foundation Year Tutor in English at Lady Margaret Hall, University of Oxford, UK.

JENNIFER HUTTON is an Affiliate Researcher at the Bristol Centre for Community Research, which looks at research into patient experience in order to improve healthcare.

STEVE KING is Professor of Economic and Social History at Nottingham Trent University, UK.

COREEN MCGUIRE is Lecturer in Twentieth-Century British History at Durham University, UK.

GEORGIA MCWHINNEY is a PhD Scholar in Modern History at Macquarie University, Sydney, Australia.

JESSICA MEYER is Associate Professor of Modern British History at the University of Leeds, UK.

ALEXIA MONCRIEFF is a Postdoctoral Research Fellow in History at the University of Leeds, UK.

JAIPREET VIRDI is Assistant Professor of the History of Medicine, Technology and Disability at the University of Delaware, US.

MICHAEL WORBOYS is Emeritus Professor, Centre for the History of Science, Technology and Medicine (CHSTM), University of Manchester, UK.

# Acknowledgements

The chapters published in this collection had their first airing during a conference held at New College, University of Oxford in September 2017, which was made possible with support from New College's Ludwig Humanities Fund and the Society for the Social History of Medicine. The staff at New College provided much-appreciated organisational support during, and in the lead-up to, the conference. Other colleagues who participated in the conference and added greatly to its vitality were Agnes Arnold-Forster, Harriet Barratt, Louise Bell, Erin Bramwell, Sally Frampton, Colin Gale, Max Gawlich, Graeme Gooday, George Campbell Gosling, Lesley Gray, Alison Moulds, Natalie Mullen, Mark Neuendorf, Caroline Nielsen, Annika Söderland and Emma Stirling-Middleton.

For the publication of this collection, we would like to thank our contributors, who have made it such a strong and unique contribution to the history of medicine and health. Several chapters were written with funding from the Arts and Humanities Research Council (AHRC) (grant no. AG/R002770/1), the European Research Council (grant no. 638694), the Wellcome Trust (grant nos 092782 and 103340), Sheffield Hallam University, and Hertford College and the Faculty of English at the University of Oxford. We and the contributors are grateful for this generous support. Thanks also to Lesley Hall and Joanna Bourke for their comments on the collection's focus and scope and to Lesley also for her help with the specifics of our chapters on sexual health. We are also grateful to Burkhart Brückner, Steve King and Michael Worboys for their comments on the collection's introduction. Thanks to David Cantor, editor of the Society for the Social History of Medicine (SSHM) edited collections, who encouraged us to submit our original proposal and who has been so supportive throughout the project. We have striven to make this a worthy addition to the SSHM's excellent series. And thank you to the production team at Manchester University Press and to the three anonymous reviewers for their comments.

The final editing and preparation of the collection happened during the COVID-19 lockdown in 2020. We are especially grateful to our families for their patience and support during that difficult time. To Lloyd Davies goes particular thanks for his careful attention to detail in editing the collection's introduction and several of its chapters and for his constant willingness to be a sounding board for new ideas and approaches.

Anne Hanley and Jessica Meyer, May 2020

# Introduction: searching for the patient

*Anne Hanley and Jessica Meyer*

In 1985 Roy Porter famously exhorted historians of medicine to 'lower the historical gaze to the sufferers' to better understand interactions between sick persons and their doctors.[1] This approach would challenge the Whiggish tendencies that had dominated the field, enabling a more fluid, nuanced historical understanding of health and medicine. 'A people's history of suffering', he believed, 'might restore to the history of medicine its human face.'[2] In many ways, Porter's work ushered in a new social history of medicine that looked beyond doctor-centred histories, opening up new methodological and conceptual approaches. In the decades since the publication of Porter's pivotal article, the theorisation of experiences of illness, pain and suffering has undoubtedly constituted a major disciplinary shift. Indeed, according to Alexandra Bacopoulous-Viau and Aude Fauvel, it has become 'not only a necessary reference but also a classic trope'.[3] The patient's perspective has become integral to historical analysis across a wide range of topics, most notably the study of medical institutions and specialisms like asylums and psychiatry.[4] And it is not just in the study of modern medicine that historians have sought to locate and amplify the voice of the patient for a richer understanding of the medical encounter. These endeavours have become just as essential to the study of medieval and early modern medicine.[5]

But despite concerted methodological efforts, patient experiences still often remain obscured in histories of health and illness. There has simply not been the degree and breadth of innovation that Porter envisaged.⁶ Flurin Condrau, for one, has noted that 'issues of how to write the patient's history, how to deal with subjectivity, experience and perhaps even choice is still very much uncharted territory for historians of medicine'.⁷ In this respect, Foucauldian theories of biopower and state authority continue to cast a long shadow. Despite Porter's seminal efforts, historians still tend to assume that patients who voiced opinions or exercised agency were exceptions to the norm and therefore of limited use in drawing wider conclusions about historical health practices, policies or infrastructure.⁸

Such assumptions about the silencing and subordination of patients are also compounded by the limitations of archival material. Porter's focus on Samuel Pepys – a noted man of letters who helpfully left to posterity a plethora of personal records – created a high bar. Subsequent generations of historians have struggled to achieve a similar patient-centredness in their work. Pepys embodied what Porter termed 'the early modern medical drama' in which affluent and privileged sick persons were cast in the 'lead role'.⁹ But Pepys was exceptional, not merely for his class, education and occupation, but also in the historical moment he occupied – one in which medical practice was at the start of a transition to its 'modern' form.¹⁰ By the mid-nineteenth century, the rise of hospital- and laboratory-based medicine had pushed patients into a supporting role, their illness experiences unfolding off-stage.

Throughout the nineteenth and twentieth centuries, medicine and medical practice were being dramatically redefined through the emergence of new institutions and ideas, increasing professionalisation, rapid economic development, far-reaching legislative change, the arrival of large-scale mechanised warfare and the recognition of public health as a political responsibility. Patients' experiences were increasingly mediated through the clinical gaze and subordinated to microscopic examinations and legislative interventions. Spurred on by developments in bacteriology and the increasing specialisation of medicine, doctors' holistic focus on their patients' subjective feelings and bodily experiences gave way to a preoccupation with collections of symptoms and biological processes.¹¹ Moreover, new bacteriological methods for diagnosing and treating illness, combined with the increased importance of public health to centralised governments, gave rise to health legislation, such as the Infectious Disease (Notification) Act 1889, which seemingly reduced patients to nameless data points.[12] The acceleration of such developments over the last two centuries, combined with medicine's tendency to construct Whiggish narratives of its own achievements, has resulted in a disproportionate historical focus on ideas and interventions that were efficacious or expedient. It is only in recent decades that medical mistakes and malpractice – and their impact on the experiences of sick persons – have become the focus of historical study.[13]

Increased access to medical treatment also led to greater demands for patient involvement in the provision of care.[14] Although historians see the post-war growth of patient activism and the emergence of 'heath consumers' as a positive refocusing on the individual, service users today remain justifiably suspicious of provisions in areas like mental health.[15] They assume that these services are focused too narrowly on controlling symptoms 'in ways that damage people's sense of empowerment and self-esteem'.[16] Indeed, in his address on health trends and projections at the Nuffield Trust's 2020 Summit, Chris Whitty, Chief Medical Officer of Health for England and Chief Scientific Advisor for the Department of Health and Social Care, insisted that medicine needs 'to be going back to an era' where illnesses were interpreted within a holistic context. Otherwise, he fears that 'people will be coming with six diseases and having to go to six specialists, none of whom talk to one another'.[17] But the problem is not just of disconnected clinical decision-making. The type of over-specialisation that Whitty warns against and that has dominated medicine for over a century also threatens to erode the personhood of patients. Certainly, long-standing preoccupations with symptomatology (rather than the complexities of a living, breathing patient) are reflected in the case notes and medical literature to which historians so often turn to understand the clinical encounter. As the medical profession increasingly scrutinises systems of integrated care and shared responsibility to tackle challenges presented by a shift from acute to chronic disease in Western society, the case becomes ever stronger for exploring the evidence of holistic practices centred on the patient as they manifested in the past.[18]

Given the enormous changes in clinical practice over the past two centuries, it should come as little surprise that the nature and identity of the patient – whether as an intellectual construction, social construction or lived reality – was also in flux, not only in Europe but across the global empires over which European nations wielded political, economic and social control. Yet historians often fail to ask a key question of the period before the birth of socialised medicine and the welfare state: what defined patienthood? Despite his calls for more patient-centred histories, Porter did not disentangle what it *meant* to be a patient. Designating historical actors as patients (rather than as 'consumers' of healthcare or as individuals with complex lives beyond their illness experiences) implies that this is the best lens through which to understand them. But as we shall see throughout this collection, the designation of 'patient' is historically problematic because it carries connotations of passivity and subordination that were often far from reality.

What it means to be a patient has undergone radical revisions in the decades since Porter's clarion call in the 1980s. Even the concept of a 'sick person' or 'sick role' has fallen out of use among many scholars in the medical humanities. This is largely because, as John Burnham observes, 'the conceptual and institutional structure of recent medical practice does not map on to key stages of the sick role as classically defined. It is that disjuncture that alerts us to a basic shift in medicine.'[19] The idea of a sick person has become too bound up with the subordinate, all-consuming role of patient as well as stigmatising assumptions that, in many cases, illness episodes result from poor decision-making or lifestyle choices.[20] Whether or not one classifies sickness events in this way, they are not the sum total of an individual's identity or health experiences. Indeed, as we have seen with the explosion of consumer-led trends in wellness and mindfulness – concepts that have been around for decades but have recently acquired considerable cultural currency – society's focus has shifted to a self-reflexive preoccupation with fulfilling, healthy lifestyles, most commonly articulated through ideas like 'self-care' and 'clean living'.[21] The British Medical Association defines self-care broadly as 'putting people in control of their own health and wellbeing' by giving them the tools to maintain their and their families' physical and mental health and, when needed, manage illnesses.[22] Of course, on 'the self-care continuum' there is a spectrum of illnesses that will require varying degrees of formal medical intervention. But the aim is to encourage Britons as far as possible to take control of their own health, not only to maintain all-round individual wellbeing but also to protect National Health Service (NHS) resources and communal health. As we shall see throughout this collection, however, there was (and remains) often a fine line between handing control to individuals and abdicating responsibility for their care.

Historians must be sensitive to what Janice Perlman terms the 'myth of marginality'.[23] Many people did not see themselves as patients, but as health users, in large part because they were actively engaged in the design and redesign of health networks, services and technologies. In their chapter on user-driven co-production of assistive respiratory technologies, Coreen McGuire, Jaipreet Virdi and Jenny Hutton remind us that historians cannot automatically assume that patients believed themselves to be marginalised in the processes of their own care. Patients and their families might have been excluded from formal committees of inquiry, but their needs and comforts were central to the design and redesign of respiratory devices. The study of such processes of design and production offer historians key access points to patient experiences. Sick persons were not simply reacting to biomedical interventions, but creating their own bodies of what Georgia McWhinney identifies in her chapter as vernacular knowledge. Like McGuire, Virdi and Hutton, McWhinney challenges the assumed disconnects and divergences in the doctor–patient relationship, showing how patients were more than just mirrors to biomedicine. As her work makes clear, self-care knowledge and practices were important coping mechanisms for soldiers facing the day-to-day trauma of life on the Western Front. Far from being marginalised, these soldier-patients – or complementary practitioners – combined medical knowledge with lay knowledge and experience in fluid ways, creating vernacular systems of care from which they derived meaning and agency.

As McWhinney's work makes clear, vernacular medical practices reflected the extent to which questions of health and illness were embedded in soldiers' day-to-day lived experience. Similarly, in his chapter Michael Worboys urges us to look past the traditional spaces and temporal limits of the clinical encounter to engage with the multiplicity of illness experiences beyond those bound up with formal healthcare structures and in so doing recognise (as Porter encouraged us to do) the importance of self-diagnosis and self-treatment. Prioritising health systems that support acute illnesses and accidents has prioritised the work of hospitals and hospital-based health professions, rather than the social care networks within communities, neighbourhoods, households and families that are so essential for long-term recovery and wellbeing.[24] And this focus has, in turn, shaped the way that historians think about illness episodes.

But the process of *becoming* and *being* a patient has been (and remains) just one small part of a person's everyday experiences of ill-health. Indeed, as we write the introduction to this edited collection, the world is in the grip of a global pandemic. In an effort to 'flatten the curve' of COVID-19 cases and alleviate pressure on health services, national and local governments across the globe are restricting their populations' freedoms by instituting varying levels of lockdown. In Britain, where test kits, ventilators and ICU beds are all in short supply, anyone with symptoms has been advised to self-isolate and not to visit hospitals or GP surgeries. To protect NHS resources, Britons were ordered (under threat of criminal sanctions) to stay at home. There were only a few exceptions to these orders, including outdoor exercise, shopping for necessities, providing care and travelling for essential work. Consequently, people are increasingly turning to self-diagnosis, not always backed up by the formal testing regime.[25] In turn, many are not seeking treatment for COVID-19 or a variety of other ailments, both minor and severe, that may befall them during lockdown. Those who are infected with COVID-19, believe themselves to be infected, or are caring for loved ones who are infected, have taken to social media and the national press to document their experiences of illness in self-isolation. Rarely has the role of self-diagnosis and self-treatment so preoccupied our national discourse.

It remains to be seen whether this vast digital collection of 'illness diaries' prompts historians to re-evaluate how they write histories of health and healthcare. But for now, the spotlight continues to be on interactions within formal healthcare structures. At present, the sources that historians use are primarily institutional and written from the perspective of the health professionals who compiled them. Using the concept of the 'symptom iceberg', Worboys estimates that such an approach misses over 80 per cent of modern healthcare events and an even higher percentage historically, since the vast majority of the sick chose not to seek formal medical help.[26] 'Doing nothing' in the event of disability or illness was (and continues to be) an active and informed choice based on experience of previous illness episodes, lay knowledge gained from social networks and formal information about symptoms and likely prognoses. As Worboys and Anne Hanley both argue, sick peoples' health priorities and ideas about disease severity and causation often differed significantly from those of health professionals and sanitary reformers. Yet the social factors that prompted their decisions to forgo professional medical interventions remain overlooked.

Fundamental to any attempt to access patient experiences of sickness and healthcare is an understanding of patient agency. But as Anne Borsay and Peter Shapley note, historians must first understand the place of personal agency within larger social, economic and political power structures.[27] Patients' agency is defined not only in relation to medical practice and practitioners. It is also bound up with an intersectional identity that cuts across class, gender, sexuality, race, socio-economic status and age. For those who could afford doctors' fees, the pre-NHS medical marketplace afforded considerable power. The poor, marginalised and institutionalised had far fewer choices, but they too were not without autonomy. In his study of pre-NHS healthcare payments, George Campbell Gosling observes that historians have rarely reflected on 'what the predecessor of a health service *free at the point of use* was, how it worked, or what it meant to hand over money to the doctor or the hospital'.[28] As chapters throughout this collection demonstrate, economic precarity fundamentally shaped the power dynamics of healthcare interactions, perpetuating inequalities in health outcomes. Under such circumstances, it is easy to see why historians assumed that patients were largely excluded from clinical decision-making and subjected to structural power imbalances.

When we think about how patients might have exercised agency, we must consider not only the therapeutic limitations of their care, but also the social and political obstacles that shaped that care. These obstacles would have seemed especially insurmountable for persons of limited means, persons who were institutionalised and persons suffering from disabling or stigmatising conditions. As Lynn M. Thomas demonstrates in her critique of agency as an analytic concept, agency was always conditional and defined within context-specific boundaries. She is right to encourage us to think about agency as a process of 'just getting by'.[29] Persons with complex or stigmatising illnesses were not overthrowing unjust systems; they were navigating those systems, attempting to achieve the best possible outcomes for themselves and their families. And those immediate necessities were fundamental to their experiences of illness and healthcare. Historians, then, need to consider not merely how we can access the elusive patient voice within or through the archive, but how we might use analytical tools to look beyond and consider patients' actions too.

Disease, according to Porter, was 'standardly the signature of wrong and could create or reinforce stigma'.[30] But some disease categories and clinical fields carried more stigma than others. In this collection, we focus primarily on military medicine, Poor Law medicine, disability, psychiatry and sexual health – all fields in which patients were thought to be especially subject to stigma or institutional authority and therefore rendered mute in the historical record. And, crucially, they are fields in which significant inequalities persist. In sexual health, for example, falling overall infection rates mask underlying inequalities in outcomes that see the vulnerable and marginalised faring worst.[31] In recent years, the freezing or reduction of spending on sexual- and reproductive-health services has been concentrated in local authorities with higher levels of social deprivation.[32] Similarly, the Care Quality Commission found that the quality and availability of mental-health services has been in consistent decline over recent years.[33] This appears to be a particular issue among military personnel, where a recent spate of suicides among veterans has highlighted the disconnected nature of the health and welfare provisions on offer to these patients.[34] As Porter observed of the history of psychiatry, 'posterity has treated the writings of mad people with enormous condescension'.[35] The same is also true of soldiers, VD sufferers and the poor and destitute, all of whom were in positions of extreme vulnerability. But stigma and vulnerability around these various states of disability and ill-health did not mean that patients were merely passive, grateful recipients of care. They quarrelled with, complained about, disregarded and even resisted heath authorities. They questioned, objected to and walked away from treatments. Doctors were pressured into particular courses of action by patients and patients' families. And on other occasions, sick persons by-passed health professionals altogether.

Indeed, complaint mechanisms, which proliferated alongside the increasing formality of nineteenth-century healthcare provisions, became an important means of generating and preserving patient voices. Through the concomitant generation of advocate voices, these mechanisms also provided opportunities for patients to finesse the art of complaint. As Paul Carter and Steve King discuss in Chapter 5, complaints increasingly involved written, rather than merely verbal, communications. This had a range of implications for the audibility of patients' voices as well as the constraints and possibilities for their expression. Even from among the very poor, complaints could not generally be ignored. Importantly, the process of investigation – the act of taking these complaints seriously – and occasional victories against institutions or persons in authority signalled to patients the extent of their individual and collective power. Crucially, complaint mechanisms *created* patients by presupposing that one defined oneself as a patient of an institution, a person or a system. Throughout the twentieth century, those mechanisms also led to the creation of support and activist groups, as Burkhart Brückner explores, that simultaneously defined people as patients *and* as members of a community with a powerful collective voice.

Yet despite these many instances of protest and resistance in the archives, it remains remarkably difficult to write nuanced histories of sick persons' experiences. As Bacopoulous-Viau and Fauvel remind us, 'calling for history from below and actually accomplishing it in any systematic and constructive fashion are different enterprises'.[36] Few of the ordinary persons studied by historians had the means or inclination to leave behind helpfully detailed accounts of their illness experiences. Even being visible in the historical record does not mean that a patient retained their voice. Historians have tended to rely far more heavily on institutional records, the majority of which were compiled by health professionals and written from their perspective. The patient is present, but their actions, voices and experiences are mediated through the clinical gaze and interpreted according to health professionals' own socially conditioned expectations and assumptions. The result has been a distorted historical picture of healthcare that subordinates patient subjectivity. This has led, in turn, to a narrow definition of the patient as a category of historical analysis. It is not enough simply to 'listen' to patients in the past. As Condrau argues, we must recognise the external forces that have shaped their representation in the archive and that these representations may not reveal the 'real' patient.[37] The challenge for us as historians is to find ways of reconciling and looking past these representations in ways that are academically rigorous, ethically reflective and avoid perpetuating harm.[38]

Without an abundance of records written by sick persons, how can their experiences be foregrounded? What is needed to recover rich, complex experiences and, importantly, to bring those experiences into conversation with the present? To begin, we need to develop concrete methods for grappling with the often-fragmentary records left by and about historical patients. This is a daunting task, and *Patient voices in Britain* goes some way towards filling this need. Focusing on the century preceding the foundation of the NHS, this collection offers a range of innovative approaches for accessing patient voices and understanding healthcare and wellbeing in the context of Britain's emerging welfare state.

## New approaches

The collection has two key objectives. The first is to reposition the patient at the centre of healthcare histories, providing a model for using new types of sources and reading familiar sources in new ways to draw out patient experiences. Its chapters use a diverse range of archives – the space in which patient voices have been collected and preserved – to explore how changes in health provisions shaped the delineation of the patient. In so doing, it demonstrates the liminal and often contested nature of patient identity. Inevitably, there are many threads of historical patient experience that we have not addressed in this collection. Among the most obvious gaps are the health experiences of Britain's BAME and LGBTQ+ communities. But our intention is that the frameworks set out here provide scope for future studies across a wider range of social and cultural spaces and with greater attention to more diverse communities. Our ambition is that it inspires other historians to integrate similar critical approaches, encourages them to tackle the ethical challenges of using sensitive archival materials and pushes them to think more carefully about the contributions that history can make to debates over the provision and direction of healthcare in Britain today. Through these explorations of archival and historical practice, each chapter reconceptualises our understanding of the patient as a historical actor. Each chapter uses case studies to make a range of points about health and illness at particular historical moments. But, importantly, each also examines how historical and archival practices interact to shape the definition of 'the patient' across time through the preservation and analysis of their voices within the historical record.

In an effort to look beyond the confines of traditionally demarcated clinical spaces and mediated views of the patient, scholars across the medical humanities have focused increasingly on the role that narrative plays in accessing patient voices. As Angela Woods observes, narrativity 'is frequently promoted as the primary vehicle through which the ill person can express her changing sense of self and identity, explore new social roles and gain membership of new communities'.[39] Illness is more than just a physiological condition. It is shaped, or even manifested, by complex webs of social networks and power structures. The ability of narratives (however fragmentary) to capture these subjective, lived experiences of illness has made them foundational source materials. But it is important to remember that health professionals also devised narrative strategies, which they used not only to organise clinical information but to process the emotional dimensions of their clinical encounters, to orient themselves in relation to their patients and to help make diagnostic and therapeutic decisions.[40] As Bryan Good and Mary-Jo Delvecchio Good put it, 'physicians talk in stories' and 'practice in stories'.[41] Indeed, the importance of these strategies for contemporary medicine was highlighted in 2015 when the *Lancet* began to allocate more space in each issue to a new narrative-rich style of case reporting that Philippa Berman and Richard Horton identify as 'an integral part of medical learning'.[42] Such didactic narrativity was equally important to historical doctor-authored accounts of patients' illnesses – accounts that were shaped by contemporary social norms and moral codes.[43] And as various chapters in this collection demonstrate, close readings against the grain, which foreground these sub-textual norms and codes, have the potential to open up important new perspectives on patients' experiences.

This leads us to an exploration of patients' inner emotional and psychological worlds, for which the history of emotions is essential to fill the gaps and understand the sick person's experiences on their own terms. In the years since Michael Roper's proposals for the centring of relationships and their emotional processes in historical studies, the history of emotions has become a significant historiographic trend.[44] The history of medicine has been, as Rob Boddice notes, at the heart of this development: 'Historians of emotions have found scientific, medical and psychological sources relating to the emotions among the principal avenues of enquiry in exploring and unpacking knowledge about the affective life of humans and animals in the past'.[45] Indeed, Boddice identifies the roots of the history of emotions in the development of psychiatry as a professional discipline, tying the theorisation of the field to the institutional and observational practices of those in medical authority.[46] Yet he goes on to suggest that the more recent development of 'neurohistory' – the history of the development of the human brain through its relationship with the cultures and societies it is responsible for creating – and its intertwining with the history of emotions has the potential to open up:

> whole new worlds [...] to be read, with particular emphasis on the material objects, spaces, places and architectures with which and in which historical actors have acted. Inferences about experiential feelings have to be situated in deep knowledge of a given historical context, encompassing everyday practice; familial life; spiritual and cosmological beliefs; social, political and racial assumptions; institutions and rituals (especially relating to the life cycle).[47]

Such an approach chimes with the concerns of this collection, with its focus on a range of archival sources and the variety of historically contingent contexts through which patient voices can be accessed.

More than this, however, a focus on what patient voices can tell us about historical affect has the potential to shift debate over the relationship between the history of emotion and the history of medicine. Historiographic discussions of this relationship have been dominated thus far by sources in which health professionals attempted to capture and record the emotions of their patients.[48] But important new work is also increasingly examining emotions associated with practices of caregiving.[49] By framing our interrogation of new sources (and the re-interrogation of familiar ones) using more inclusive definitions of 'the patient', this collection explores the multiple ways in which emotional experiences of health and illness, suffering and relief, were articulated in the past. Such voices have traditionally been classed as unreliable, particularly those of mental-health patients. As Brückner and Sarah Holland show in Chapters 3 and 4 respectively, however, personal experience and emotional responses, including grief, anger and fear, formed the basis of much of the complaint upon which such patients could build a sense of agency. Reading these voices as articulations of emotional experience subverts the very grounds on which they were historically dismissed, reaffirming Porter's own studies on the history of psychiatry.[50] Exploring emotional relationality, meanwhile, as in the correspondence discussed by Lloyd (Meadhbh) Houston in Chapter 8, enables a fuller exploration of the carer as emotional actor rather than dispassionate observer.

Nor is it only the emotions of patients and caregivers that are at stake. As Katie Barclay has pointed out in her discussion of historians' emotional relationship with their subjects, work on ethical engagement in historical practice 'has highlighted the ethical obligations of our role as witnesses and storytellers, not just as objective bystanders, but as implicated in the production of meaning through our witnessing, through our storytelling, through the political engagements of our research as it goes out into the world'.[51] Chris Millard goes even further, exploring how, as part of an increasingly established intellectual tradition, historians might draw on their own health experiences to position their research.[52] Barclay demonstrates how such ethical obligations apply across a variety of approaches in social and cultural history. But as discussed by Jessica Meyer and Alexia Moncrieff in Chapter 2, this presents particular challenges to historians of medicine. The mapping of patient experience in ways that challenge definitions and demarcations of patienthood exposes individuals to scrutiny in ways that they may have neither desired nor consented to when their stories were archived.

This in itself forms part of wider debates over the use (and potential misuse) of historical patient data. But these debates have tended to take place within medical and scientific disciplines. Although a number of historians have mulled over these challenges, there are as yet no satisfactory guidelines. Historians have, all too often, been left to make these fraught decisions based on their own professional judgement.[53] They are faced with an ethical conundrum. On the one hand, historical patients or health users might be classed as vulnerable subjects. As such, issues of consent become especially important if we are considering using their stories in our historical analyses. On the other hand, these patients and health users cannot give consent from beyond the grave and to forgo incorporating their voices in our work may perpetuate the marginalisation of groups whose histories deserve to be told. The best model thus far for ethical historical research has come from historians of psychiatry, who seek to balance the privacy of patients burdened by historically stigmatising diagnoses with a desire to allow those patients a voice as historical actors with claims to agency. As Jennifer Wallis argues, 'there is something particularly dehumanising about taking away the patient's real name and replacing it with a pseudonym'.[54] The creative and compassionate approaches pioneered by historians in this field demonstrate why we should not shy away from drawing on sensitive source materials. Although they can be used to identify patients and present in minute detail the traumatic experience of their health encounters, such sources also play a vital 'rehumanising' role. As Holland explains in her chapter on asylum farm labour, such information can be included as a means of nuancing our understanding of patients' lives before their sickness or institutionalisation and, by extension, their experiences while in the institution.

## Lessons from history?

Creative and compassionate approaches to the use of the patient voice have relevance not only to historians' professional practice. Porter wrote his seminal article at a time of growing patient-centred activism and it was in the context of this movement that he called for greater historical attention to the voices of patients.[55] It is therefore fitting that our collection, which has been so greatly inspired by Porter's work, also highlights the central role that patients should play in decisions about their health and healthcare. Although often mediated through the clinical gaze, patient voices in the archive constitute points of resistance and negotiation. And by engaging with them as such, the collection also highlights how these historical case studies might speak to contemporary health challenges. In examining patient experiences, this collection shines a light not only on the recipients of care but also the structures and dynamics of caregiving, infrastructural (re)organisations, clinical practices and policy shifts that had far-reaching consequences for the provision of care in Britain. And it is with these wider contexts of care that the collection's second focus is concerned: namely, the important role that history can play in understanding contemporary healthcare challenges.

As demonstrated by the work of organisations like History & Policy, historical research has the potential to contribute in a variety of ways to current conversations about health and wellbeing. Indeed, the regularity with which history is invoked (albeit often bluntly) to lend support to new health policies is testament to both its popularity and its importance.[56] The second aim of *Patient voices* is therefore to explore ways in which history resonates with contemporary health challenges while also deepening our understanding of what this means for our historical practice.[57] Our aim is that, by bringing our historical studies into conversation with contemporary health issues, the collection will prompt other historians to think more carefully and creatively about how their historical perspectives might usefully be brought to bear on health challenges today. We are not proposing a one-size-fits-all blueprint. Rather, our aim is to help historians locate and capitalise on those points in their own research that speak to current health policies, infrastructure, service delivery or service-user experiences.

Considerations of how the patient and their agency can be located in ethical historical practice by historians and archivists perhaps most clearly brings together the two objectives of this collection to demonstrate its methodological significance to academia and beyond. But the potential for nuanced analysis of the historical patient voice goes beyond questions of ethical usage. Among the current and emerging health priorities identified by Whitty are multi-morbidity, mental health and antimicrobial resistance.[58] The focus of this collection on Poor Law medicine, psychiatry and sexual health all point to ways in which the historical voice can nuance government, institutional and community approaches to these and other health challenges. This is not to suggest that there are any simple 'lessons from history' that might be adopted. Rather, by listening to patients' voices from the past – voices that resisted, acquiesced, challenged and redefined medical practice – we might avoid potential pitfalls in current health interventions and even discover unexpected routes to desired outcomes. The collection demonstrates how history might offer enriched perspectives on a diverse range of healthcare issues, including general practice, military medicine, disability and sexual and mental health. Each chapter locates patient or user experiences within those historical moments when individual autonomy was brought into conflict with state authority and collective interest. But, importantly, each chapter also reflects on how these historical tensions continue to shape attitudes towards health, illness and the clinical encounter.

As the chapters in this collection demonstrate, the historian's most obvious contribution to contemporary health challenges is their ability to identify and analyse long-term trends. Only by looking at health data over these longer periods of time can we hope to recognise meaningful patterns. In Simon Szreter's view, quarter-century units should constitute a *minimum* timeframe for developing health initiatives and assessing their effectiveness.[59] As historians, our training and knowledge enables us to assess complex webs of interconnected health impacts stretching across these longer time periods. In so doing, we can use our knowledge of the past, and its echoes in the present, to help map potential directions for the future.

But to do so, we must, as Virginia Berridge urges, become more adept at articulating our work for audiences beyond academia.[60] Taking our cue from Bacopoulous-Viau and Fauvel, we aim to show that histories of patient experience are best understood through 'myriad personal stories'.[61] But conscious of Condrau's criticism that the historiographical turn towards patient experiences has given rise to personal stories defined by their subjectivity and singularity, we have sought to demonstrate the value of such case studies to current reflections on healthcare.[62] Indeed, these stories are more than just engaging sources. Patient activists and medical-humanities scholars alike have made the case for 'expertise through lived experience' – that personal experiences of illness grant the individual a form of expertise that should be acknowledged and respected in clinical decision-making.[63] Contrary to Condrau's insistence, patients' experiences are never merely interesting anecdotes or picturesque detail. In recent years, health charities and think-tanks have called for the prioritising of local cultural contexts to ensure the sustainability of NHS initiatives.[64] And in view of this focus on scaling and adapting initiatives to reflect the cultural specificities of local health needs and services, such personal stories no longer seem quite so irrelevant to bigger conversations about past or future healthcare provisions. Given that local context can 'often represent significant barriers to success', historians, healthcare providers and policy-makers would all do well to think more carefully about how personal stories can inform the implementation of new initiatives. As we are seeing in the responses to the COVID-19 pandemic, individual stories viewed collectively constitute a rich, nuanced history of health, illness and medical care. In particular, they illustrate the challenges of negotiating the rollout of health interventions at a local level. As David Hall-Matthews insists, 'by embracing complexity, historians may be able to foresee possible ranges of outcomes or, with a little more certainty, warn of likely adverse reactions to healthcare interventions that have chimed negatively with local populations in the past'.[65] When properly contextualised and carefully read, patient experiences open up important perspectives on the impact of historical medical practices, cultural attitudes and policy interventions for communities and individuals.

Embracing such complexity also means recognising the heterogeneity of past patient experiences, which in turn makes the historian uniquely sensitive to the inherent challenges of standardising healthcare interventions, both then and today. Indeed, the heterogeneity of sickness and disability experiences has posed (and continues to pose) serious challenges for a society that has prioritised centralised health initiatives and standardised diagnostic practices and treatments. Understanding what has previously worked or not worked for health users and, importantly, *why* it has or has not worked, is necessary for identifying potential problems in the development of health services today. We may use our historical analysis and interpretations to push against received public understandings of the nation's health history, especially stale and often decontextualised vignettes of healthcare provisions predating the establishment of the NHS.[66] As this collection demonstrates, historical tropes and Whiggish visions of cumulative improvement mask a host of persistent inequalities in healthcare accessibility and outcomes – inequalities that are recognisable only through an analysis of long-term trends and an understanding of the shortcomings in historical health provisions.[67]

Positive, sustainable health interventions require an understanding of where ideas about health and illness have come from and being able to identify where and why certain attitudes towards sickness and sick persons have persisted.[68] For example, shame and stigma have been (and remain) monumental barriers to achieving positive health experiences and outcomes. As we see throughout this collection, by nuancing understandings of shame and stigma historians can begin to identify ways to push successfully against the embarrassed silences that shape experiences of disability, mental illness and sexual health. Moreover, historical critique has the potential to show how and why previous provisions have failed to address – or have even exacerbated – these barriers to effective healthcare. And by remaining sensitive to past failings, we may avoid repeating mistakes.[69] Similarly, close investigations of resistance to medical care, particularly provided by institutions with ties to the state, can address the challenges of the provision of such care. As Brückner, Holland and Carter and King all suggest, the power of patients' complaints in resisting institutional dominance was complex and, crucially, often effective in unexpected ways. Such analysis has the potential to inform contemporary approaches to complaint, enhancing the effectiveness of institutional response.

Historians are also sensitive to the complex and often-fraught personal relationships that determined an individual's health outcomes as well as their experiences of illness and the clinical encounter. For example, as Houston and Hanley reveal, patients' positive experiences of VD treatment were dependent on the attitudes of the people responsible for their care. The positive experiences of Thomas Kirkpatrick's patients were not the norm during the interwar years when syphilis and gonorrhoea still carried profound stigma. In the decades before the establishment of the NHS, patient–carer relationships often had a strong financial dimension. This was nowhere more acute than in cases of stigmatising illness, where sick persons may have doubted or resisted the willingness of friends and family to take on the emotional labour of caregiving. The care-based relationships that patients formed with family, doctors, communities, institutions and even inanimate objects were shaped and sustained by less-quantifiable forms of what Pierre Bourdieu identified as social capital.[70] Fearing condemnation, ostracism, social ruin, institutionalisation and even imprisonment, persons with VD were driven underground, away from these forms of social capital and formal medical care. In the absence of such networks of support, sick persons – regardless of their financial resources or social status – have often had to rely on the beneficence or open-mindedness of a single individual or philanthropic institution. By drawing attention to the precarity and unreliability inherent in such power relations, this collection also highlights the centrality of social capital to the achievement of positive health outcomes on an individual and collective level.

The pressures placed on our society and its healthcare infrastructure by COVID-19 are not only highlighting the cracks in that infrastructure. As the weaknesses and shortfalls in health provisions are exacerbated, reliance on social networks for support and, indeed, survival, become all the more essential. Worboys's study of the social factors that have shaped people's decisions either to forgo or to seek out formal medical care demonstrates precisely how essential social capital has been to the maintenance of health. Sensitivity to these historical networks is important in light of the market forces increasingly shaping caregiving practices. Economic rationality has, according to Arthur Kleinman, 'infiltrated' every aspect of medicine at the expense of interpersonal relationships that prioritise selfhood, dignity and emotional subjectivity.[71] Kleinman insists that: 'If caregiving is absent from the political and economic discourse on health care, then nothing but institutional and monetary issues seem to matter. Even questions of "quality" in health care become distorted.'[72] As the British Medical Association (BMA) observed in 2019, even in the case of self-care there is a risk that, without accessible support structures embedded within communities, the health advantages will be felt only by 'higher socioeconomic groups'.[73] To resist the reduction of caregiving to a series of financial considerations requires us to appreciate its less-quantifiable value to patients, doctors, families and communities. And this is where history becomes so essential.

As each chapter in this collection demonstrates, to improve individual- *and* population-health outcomes, it is not sufficient to rely on material interventions or what Szreter terms 'technological fixes'. It also requires networks of reciprocal support: 'attention to the quality and quantity of relationships that carry and make interpretable any such material or technological transfers'.[74] As McGuire, Virdi and Hutton reveal in their examination of the co-production of assistive respiratory technologies, these types of reciprocal, collaborative relationships were (and remain) central to the formation of positive healthcare experiences and outcomes. The rapid development and diversification of health technologies (one of the fastest growth areas in health spending) poses ever new challenges to which health services and service users will both need to adapt.[75] And the success of these developments, such as the reduced invasiveness of assistive technologies in daily life, depends very much on the extent to which they are user-driven. An individual's positive experiences of living with oxygen machines or ventilators required collective sensitivity to the stigma associated with reliance on such technology as well as the reciprocal processes of knowledge exchange that enabled their development. Such networks required self-conscious awareness on the part of all involved that they were working towards shared, mutually beneficial objectives.[76] By using frameworks like Bruno Latour's actor–network theory to scrutinise these relationships, we can begin to map the fundamental connections joining patients, families, communities, health professionals and even the material culture of healthcare.[77] Understanding the nature of the kin networks and professional relationships through which social capital was generated and sustained historically not only opens up opportunities for locating patient experiences. It also allows historians to recognise and respond to the inequalities in, and fragility of, similar networks today as well as the potentially harmful consequences should they be dismantled.

## Patient voices in Britain

The chapters in this collection thus recentre the patient as a complex historical actor and, in so doing, aim to illustrate just some of the many ways in which nuanced historical understandings might speak to similar health challenges facing us today. The collection opens with the examination of current historical practice in relation to definitions of the patient. Part I – Locating the patient – offers readers a series of theoretical reflections on some of the ethical and methodological challenges that beset attempts to access patient voices in historical records. Worboys considers in Chapter 1 how our understanding of the status of 'patient' changes when the historical gaze centres on states of illness rather than the formal structures through which illness is often managed. In so doing he pushes beyond Porter and Condrau's calls to reposition or redefine the 'patient' and their arenas, arguing that 'non-patients' and 'pre-patients', who may have suffered pain and discomfort without seeking formal medical interventions, have much to tell historians. Meyer and Moncrieff, meanwhile, interrogate the role of the historian in constructing the historical patient. They engage, in Chapter 2, with the ethical challenges arising from the increased digitisation of sensitive archival materials and encourage other historians to tackle these challenges in more considered ways. Interrogating the ethical implications of using medical records created and preserved by the state outside of formal medical systems, they question the historian's role in the medical surveillance of historical actors who may or may not have had the capacity to consent to the use of their data.

Building on this problematising of the patient and the location of their voices in the historical record, Part II – Voices from the institution – re-examines how historians might access patient experiences and even patient 'voices' from the archives of very different psychiatric and custodial institutions. An inverse form of agency can be seen in the resistance articulated by psychiatric patients, who often rejected the identity of patient. In his comparative analysis, in Chapter 3, of patient experiences in psychiatric institutions in Britain and Germany, Brückner demonstrates the continuities of such resistance across European cultures in the nineteenth century, pointing to transnational practices of organisation and advocacy in this rapidly developing field of medicalisation and specialisation. Holland, meanwhile, in Chapter 4, shows how the specific space of asylum farms were used to define and control mental-health patients, as well as how patients attempted to subvert these efforts. In these two very different spaces, individuals sought to challenge the (often stigmatising) definitions of patienthood that were imposed on them by health professionals.

Letters are an archival source traditionally used to access patients' voices. Yet their flexibility, and the range of potential constructions of patienthood that may emerge from them, is often underestimated. By examining letters written by people more usually identified in ways other than as patients, in Chapter 5 Carter and King take us beyond the immediate medical encounter, complicating readings of the patient as a relational status. Letters from Poor Law patients recount the lived experiences of health and the clinical encounter. The exposure of these letters to historical scrutiny gives voice to the intersections of poverty and illness in ways that other official records could not or would not capture. Again, they nuance the definition of 'patient' by highlighting the ways that this identity was mobilised as a form of social resistance.

In contrast to these studies of the patient voice as resistant, Part III – User-driven medicine – explores the dynamics of the medical encounter when patients and their voices have taken centre ground in practice as well as in the historical record. In Chapter 6, McGuire, Virdi and Hutton discuss medical co-creation, specifically the role of patient voice and experience in the development of breathing technologies in the early and mid-twentieth century. McWhinney, meanwhile, looks, in Chapter 7, at the vernacular medical practices of soldiers during the First World War to demonstrate the on-going importance of maintaining health outside the formal practices of the military medical system. In doing so, she reunites us with Worboys's notions of non-patients and pre-patients – individuals engaged in day-to-day behaviours and practices designed to maintain health apart from, if not incidental to, the medical encounter. Patients such as these deserve to have their voices recorded and heard, as do those who used the medical encounter as a means of defining themselves as something other, or more than, medicalised minds and bodies. Such voices highlight the multiple ways in which individuals engage with medicine and caregiving, beyond the passivity or resistance which tend to form the centre of official and institutional narratives.

The collection concludes in Part IV – Negotiating stigma and shame – with an examination of the methodological challenges historians face when trying to access patient experiences of illnesses that carried (and continue to carry) profound stigma. In Chapter 8, Houston considers the relationships between VD patients and their doctors, using letters to show how medical encounters did not necessarily define patients negatively and could, in fact, be used by patients to address wider social problems. By contrast in Chapter 9, Hanley examines how shame and stigma became powerful and pernicious factors in the social construction of disease and experiences of illness. She demonstrates the range of historical sources that can be read successfully and ethically to build up a picture of patient experiences. For this picture to be nuanced, she argues, historians need to be flexible and creative in the varieties of sources upon which they draw.

*Introduction* 23

Taken together, the chapters that make up this collection point to the ongoing potential for methodological development in the history of medicine through the continued, nuanced use of the patient voice. There will always be a degree of unknowability shrouding historical patient experiences. But, as Julia Laite explains, 'history's most unknowable, disconnected, almost invisible threads' are often those that call most seductively to the historian.[78] We will never completely know the experiences of institutionalised men and women, or those sidelined and shunned by the stigma surrounding their ill-health. But by thinking broadly about how patients' voices can be located in the historical record and how historians can ethically interpret the range of voices found there, this collection reasserts the urgency of foregrounding past health encounters and experiences. Patient voices are there, in the archive. To better understand health practices today, we need to listen to them.

## Notes

1 Roy Porter, 'The Patient's View: Doing Medical History from Below', *Theory and Society* 14:2 (1985), 175–98, 192.
2 Ibid., 194.
3 Alexandra Bacopoulous-Viau and Aude Fauvel, 'The Patient's Turn: Roy Porter and Psychiatry's Tales, Thirty Years On', *Medical History* 60:1 (2016), 1–18.
4 John V. Pickstone, *Medicine and Industrial Society: A History of Hospital Development in Manchester and its Region, 1752–1946* (Manchester: Manchester University Press, 1985); Guenther B. Risse, *Mending Bodies, Saving Souls: A History of Hospitals* (Oxford: Oxford University Press, 1999); Joel D. Howell, *Technology in the Hospital: Transforming Patient Care in the Early Twentieth Century* (Baltimore: Johns Hopkins University Press, 1995); Kerry Davis, 'Silent and Censured Travellers? Patients' Narratives and Patients' Voices: Perspectives in the History of Mental Illness since 1948', *Social History of Medicine* 14:2 (2001), 267–92.
5 Michael R. McVaugh, *Medicine Before the Plague: Practitioners and their Patients in the Crown of Aragon, 1285–1345* (Cambridge: Cambridge University Press, 1993); Michael Stolberg, *Experiencing Illness and the Sick Body in Early Modern Europe* (Basingstoke: Palgrave, 2011); Lucinda McCray Beier, *Sufferers and Healers: The Experience of Illness in Seventeenth-Century England* (Abingdon: Routledge, 1987); Hilary

Marland, *Medicine and Society in Wakefield and Huddersfield 1780–1870* (Cambridge: Cambridge University Press, 1987); Anne Digby, *Making a Medical Living: Doctors and Patients in the Market for Medicine, 1720–1911* (Cambridge: Cambridge University Press, 1994); Jennifer Evans and Ciara Meehan (eds), *Perceptions of Pregnancy from the Seventeenth to the Twentieth Century* (Basingstoke: Palgrave, 2017).

6   Among only a handful of exceptions are the edited collections by Anne Borsay, Peter Shapely, Jonathan Reinarz and Rebecca Wynter. See Anne Borsay and Peter Shapely, *Medicine, Charity and Mutual Aid: The Consumption of Health and Welfare in Britain, c.1550–1950* (Farnham: Ashgate, 2007); Jonathan Reinarz and Rebecca Wynter, *Complaints, Controversies and Grievances in Medicine: Historical and Social Science Perspectives* (Abingdon: Routledge, 2015).

7   Flurin Condrau, 'The Patient's View Meets the Clinical Gaze', *Social History of Medicine* 20:3 (2007), 525–40, 526.

8   Bacopoulous-Viau and Fauvel, 'The Patient's Turn', 3.

9   Roy Porter, *Bodies Politic: Disease, Death and Doctors in Britain, 1650–1900* (London: Reaktion Books, 2001), 150.

10  Roger Cooter, 'Medicine and Modernity', in Mark Jackson (ed.), *The Oxford Handbook of the History of Medicine* (Oxford: Oxford University Press, 2011), 100–17.

11  N.D. Jewson, 'The Disappearance of the Sick-Man from Medical Cosmology, 1770–1870', *International Journal of Epidemiology* 10:2 (1976), 225–44. See also, Andrew Cunningham and Perry Williams (eds), *The Laboratory Revolution in Medicine* (Cambridge: Cambridge University Press, 1992); Christopher Lawrence, 'Incommunicable Knowledge: Science, Technology and the Clinical Art in Britain 1850–1914', *Journal of Contemporary History* 20:4 (1985), 503–22.

12  Dorothy Porter, 'Introduction', in Dorothy Porter (ed.), *The History of Public Health and the Modern State* (Amsterdam: Rodopi, 1994), 1–44; Graham Mooney, *Intrusive Interventions: Public Health, Domestic Space, and Infectious Disease Surveillance in England, 1840–1914* (Woodbridge: Boydell & Brewer, 2015).

13  See, for example, Susan Lederer, *Subjected to Science: Human Experimentation in America before the Second World War* (Baltimore: Johns Hopkins University Press, 1994); Susan Lederer, 'Experimentation and Ethics', in Peter Bowler and John Pickstone (eds), *The Cambridge History of Science: The Modern Biological and Earth Sciences* (Cambridge: Cambridge University Press, 2009), 583–601; Kim Price, *Medical Negligence in Victorian Britain: The Crisis of Care under the English Poor Law, 1834–1900* (London: Bloomsbury, 2015); Anne Hanley, 'Syphilization and Its Discontents: Experimental Inoculation against Syphilis at the London Lock Hospital', *Bulletin of the History of Medicine* 91:1 (2017),

1–32; Molly Ladd-Taylor, *Fixing the Poor: Eugenic Sterilization and Child Welfare in the Twentieth Century* (Baltimore: Johns Hopkins University Press, 2017).

14  See, for example, Fiona Reid, *Medicine in First World War Europe: Soldiers, Medics, Pacifists* (London: Bloomsbury, 2017), 198.

15  For more on these post-war changes, see Alex Molds, *Making the Consumer Patient: Patient Organisations and Health Consumerism in Britain* (Manchester: Manchester University Press, 2015), 5; David Armstrong, 'The Patient's View', *Social Science and Medicine* 18:9 (1984), 737–44; David Armstrong, 'Actors, Patients and Agency: A Recent History', *Sociology of Health and Illness* 36:2 (2014), 163–74.

16  Ben Collins, 'Outcomes for Mental Health Services: What Really Matters?', The King's Fund (March 2019), www.kingsfund.org.uk/sites/default/files/2019-03/outcomes-mental-health-services_0.pdf (accessed 10 March 2020), 4.

17  'Summit 2020 Session: Prof Chris Whitty on Health Trends and Projections Over the Next 20 Years', The Nuffield Trust (27 February 2020), www.nuffieldtrust.org.uk/media/summit-2020-session-prof-chris-whitty-on-the-direction-of-health-trends-over-the-next-20-years (accessed 10 March 2020).

18  Dan Wellings, 'Joined-Up Listening: Integrated Care and Patient Insight', The King's Fund (August 2018), www.kingsfund.org.uk/publications/joined-up-listening-integrated-care-and-patient-insight (accessed 11 March 2020); Chris Ham, Anna Charles and Dan Wellings, 'Shared Responsibility for Health: The Cultural Change We Need', The King's Fund (November 2018), www.kingsfund.org.uk/publications/shared-responsibility-health (accessed 11 March 2020).

19  John C. Burnham, 'The Death of the Sick Role', *Social History of Medicine* 25:4 (2012), 761–76, 761.

20  Ibid., 772.

21  For the psychotherapeutic history of mindfulness, see Matthew Drage, 'Of Mountains, Lakes and Essences: John Teasdale and the Transmission of Mindfulness', *History of the Human Sciences* 31:4 (2018), 107–30. See also Anna Alexandrova, *A Philosophy for the Science of Well-Being* (Oxford: Oxford University Press, 2017); Carl Cederström and Andre Spicer, *The Wellness Syndrome* (Cambridge: Polity Press, 2015); Colleen Derkatch, 'The Self-Generating Language of Wellness and Natural Health', *Rhetoric of Health and Medicine* 1:1–2 (2018), 132–60.

22  British Medical Association, *Selfcare: Question and Answer* (November 2019), 1.

23  Janice E. Perlman, *The Myth of Marginality: Urban Poverty and Politics in Rio de Janeiro* (Berkeley: University of California Press, 1976).

24 Robert H. Blank, Viola Burau and Ellen Kuhlmann, *Comparative Health Policy*, 5th edition (London: Red Globe Press, 2018), 181.
25 COVID-19 testing in England and Wales was made available to those over five years old with symptoms on 18 May, a month and a half after the government instituted lockdown measures. 'Matt Hancock MP Gives Update on Covid Response', www.parliament.uk/business/news/2020/may/matt-hancock-mp-gives-update-on-covid-19-response (accessed 27 July 2020).
26 Alison M.I. Elliott, Anne McAteer and Philip C. Hannaford, 'Revisiting the Symptom Iceberg in Today's Primary Care: Results from a UK Population Survey', *BMC Family Practice* 12 (2011), 1–11. See also Michael Worboy's chapter in this collection.
27 Borsay and Shapely, *Medicine, Charity and Mutual Aid*, 2.
28 George Campbell Gosling, *Payment and Philanthropy in British Healthcare, 1918–48* (Manchester: Manchester University Press, 2017), 2.
29 For more on the conceptual challenges of understanding historical agency, see Lynn M. Thomas, 'Historicising Agency', *Gender & History* 28:2 (2016), 324–39.
30 Porter, *Bodies Politic*, 92.
31 House of Commons, Health and Social Care Committee, 'Sexual Health: Fourteenth Report of Session 2017–19. Report, Together with Formal Minutes Relating to the Report', HC 1419 (House of Commons, 2019).
32 Anne Hanley, 'Protection or Control? The Debate over Emergency Contraception', *History & Policy*, www.historyandpolicy.org/opinion-articles/articles/protection-or-control-the-debate-over-emergency-contraception (accessed 18 February 2020); Advisory Group on Contraception, *At Tipping Point: An Audit of Cuts to Contraceptive Services and Their Consequences for Women* (November 2018), http://theagc.org.uk/wp-content/uploads/2018/11/At_tipping_point_AGC_Nov_18.pdf (accessed 14 January 2020).
33 Care Quality Commission, '2019 Community Mental Health Survey: Statistical Release' (2019), www.cqc.org.uk/sites/default/files/20191126_cmh19_statisticalrelease.pdf (accessed 10 March 2020).
34 Simon Harold Walker, 'We Need to Talk About Suicide in the Military', *The Conversation*, https://theconversation.com/we-need-to-talk-about-suicide-in-the-military-119219 (accessed 11 March 2020).
35 Roy Porter, *A Social History of Madness: Stories of the Insane* (London: Weidenfeld & Nicolson, 1987), 2.
36 Bacopoulous-Viau and Fauvel, 'The Patient's Turn', 12.
37 Condrau, 'The Patient's View Meets the Clinical Gaze', 536.
38 For further reflections on the ethical implications of archival research and the researcher's ethical obligations to their dead subjects, see Jelena

Subotić, 'Ethics of Archival Research on Political Violence', *Journal of Peace Studies* (2020), 1–13.

39 Angela Woods, 'The Limits of Narrative: Provocations for the Medical Humanities', *Medical Humanities* 37:2 (2011), 73–8, 73.

40 Brian Hurwitz and Victoria Bates, 'The Roots and Ramifications of Narrative in Modern Medicine', in Anne Whitehead, Angela Woods, with Sarah Atkinson, Jane McNaughton, Jennifer Richards (eds), *The Edinburgh Companion to the Critical Medical Humanities* (Edinburgh: Edinburgh University Press, 2016), 559–60.

41 Bryan J. Good and Mary-Jo Delvecchio Good, '"Fiction" and "Historicity" in Doctors' Stories: Social and Narrative Dimensions of Learning Medicine', in Cheryl Mattingly and Linda C. Garro (eds), *Narrative and the Cultural Construction of Illness* (Berkeley: University of California Press, 2000), 50–69.

42 Philippa Berman and Richard Horton, 'Case Reports in *The Lancet*: A New Narrative', *Lancet* (4 April 2015), 1277.

43 Hurwitz and Bates, 'The Roots and Ramifications of Narrative in Modern Medicine', 561.

44 Michael Roper, 'Slipping Out of View: Subjectivity and Emotion in Gender History', *History Workshop Journal* 59:1 (2005), 57–72.

45 Rob Boddice, 'Medicine, Science and Psychology', in Katie Barclay, Sharon Crozier-de-Rosa and Peter Stearns (eds), *Sources for the History of Emotions: A Guide* (Abingdon: Routledge, 2020).

46 Rob Boddice, 'The History of Emotions', in Sasha Handley, Rohan McWilliam and Lucy Noakes (eds), *New Directions in Social and Cultural History* (London: Bloomsbury, 2018), 45–64, 47.

47 Boddice, 'The History of Emotions', 57–8.

48 Boddice, 'Medicine, Science and Psychology'; on the study of emotions in the history of sexuality and medicine, see Caroline Rusterholz, 'You Can't Dismiss that as Being Less Happy, You See it is Different': Sexual Counselling in 1950s England', *Twentieth Century British History* 30:3 (2019), 375–98.

49 See, for example, Agnes Arnold-Foster, '"A Small Cemetery": Death and Dying in the Contemporary British Operating Theatre', *Medical Humanities* (Advanced Access 2019), 1–10; Michael Brown, 'Surgery, Identity and Embodied Emotion: John Bell, James Gregory and the Edinburgh "Medical War"', *History* 104:359 (2019), 19–41; Jessica Meyer, *An Equal Burden: The Men of the Royal Army Medical Corps in the First World War* (Oxford: Oxford University Press, 2019), chapter 3.

50 See, for example, Roy Porter, *A Social History of Madness*; Roy Porter, *Mind-Forg'd Manacles: A History of Madness in England from the Restoration to the Regency* (Harvard: Harvard University Press, 1987).

51 Katie Barclay, 'Falling in Love With the Dead', *Rethinking History* 22:4 (2018), 459–73.
52 Chris Millard, 'Using Personal Experience in the Academic Medical Humanities: A Genealogy', *Social Theory & Health* (Advanced Access 2019), 1–15.
53 These problems were the focus of 'Supporting Researchers Working on Sensitive Histories' – a workshop held in January 2020 at Birkbeck, University of London.
54 Jennifer Wallis, *Investigating the Body in the Victorian Asylum: Doctors, Patients and Practices* (Basingstoke: Palgrave, 2017), 34.
55 For more on the rise of patient-led campaigns, see Molds, *Making the Consumer Patient*; Alex Mold, 'Complaining in the Age of Consumption: Patients, Consumers or Citizens?', in Jonathan Reinarz and Rebecca Wynter (eds), *Complaints, Controversies and Grievances in Medicine: Historical and Social Science Perspectives* (Abingdon: Routledge, 2015), 167–83.
56 Sally Sheard, 'History Matters: The Critical Contribution of Historical Analysis to Contemporary Health Policy and Health Care', *Health Care Analysis* 26 (2018), 140–54, 140.
57 Here, we are using policy-making to describe general statements of intent by governments, health authorities and health organisations; tangible actions taken on specific health issues; and sets of guidelines for the protection and management of health. For further discussion of these different aspects of policy-making, see Blank, Burau and Kuhlmann, *Comparative Health Policy*.
58 'Summit 2020 Session: Prof Chris Whitty on Health Trends and Projections over the next 20 Years'.
59 Simon Szreter, *Health and Wealth: Studies in History and Policy* (Rochester: Rochester University Press, 2005), 19–20.
60 Virginia Berridge, 'History Matters? History's Role in Health Policy Making', *Medical History* 52:3 (2008), 311–26, 325. See also Virginia Berridge, 'Why Policy Needs History (and Historians)', *Health Economics, Policy and Law* 13 (2018), 369–81.
61 Bacopoulous-Viau and Fauvel, 'The Patient's Turn', 12.
62 Condrau, 'The Patient's View Meets the Clinical Gaze', 536.
63 For more on 'experts by experience' in healthcare, see Millard, 'Using Personal Experience in the Academic Medical Humanities', 1–15.
64 Nina Hemmings, Rachel Hutchings, Sophie Castle-Clarke and Dr William Palmer, 'Research Report March 2020. Achieving Scale and Spread: Learning for Innovators and Policymakers', The Nuffield Trust (2020), www.nuffieldtrust.org.uk/files/2020-03/achieving-scale-and-spread-report-final.pdf (accessed 10 March 2020).

## Introduction

65  David Hall-Matthews, 'Can Historians Assist Development Policy-Making, or Just Highlight its Faults?', in C.A. Bayly, Vijayendra Rao, Simon Szreter and Michael Woolcock (eds), *Historians and Development Policy: A Necessary Dialogue* (Manchester: Manchester University Press, 2011), 169–74, 169.
66  Berridge, 'History Matters?', 313.
67  Sheard, 'History Matters', 144.
68  Hall-Matthews, 'Can Historians Assist Development Policy-Making', 171.
69  For further discussion of this, see Sheard, 'History Matters', 154.
70  Pierre Bourdieu, 'The Forms of Social Capital', in Imre Szeman and Timothy Kaposy (eds), *Cultural Theory: An Anthology* (Malden: Wiley-Blackwell, 1986), 81–93; Robert Putnam, 'Social Capital: Measurement and Consequences', *Canadian Journal of Policy Research* 2 (2001), 41–51. For further discussion of the role of social capital in shaping health outcomes, see Nikolas Rose, *Our Psychiatric Future: The Politics of Mental Health* (Cambridge: Polity Press, 2019), 53–57; Szreter, *Health and Wealth*, 376–412; John Welshman, 'Searching for Social Capital: Historical Perspectives on Health, Poverty and Culture', *Journal of the Royal Society for the Promotion of Health* 126:6 (2006), 268–74.
71  Arthur Kleinman, 'The Art of Medicine: Caregiving as Moral Experience', *Lancet* (3 November 2012), 1550–1.
72  Ibid., 1551.
73  British Medical Association, *Selfcare: Question and Answer* (November 2019).
74  Szreter, *Health and Wealth*, 411.
75  Blank, Burau and Kuhlmann, *Comparative Health Policy*, 17–23.
76  Szreter, *Health and Wealth*, 391.
77  For more of the structure and dynamics of such networks, including the role of material culture, see Bruno Latour, *Reassembling the Social: An Introduction to Actor-Network-Theory* (Oxford: Oxford University Press, 2005); Hans K. Klein and Daniel Lee Kleinman, 'The Social Construction of Technology: Structural Considerations', *Science, Technology and Human Values* 27:1 (2002), 28–52.
78  Julia Laite, 'Radical Uncertainty', *History Workshop Online* (16 September 2020), www.historyworkshop.org.uk/radical-uncertainty (accessed 20 September 2020). See also Julia Laite, 'Choose Your Own Adventure History', Storying the Past: A blog for creative histories and the #storypast virtual reading group (18 October 2017), https://storyingthepast.wordpress.com/2017/10/18/choose-your-own-adventure-history-by-julia-laite (accessed 24 September 2020).

# I

Locating the patient: new approaches

# 1

# The non-patient's view*

## Michael Worboys

Roy Porter's article 'The Patient's View' stimulated a major change in medical history. In many ways it defined the new social history of medicine, which since the 1970s had been challenging doctor-centred histories and opening new approaches and topics. Many historians took up Porter's invitation to rewrite medicine's past 'from below', but I argue in this chapter that they have not been radical enough and have missed one of his major challenges. The overlooked item is the last on his agenda for future research:

> We should stop seeing the doctor as the agent of primary care. People took care before they took physick. What we habitually call primary care is in fact secondary care, once the sufferer has become a patient, [and] has entered the medical arena.[1]

Porter is pointing to the importance of self-diagnosis and self-treatment – the beliefs, behaviours and actions of sick people who did not go to the doctor and remained 'non-patients'. In time and if symptoms persisted, they might have seen a medical practitioner. Though not addressed in this chapter, an important question therefore is what it took, in terms of beliefs, symptoms, opportunities and resources, for a person to move from being a 'non-patient' to a patient. This issue has become an important policy issue in the early twenty-first century, in terms of demand on health services.

Exploring this new area of ignorance requires historians to explore familiar sources in new ways and to find new sources, many of which have previously been regarded as non-medical. Historians of medicine have been quite presentist in only rarely exploring prayer as an aid to healing, which was and remains a common response to illness. It also requires the creative reading of absences. For example, 'doing nothing' about an illness should be approached, not as passive or negative, but as a positive action, based on knowledge, opportunity and experience.

One indication of the scale and importance of the 'non-patient' for medical history is suggested by contemporary sociological studies of the so-called 'symptom iceberg': 'the phenomenon that most symptoms are managed in the community without people seeking professional healthcare'.[2] The 'iceberg of illness' had been identified as early as 1949 by Percy Stocks and then by John and Elizabeth Horder in 1954.[3] In 1972, Karen Dunnell and Ann Cartwright published a study of medicine-taking in Britain, based on surveys over a two-week period.[4] The context was concern that people were not going to the doctor, rather preferring to take the growing range of proprietary medicine. They found 91 per cent of those questioned reported 'abnormal symptoms' in the previous fortnight, with just 16 per cent consulting a doctor.[5] More detailed studies were undertaken in the 2000s. The most comprehensive study sent questionnaires to 8,000 randomly chosen adults aged eighteen to sixty.[6] Of these, 33.2 per cent returned a completed questionnaire, describing a total of 7,994 symptoms. Their actions – which are not mutually exclusive – are summarised in Table 1.1 and illustrated in Figure 1.1.

The key finding of the study was that only 8.3 per cent of symptom episodes led to the sufferer seeing their GP, with a further 3.1 per cent seeing another type of orthodox practitioner (e.g. nurse or pharmacist) or proxy (e.g. NHS24/NHS Direct). A further 11.1 per cent were already 'patients' and took a prescribed medicine. Thus, around 80 per cent of people in the sample with symptoms can be regarded as 'non-patients'. The survey focused on responses to symptoms not illnesses per se, though this was allowed for by ranking the seriousness of symptoms defining specific illnesses. The four most serious (and corresponding percentages of respondents seeing the GP) were shortness of breath (18.2 per cent), blood in stool (23.1 per cent), unintentional weight loss (27 per cent) and chest pain (15.7 per cent).[7]

Thus, in the early twenty-first century, in a country where access to care through the National Health Service (NHS) is free at the

Table 1.1 Actions taken by survey participants for each symptom experienced in the preceding two weeks

| Action | % |
| --- | --- |
| Did nothing at all | 48.6 |
| Looked for information | 2.6 |
| Discussed with family and friends | 9.8 |
| Took over-the-counter medicines | 25.0 |
| Phoned NHS24/NHS Direct | 0.5 |
| Consulted nurse | 0.8 |
| Consulted pharmacist | 1.8 |
| Consulted complementary therapist | 1.8 |
| Consulted GP (on phone or in person) | 8.3 |
| Took prescribed medicines | 11.1 |

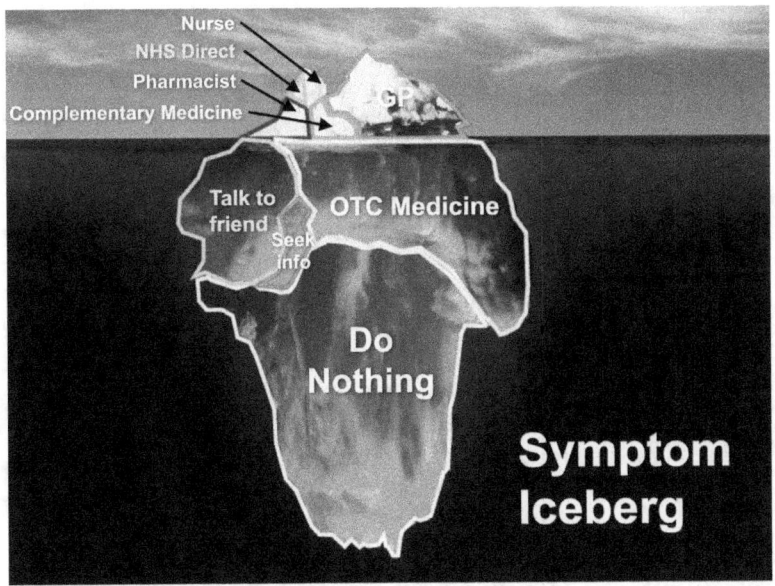

1.1 Graphic representing the 'symptom iceberg'

point of delivery, and after a century of great advances when public confidence in medicine's ability to cure is very high, only one in five symptom episodes involves the sufferer becoming a patient. The obvious question for historians is, what would the proportion have been before the introduction of the NHS and the 'therapeutic revolution' of the twentieth century? The answer in all probability is a very much lower percentage.[8] Also, the proportions were likely to have differed between men, women and children. Where and when medical treatment was seen to be more effective, priority would have been given to men as the main breadwinner and to children.[9] Anne Hanley's chapter in this volume points to other ways responses were patterned.[10] The stigma of venereal infection meant that self-treatment was tried for longer, and with gonorrhoea, there was the belief that the infection was like a head cold's runny nose 'down there' and would be self-limiting.

In this chapter, I make the case for historians to give greater attention to the 'non-patient's view' and especially to their actions. While records of their views are likely to be scarce, those of their actions, such as buying products and literature for self-treatment, should be less so. My focus is on Britain in the century before the establishment of the NHS. I begin with a brief review of where I have explored this topic in my own work, which was largely framed as the 'public's view', now changed in this chapter to 'non-patient's view'. I then deal in turn with the main categories of action from the 'symptom iceberg' study: doing nothing; looking for information; discussing with family and friends; and taking over-the-counter medicines. I finish with a discussion of sources as this is a major challenge for the approach and subject matter I am advocating. In the conclusion I discuss briefly the policy implications for healthcare in the twenty-first century. The advice to 'Not see the doctor' was advocated directly in the winter of 2017–18 and again in the early months of the COVID-19 pandemic in 2020 to help ease demand on the NHS. More positively, the Self Care Forum, founded in 2011, has been lobbying for greater investment and education for 'empowering people with the confidence and information to look after themselves when they can'.[11]

My time frame means that I will not be exploring historical antecedents, nor parallels with the extension of the late twentieth-century doctor's gaze on the 'potential patient', as defined by their risk factors.[12] And although I discuss only physical illnesses in this chapter, it will be clear that the same arguments and wider historical lenses are needed for mental illnesses. I also see this chapter as a contribution to the new interest in 'Medicine in the Household', which was the subject of a special issue of *Social History of Medicine* in 2016 in which its editors explored more imaginatively what counted as 'medical' in history.[13] There are also possible links to work on the 'patient-consumer'. Alex Mold's review of the uses of the term in Britain shows that it has been framed, no doubt because of the NHS, largely in terms of consuming state medical services.[14] However, Nancy Tomes's work on patient-consumers in the United States necessarily has a wider focus given the country's different history of healthcare infrastructure and can be read as a study of the transition from 'non-patient' to patient.[15]

## The public's view

I was a ready subscriber to Porter's manifesto for 'The Patient's View' and first attempted to capture what I now term the 'non-patient's view' in an article published in 1994, co-authored with Michael Sigsworth, on 'The Public's View of Public Health' based on a study of Yorkshire towns.[16] We explored the public's view of early nineteenth-century sanitary reform. Our main point was that 'the Great Unwashed' had different ideas and priorities to sanitary reformers, and that these were more economic than environmental, and based on different ideas of the nature and causes of disease. For example, the working class in Leeds wanted decent wages to buy the food that would build strong, disease-resistant bodily 'frames', ahead of clean water. Improved wages would additionally allow them immediate escape from overcrowding in slum dwellings by moving to the healthier streets that they recognised only too well. However, in their new dwellings they would still want to keep pigs, which far from being filthy sources of disease, were valuable scavengers that cleared up and recycled waste, provided manure to sell or fertilise land, and a good Christmas dinner in mid-winter. Second, in the 2007 book on rabies in Victorian Britain, co-authored with Neil Pemberton, we considered the responses of victims and their families to dog bites, and the calculations they made about the risks and benefits of different actions.[17] The options ranged widely. Assuming that the dog was unlikely to be rabid or that a harmless amount of poison had been inoculated, many chose to wait and see. Others employed a range of preventives and curatives, from applying the hair of the dog to the wound, hand-me-down herbal potions and patent medicines, and vapour baths to sweat out the poison, to the medical option of cauterisation or excision of wound tissue. Doctors at the time were clear that the chance of any biting dog having rabies was very small, hence their frustration over lay beliefs that almost all remedies 'worked' most of the time. Finally, in the 2013 book on fungal diseases, co-authored with Aya Homei, we discussed responses to infections like athlete's foot, which caused irritation rather than illness: from accepting irritation and trusting to the healing power of nature, through applying patent ointments (what one doctor termed 'the unbelievable chemical abuse' of the nation's feet).[18]

Also interesting for the argument advanced in this chapter is the doctoral thesis of Rachael Russell on nausea and vomiting in nineteenth-century Britain.[19] The most severe forms of nausea and sickness, seasickness and morning sickness, were temporary and therefore mostly endured with stoicism and the knowledge of eventual certain relief. However, many precautions and remedies were proposed, from mental disciplines to medicinal compounds, patent and prescription. Most episodes of vomiting were transient, usually explained by something eaten, over-indulgence, something catching, or as ancillary to another illness. The very nature of the symptoms meant that taking something by mouth was largely redundant, hence, wait-and-see was the commonest action. With nausea, measures taken, if any, depended on many things: past experiences, the duration and intensity of symptoms, the frequency of fainting, associations with pain and other signs. Russell's thesis shows that throughout the nineteenth century and across social classes, people had highly developed understandings of their body's normal and abnormal functioning, and of likely linkages between prognoses and various remedial measures. These were drawn from experience, knowledge and help drawn from social networks, and from a variety of information sources.

In the following sections of this chapter, I discuss in turn the four 'non-patient' responses identified in 'symptom iceberg' studies:

doing nothing; looking for information; family and friends; taking over-the-counter medicines; and then ending with a discussion of sources.

## Doing nothing at all

For the most serious symptoms in the 'symptom iceberg' survey, the percentages for 'doing nothing at all' were shortness of breath (47.2 per cent), blood in stool (57.7 per cent), unintentional weight loss (59.9 per cent) and chest pain (52 per cent). What do we make of these surprising figures? Surely, it is that 'doing nothing at all' does not capture people's responses, as it implies passivity or fatalism. Put another way, it makes 'doing nothing at all' a residual. It assumes a 'deficit model' where medical intervention is normal and necessary and that anything less is considered to be negligent. I argue that 'doing nothing at all' is (and was) an active and informed choice, based on experience, lay understandings of the meaning of symptoms and likely prognoses. More simply, 'doing nothing at all' is doing something. Wait-and-see shows faith in the healing powers of nature and points to the issue of the threshold for the move from 'non-patient' to patient. In his 1977 essay on 'The Therapeutic Revolution in Nineteenth-Century America', Charles Rosenberg suggests that this move became easier from the late nineteenth century, due to changed social, economic and cultural factors, and also because doctors and the public increasingly shared the same view of the body and had growing confidence in medicine's powers.[20]

The 'symptom iceberg' survey was thoroughly materialist. It only asked about physical, material and social responses to illness, not spiritual and psychological ones. Yet there is evidence that prayer is a very common response to symptoms and illness. In the early twenty-first century church attendances in Britain are low. None the less, a survey of 2,069 people, across all ages in 2017, found that 51 per cent still prayed; indeed, a fifth of non-believers prayed.[21] Among those who prayed in a group that included non-believers, 40 per cent did so for healing, with the figure similar across all religions.[22] If these levels are found today, it is almost certain they would have been higher historically when religious observance and belief were the norm.

Such is the implicit materialism of medical historians today, that very few have even considered prayer as a rational, let alone possibly effective, response to symptoms. One exception is Joanna Bourke in her book *The Story of Pain: From Prayer to Painkillers*.[23] While the subtitle might be teleological, carrying the implication of progress from faith in God to effective pharmaceuticals, the narrative shows the changing religious meanings given to pain. If it was a punishment, then perhaps relief should not be sought, but if it was due to malign forces then prayer was legitimate. Bourke's narrative shows the complexities of responses to pain, lay and medical, with spiritual, psychological, material and social actions combined and intertwined. An important point is that many prayers would have been social as well as private, and offered solace and hope, with shared meanings and experiences. Lastly, and perhaps most importantly, prayers would have been experienced to 'work'. The great majority of symptoms and illnesses are self-limiting, with individual experience unable to distinguish whether the association between prayer and their recovery was cause and effect, or coincidence.

Evidence for the role of prayer in responses to illness are to be found in private diaries, but there were also public demonstrations of prayer and its success in healing. Historians have been interested in the seeming increase in public acts of worship in response to crises in Victorian Britain.[24] With regard to disease and medicine, these studies have been mostly framed in terms of changing relations between science and religion, yet, the efficacy of prayer was the immediate issue.[25] The most celebrated instance was in the winter of 1871, prompted by the Prince of Wales suffering from suspected typhoid fever. Government ministers and church leaders organised national prayer days for his return to health, and when this was successful, arranged nationwide services of thanksgiving. There had been no large-scale public turn to prayer ten years earlier, when the Prince's father died of the same disease, but during the 1860s prayers came into favour for relief from disease. Frank Turner's discussion of the episode is in terms of the struggle for cultural authority between scientists and the clergy, with the latter winning when the Prince recovered four days after prayers were read out in churches across the nation.[26] Turner quotes a letter to *The Guardian* from a vicar who wrote that 'The wonderful change in the condition of the Prince of Wales will surely impress many hitherto doubtful of the efficacy of prayer'.[27] To rub salt in the wound of the medical profession, there were three further religious observances of thanksgiving for divine intervention with the Prince's illness. Reports on the episode in *The Guardian* spoke of 'the direct and personal working of the Hand of God', and that the Prince's recovery 'was not by some abstract "Law of Health", not merely by human skill and tenderness, but by the mercy of God who hears and answers prayers'.[28]

Turner shows that the reaction of the medical profession was to argue that religion and science were complementary. An editorial in the *Lancet* recognised 'the hand of Providence', but also contended that modern medical science had 'signally won fresh laurels in the recovery of the Prince of Wales'.[29] For nineteenth-century America, Rosenberg makes the same point, observing that for most doctors and patients, 'There was no inconsistency between [the medical] world of rationalistic explanation and traditional spiritual values.'[30] However, some scientists were less accommodating. Indeed, Francis Galton was moved to undertake statistical analyses on the efficacy of prayer, finding that 'sick persons who pray, or are prayed for, on the average' did not recover more quickly.[31] Given the power of churches in Victorian Britain, if calls to prayers for recovery from illness and questions about its efficacy were so public, then in private it is almost certain that prayers for the recovery of the sick were pervasive across society.[32] Indeed, every hospital had a chaplain and while their formal role was to serve the spiritual rather than the material needs of patients, prayers for divine intervention to aid recoveries were customary.[33] The chapters in this volume by Hanley and Houston both discuss the notion that patients' engagement with doctors was a type of 'lay confession', where they might acknowledge how their behaviour contributed to their condition. Regular evening prayers on wards fostered a spiritual ambience, which was manifest in some institutions by the religious affiliation of nursing orders. The only conflict evident in the medical press was of doctors' complaints that chaplains were paid more, enjoyed better conditions, and were, perhaps, more valued.[34]

## Looking for information

*Medicine Without Doctors* was a pioneering collection of essays published in 1977, edited by Guenther Risse, Ronald Numbers and Judith Leavitt.[35] In many ways it anticipated Porter's 'patient's view' manifesto. Like Porter, Risse's 'Introduction' observes that the importance of 'do-it-yourself healing' was not reflected in medical historiography and argues that those taking up its investigation should be open to the varieties and eclecticism of self-care and self-treatment. He set out an agenda that emphasised the need to consider prevention, as well as diagnosis and treatment: to look at physical and mental problems; to recognise that actions were shaped by the traditions and experiences of family, friends and wider groups; to take cognisance of the healing powers of nature in resolving many illnesses; and to not forget the placebo effect. However, most of the contributors to *Medicine Without Doctors* wrote on 'alternative' healthcare systems and the information they provided for self-help. They tended to assume a version of the 'deficit model', where orthodox medicine was unavailable or spurned, with the gap filled by movements, such as Thomsonianism and homeopathy, or by patent medicines and quackery. Much of the work promoted by Porter's 1985 essay on British healthcare has been on similar topics.[36] One wonders if the link between the patient's view and 'medicine' is ingrained to such an extent that historians could only think in terms of systems: orthodox or non-orthodox alternative?

Two essays in *Medicine Without Doctors* do go beyond medical systems and quackery to consider self-reliant responses to illness. Risse highlights the importance of the sick person's knowledge and experience of their own body, its past illnesses, how responses were shaped by religious beliefs and practices, and a commitment to self-reliance. James Harvey Young shows the need for relativism in considering what 'worked', be that treatments or 'wait-and-see'. He also stresses the importance of emotion and feelings, concluding with a nod to the healing powers of nature and the placebo effect that, 'Self-help, of course, has a high enough percentage of success to build confidence in the means of employed', and any measure might help 'by furnishing a sense of relief through the sheer act of doing something, by encouraging mood'.[37]

## Family and friends[38]

The 'Introduction' to *Medicine Without Doctors* did look beyond systems to 'orally transmitted folk traditions', but these mostly remained tied to systems.[39] British historians and social scientists have followed the same trajectory, taking folk medicine to be 'all those practices which lie outside the "normal" sphere of operations of orthodox western medical practice'; in other words, quacks, alternative, complementary and fringe medicine.[40] Such studies, which were presented as a radical turn, still neglected 'non-patient' healthcare. None the less, I want to take the notion of 'orally transmitted folk traditions' and develop it differently. My suggestion is to take the 'folk' in folk medicine in the colloquial sense of 'folks' and specifically the ideas and practices that circulated in families, neighbourhoods and communities.[41] Dunnell's and Cartwright's study of medicine-taking in Britain in the early 1970s found that 'only a small proportion, a tenth, of the non-prescribed medicines taken by adults had been first suggested by a doctor; most were the suggestions of parents, friends, neighbours, husbands or wives or other relatives'.[42]

For the same period in Britain, there is one seminal study of folk medicine, namely Cecil Helman's '"Feed a Cold, Starve a Fever"'.[43] Helman was a general practitioner, who also qualified in anthropology and combined the two disciplines in a study of the belief systems and practices of his patients regarding the causes and cures of colds and fevers. Over four years, he undertook interviews with selected patients from his practice in the West London suburb of Stanmore. The prime puzzle he sought to solve was the persistence of humoral ideas about colds and fevers in the age of modern biomedicine and particularly bacterial and viral explanations of infection. He showed that patients and, importantly, doctors too, worked across the two seemingly contradictory registers of humoral and infective models of disease causation and treatment. Sometimes they were in conflict, but more often they were found in parallel, or in innovative, *ad hoc* syntheses. His findings echoed those of anthropologists' studies on non-Western cultures, were the norm was so-called medical pluralism.[44]

Helman acknowledged one important weakness in his study: 'Only those cases of illness brought to the GP's attention could be included.'[45] Thus, he ignored illnesses that were self-treated or untreated. Nonetheless, his findings offer valuable insights into the ideas and actions of 'non-patients'. Helman paid particular attention to coughs, then the most commonly complained of symptom in general practice. In fact, after aspirin and similar analgesics, the combination of prescribed and over-the-counter cough remedies constituted the second most common class of medicines consumed in the country.[46] He concluded that the use of over-the-counter medicines, in the face of medical evidence that these mixtures had no value in treating infection, 'can be explained (if only in part) by the patients' need to "make sense" of treatment for their illness in terms of their indigenous medical system'.[47] It is interesting that he posits that his patients in Stanmore had 'indigenous medical systems' in the same manner as anthropologists had talked about the beliefs and practices of groups in non-Western cultures. However, in West London and as often elsewhere 'indigenous medical systems' had been infected with orthodox, Western medicine. Thus, Helman found that humoral notions of removing excess fluid and 'muck' from the lungs and chest had been combined with germ theories of infection, to make sufferers seek to expel or kill invading agents and their poisons.

One disease for which 'folk medicine' in my familial sense has been explored is whooping cough (pertussis), a childhood infection characterised by severe (whooping) coughing fits. Its distinctive symptoms meant it was defined as a specific disease from the early modern period, with many remedies tried by parents, following family traditions, or the advice of neighbours and friends. Those remedies common in Britain, according to Samuel Radbill's quarrying of the folklore literature, included tying a spider or wood louse in a bag for the suffer to wear round their neck or nearby; wearing red or blue cloth; three-times protocols (drinking milk stood for three hours, three times for three mornings, and wearing a string with nine knots); crawling under a bramble bush; and passing children through a tunnel or similar hollow.[48] Donkeys and other animals were variously used in passing, seemingly hoping that passage under their body would allow the disease to be passed to the animal. Remedies were also combined. Thus, children were passed under a donkey or ass three times, or taken for a ride, preferably to a crossroads and back, and the hair of a donkey eaten or worn round the neck.[49] Many concoctions were made with parts of animals, such as frogs in the hope that croaking would be passed on, or that the smell of sheep and donkey dung would break the cycle of paroxysmal coughing. Whooping cough had a relatively low mortality rate in children over a year old. Therefore, for most sufferers most of the time, these treatments worked.[50]

In a survey of late nineteenth- and early twentieth-century cough remedies, Radbill found that a change of air was often recommended to 'break the cough'. In Hull, parents took their children across the Humber and in Scotland to distilleries and gasworks. Taking children to gasworks grew in popularity with germ theories of infection and the profile given to carbolic acid in antiseptic and antigerm measures after 1870.[51] This is another example of Helman's point about the synthesis of 'indigenous' and orthodox medical cultures, seen in the practice of families taking sufferers to inhale presumed chemicals antidotes – the waste gases released by factories and works. This practice was tried during cholera outbreaks in Leeds and more widely for pulmonary tuberculosis, with children taking the air by playing near creosoting or tarmacking gangs.[52] With whooping cough, one practice was to take the sick child 'for a walk round the gasworks every day for a week, and he'll be as right as rain in a very short time'.[53] During the outbreak of the disease in the winter of 1925–26, the South Suburban Gas Co., Ltd., whose chief engineer and manager George Livesey was an active philanthropist, made their works in Lower Sydenham available to local families. The company turned its 'pump-room into a clinic, where children could go and "take the smells"'.[54] The 'smells' were 'ammonia, sulphuretted hydrogen – that obnoxious gas which makes one think of rotten eggs – naphthaline [sic] and tar'.[55] Ammonia and tar were said to be the key agents: 'It is more or less a case of killing to cure, for in most instances the fumes from the gas liquor bring on violent fits of coughing. But the trouble in the throat, which causes the whoop, is often removed in this manner.'[56] This rationale combines humoral notions of clearing phlegm, with modern ideas of chemical disinfection.

## Taking over-the-counter medicines

A common assumption in most historical studies of over-the-counter or patent medicines is that their sellers made exaggerated, even fraudulent, claims about their effectiveness; put simply, they did not 'work'. This view is most evident in studies by pharmacist-historians, who have been fascinated by the ingredients of patent remedies and the seeming gullibility of the people who bought and took them.[57] However, they also recognise that these medicines often contained substances like opium, alcohol, emetics and purgatives. Thus, they would, if taken in large enough doses, have produced physiological changes and altered symptoms. Yet, the charge remains that manufacturers and sellers were wrong to claim that their medicines 'worked', hence, they were and are appropriately labelled quackery. Such claims are based on modern pharmacology's ability to demonstrate that the component compounds of patent medicines could not have altered the underlying pathology and in many cases had side-effects that were deleterious to health.

I argue, as with prayers, the case for being relativistic about what 'worked' and developing a fuller, more nuanced understanding of the experiences of health and illness. Consider the experience of a nineteenth-century consumer of Holloway's Pills, the most popular patent remedy by market share.[58] Pharmacist-historians have followed the lead of the British Medical Association's (BMA) exposés of 'Secret Remedies' in the 1900s, in disparaging the man and his medicines. The pills were revealed to be mostly composed of ineffectual ingredients: aloes, powdered ginger and soap.[59] Edwardian doctors often wrote of public gullibility in repeat purchases of such concoctions, though as Harvey Young presumed, much of their efficacy and market success must be due to placebo effects.[60]

The fortunes built by entrepreneurs such as Thomas Holloway and Thomas Beecham indicate that customers felt that they were getting value for money, so it is worth looking beyond any presumed placebo effect.[61] One typical advertisement for 'Holloways Pills and Ointment' in 1869 recommended they be taken for the following conditions:

> Bad legs, Bad breasts, Burns, Bunions, Bite of Mosquitoes and sandflies, Coco-bay, Chicago-foot, Chilblains, Chapped Hands, Corns(soft), Cancers, Contracted and stiff joints, Elephantiasis, Fistulas, Gout, Glandular Swellings, Lumbago, Rheumatism, Scalds, Sore Nipples, Sore-throats, Skin Diseases, Scurvy, Tumours, Ulcers, Wounds, Yaws, &c., &c., &c.[62]

Lists such as these were often printed in small type and would have been hard to read given the state of indoor lighting and contemporary optometry. None the less, it is interesting to speculate on the meanings that customers would have taken from the marketing. First, the listing gained authority in mixing medical and lay terms, while its length and indication of multi-valency could have indicated the pills' potency. Second, Holloway's Pills and Ointment were promoted as both a specific and general remedy. Their action was described in humoral terms that were congruent with popular understandings of the body: 'A course of this admirable medicine clears *the blood* of impurities and improves its quality. The *whole system* is thus benefited through the usual *channels* without reduction of strength, shock to the *nerves*, or any other inconvenience.'[63] Third, many of the conditions would have been self-limiting, resolved by what contemporaries would have described as the healing powers of nature, nowadays expressed as immune responses, anti-inflammatory mechanisms, physiological adaptations and, perhaps, behavioural changes induced by symptoms. For example, lumbago, if the demands of work permitted, would have led sufferers to try and change their behaviour, seek rest, or find new ways of coping. Fourth, customers were encouraged to use the medicines for prevention as well as cures, hence, not suffering from any of the complaints listed would have been seen as the pills 'working'. All four considerations were congruent with popular understandings of the body that was part humoral, part physiological and part anatomical, and the experience of those taking the pills was that more often than not they were effective. One imaginative use of this source is to speculate on whether those taking Holloway's Pills regarded themselves as patients, their own doctor, or more likely both. The next step is to consider what might have happened if their illness persisted or worsened and when to seek a second opinion, to become what should rightly be called 'a medical patient'?

Such remedies seem to have been no less popular a half-century on in the years immediately before the NHS. For this later period we no longer have to rely on proxies and speculation as this was the era of new types of social surveys.[64] In 1944, Jack Davies, then in the Physiology Department at the University of Bristol, published the results of a survey of 'the medicines not taken under medical advice', by participants of the Medical Research Council's haemoglobin survey.[65] This was a nominally healthy group of 277 people (149 male and 128 female), aged 15 to 45+ years and from a variety of occupations. The headline finding was that 75 per cent (71 per cent males and 83 per cent female) were taking non-prescribed medicines, the commonest were laxatives (saline and vegetable) and aspirin. Davies was disappointed that 'after the propaganda of the last few years', few people were taking iron, vitamins and other preventives proven by science to be effective. However, his conclusions were mixed. On the one hand he was pleased that Victorian patent medicines, described as 'the most extravagant and exotic remedies', were no longer widely used and that 'there was a widespread desire for information among those questioned'. Tellingly, he observed of his survey group that:

> They desired good health, and many quite sincerely thought that they were ensuring it by taking these medicines. The majority of those surveyed were ostensibly healthy people, and when the high proportion taking drugs is noted we may well wonder at the probable extent of self-medication among the sick folk.[66]

On the other hand, Davies was sure that, though consumers benefited from 'the therapeutic powers of hope and faith', they were swindled. He was doubtful that education was the answer and worried that advertisers were becoming more sophisticated and effective; hence, his conclusion was that 'to prevent much public exploitation and ill-health, restrictive legislation is imperative'.[67] My argument is that the public were not being exploited through ignorance, but rather were making informed decisions based on experience as much as manufacturers claims, and shaped by the healthcare options available, economics and cultural values. Needless to say, Britain, the landscape in which Davies set his views, was about to change radically with the establishment of the NHS.

## Sources

How do historians recover the views and actions of 'non-patients'? Information on most short-term, self-limiting and resolved symptom episodes will not have been recorded, let alone kept. Yet there are sources that can be tapped. The first thing to say is, if I am correct about the scale and prevalence of the sick remaining 'non-patients', then there is potentially an awful lot of self-help healthcare to look for. In seeking the 'patient's view', historians have necessarily been led to look at 'medical records' in the broadest sense. These have been read in patient-centred ways, but they remain 'medical'; recorded by doctors and other medical actors. For example, the many studies based on patient letters to doctors in the eighteenth century are, by definition, from people who became 'patients', though teleology can be avoided by looking at the early stages of a correspondence to recover the 'pre-patient's' view. What actions did they take as 'non-patients' and what led them to become patients? In this chapter, I have given other examples of how well-known and well-hewn sources can be interrogated in new ways.

One source that can be looked at again is diaries. Emma Griffin has recently used working-class diaries and what they say about diets to look again at debates over the standard of living.[68] Similar studies could be made for illness and healthcare. There is much on healthcare and medicines in the working autobiographies collected by John Burnett, David Mayall and David Vincent.[69] The reminisces of Mary Jones tell of her sister reacting badly to smallpox vaccination. As her condition worsened, the doctor reportedly gave up hope, stating that, 'if she lived, she would be either a cripple or an imbecile'. However, her mother Elizabeth did not give up and nursed her back to health with an eclectic mix of measures:

> She went to the farmer to get milk twice a day from one cow, his healthiest, she got the butcher (?) send a small amount of fresh blood each day She went to the builder yard for a piece of rock lime which she (?) daily, she got cod liver oil and oranges. these she administered in very small doses (?) large amounts of love, her little limbs were (?) with olive oil and she carried the baby lying on a pillow for small doses of sunshine into the garden.[70]

Perhaps there is another type of 'non-patient' to explore: the 'post-patient' who is no longer under medical supervision. Indeed, this group is likely to have been larger historically, when recoveries were likely to have taken longer and been based largely on constitutional support, perhaps a change of air and often long periods of convalescence. Medical historians have begun to examine convalescence and the proliferation of medical advice and convalescent homes.[71] The corollary from the argument of this chapter is that most 'getting better' was self-managed and in circumstances that likely did not have exemption from family and work. Moreover, 'post-patients' would not only have been recovering physically, but also mentally with continued anxiety about their future.[72]

For Britain in the twentieth century, there is the rich material collected by Mass Observation (MO). The diaries, survey reports and other material collected are an excellent resource: practically because many records have been digitised and are searchable, and empirically because they capture health and illness in the context of everyday life, not medical ideas and actions. On 'non-patients', particularly instructive is the 1943 *Report on Taking Medicines in War-Time* for what it says about MO's interest in public morale. Were more medicines being sold and, if so, was this due to poor dietary, anxiety, or both.[73] The main finding, based on self-reporting, was that there had been no increase in the number or quantity of non-prescription medicines being taken. Incidentally, the report's narrative reveals the reasons people gave for their consumption of medicines. One person in seven was taking something regularly as a preventative. Those people taking a prescribed medicine were often also taking a non-prescribed medicine in addition. In 1943, one respondent wrote:

> Last winter and this I have taken iodine solution internally as a cure for chilblains, and this winter I have taken matetone [a tonic] for a few days at a time when I have been feeling run down or tired. Last winter I had injections to keep me free from colds, but I am one of the unfortunate beings with whom this method is of no use. Having heard very good reports from two friends of Serocalcin as a preventative of colds, I have tried that this winter and it seems to have been fairly successful so far.[74]

Oral vaccines for the common cold were controversial and expensive, as with 'Buccaline', sold by Hayman and Freeman chemists of Piccadilly, London.[75] The other medicines being taken by those surveyed were: sedatives (Aspro, Aspirin, Veganin, Luminal), laxatives (Liver Salts including Andrew's, Epsom's, Eno's, Paraffin, Taxol, Senna Pods, All Bran) and digestives (McLean's Stomach Powder, Milk of Magnesia). The number of popular brands is an indication of the size of the market.

In August 1943, the journal the *Manufacturing Chemist and Manufacturing Perfumer*, published a report by MO's National Panel of Voluntary Informants titled 'What the Consumer Thinks of Self-Medication'.[76] Its subtitle set out that it was 'the middle-class reaction', later qualified by the authors to be that of the 'more than averagely

## ARE YOU FIGHTING a cold?

YOU may be the type of person in whom a cold is of short duration but severe in character, or you may suffer from an "everlasting" cold—one which returns over and over again. In both cases the ultimate defeat of the attack depends upon the natural defence powers of the body. SEROCALCIN is successful in dealing with colds because it stimulates these natural powers of resistance.

**A SIMPLE TREATMENT**
SEROCALCIN is taken in tablet form and the dosage for treating an existing cold is 3 tablets three times daily. It contains no "drugs" and gives excellent results with children.

**FOR PREVENTION, TOO**
An immunising course of SEROCALCIN gives complete protection against colds for 3 to 4 months in 80% of cases. For this purpose, 60 tablets are taken at the rate of 2 daily.

**SUPPLIES AND PRICES**
War Factories, Hospitals, Schools and Export have priority claims on the supply of SEROCALCIN (Registered Trade Mark) but it is now obtainable from most Chemists. The cost is:—

20 Tablets 3/4½—for intensive treatment of an existing cold.

60 Tablets 8/5½—the immunising course for preventing colds.

Prices include Purchase Tax.

*A booklet "Immunity from Colds" will gladly be sent to doctors, nurses and interested members of the public on receipt of 1d. stamp (as required by Control of Paper Order).*

**SEROCALCIN DEFEATS COLDS**

HARWOODS LABORATORIES LTD., RICKMANSWORTH ROAD, WATFORD, HERTS.

1.2 Advertisement from the *Yorkshire Post* (13 February 1943)

informed and thoughtful section of the community'. The enquiry was also to look at 'the patent medicine trade', where both the terms 'patent' and 'trade' would have been pejorative.[77] Among those consulted, 70 per cent said they were opposed to the patent trade, though it is clear from this and other surveys that many of these were taking patent medicines.[78] One complicating factor was the public were uncertain over what was and was not a patent medicine, because of the convergence in styles of packaging and marketing across the pharmaceutical industry.[79] Most prejudice was against the heavily advertised, high-priced remedies that made bold, curative claims. Cheaper patent medicines were more acceptable if thought to be 'harmless', or as only offering 'psychological cures'. In other words, placebo effects.

## Conclusions

On 29 December 2017 the Royal College of General Practitioners (RCGP) issued a statement urging the British public 'Not to call the doctor'. There was a specific context: the long Christmas break, but more significant were the longer-term pressures on the NHS's frontline services due to funding not keeping up with inflation, increased demand and the specific pressure of winter illnesses.[80] The RCGP urged people to think '3 before GP'.[81] The RCGP produced a poster for display in surgery waiting rooms. It was, needless to say, too late to change patients' behaviour, so it was presumably aimed at encouraging those attending to remain 'non-patients' in the future. There was a similar appeal to adopt self-care in the early stages of the COVID-19 pandemic.

The RCGP advice was, first, to see if the illness could be dealt with by self-care; second, to seek help from reputable online resources; and third, to consult a pharmacist. It is not clear how successful this attempt to manage demand was, but what is certain is that it was unnecessary. The leaders of the RCGP were apparently unaware of the published work on the 'symptom iceberg'. Nor, from their own practice experience, had GP leaders seemingly thought about the actions people had taken before arriving at their surgery for an appointment, though determining previous self-care measures is an important element in patient history taking. Questions about self-care are, of course, routine. Doctors need to know what, if any, medications have been taken as these could affect the presentation of signs and symptoms.

In the context of the problems in the NHS and the likely waiting time for a GP appointment, it is likely that self-care had been extensive. Interestingly, the RCGP has run an e-learning course, available to GPs and the public, on 'Self Care for Minor Ailments'.[82] The course is run in partnership with the Self Care Forum, a campaign and lobby group that 'aims to further the reach of self-care and embed it into everyday life'. Self-Care is defined as 'the actions that individuals take for themselves, on behalf of and with others to develop, protect, maintain and improve their health, wellbeing or wellness'. Their approach is framed as the self-care continuum, from 'pure self-care', with the individual responsible at one pole (essentially 'non-patient' actions), to 'pure medical care' and professional responsibility at the other.[83] There was a similar injunction to self-care in the early stages of the COVID-19 pandemic in the spring of 2020. People who believed they had the infection but with mild symptoms, were told to stay at home and manage their condition with antipyretics and rest. The aim was two-fold: to isolate the infected to prevent the spread of the disease; and to ease demand on health services.

There are important policy issues at stake if the RCGP, and the NHS more widely, is trying to change the terms of when, if indeed at all, people should see the doctor. And confusion too, because with cancers, mental illness and other conditions, people are told not to delay, as this makes the disease more difficult to treat. Clearly, those working in the health professions and its policy-makers, as well as medical historians, need to know more about the 'non-patient', their views and their actions, and the transition from 'non-patient' to patient. Such analyses ought to be informing initiatives such as the NHS 10-year plan announced at the beginning of 2019, a principal aim of which is making people healthier, more self-reliant for their healthcare, and not have to see their GP.[84]

In this chapter I have argued that historians writing the 'medical history from below' need to be more radical and widen their gaze to consider self-care and self-treatment. Moreover, they should not regard this teleologically as a precursor to becoming a patient, but as an end in itself. One question raised in this chapter, and again which has been strangely neglected by historians of medicine, is the timing of the decision to seek a medical encounter and become a patient. That said, becoming a patient has been (and remains) a small part of the everyday experience of ill health. Nearly half-a-century on from Porter's manifesto, historians of medicine are still writing 'doctors' histories', in the sense that they use sources that focus on the interactions of a specific group of sick people – patients – with the medical profession and its institutions. This approach misses over 80 per cent of healthcare today and no doubt a higher percentage historically. Furthermore, historians have tended to study the diseases that medicine prioritises. Histories are biased in favour of mortality over morbidity, acute over chronic disease, and serious over slight complaints. With each of these pairs, the latter was and is overwhelmingly the lived experience of illness and disease.

It would help too if there were more historical studies of minor and chronic diseases, far and away the common experience of illness, and fewer on serious, acute diseases. With the latter, medical sources and perspectives are almost always bound to predominate, while the view from below will necessarily be that of patients. If there were more studies of minor and chronic illnesses, as in this volume in the chapters by Georgia McWhinney and Coreen McGuire, Jaipreet Virdi and Jenny Hutton, there would be more opportunity to explore non-patient views and actions. As I have shown, the typical experience of minor illnesses is not to see the doctor. But that might still be considered a 'deficit model' framing. It would be more useful and accurate to say the experience of minor illness was (and remains) self-diagnosis and self-management, then perhaps self-treatment, and in one-in-twelve instances to see the doctor. The management of chronic conditions, where the notion of the 'post-patient' might be useful, is care as much, if not more than, treatment. With minor illnesses and chronic conditions there are opportunities for a new social history of medicine, where the 'social' is about the 'parents, friends, neighbours, husbands or wives or other relatives'.

## Notes

\* I would like to thank the editors of this volume, Anne Hanley and Jessica Meyer, for their comments on this chapter and for bringing the collection together. The discussions of my work at two meetings were extremely helpful: 'Patient Voices' in Oxford, September 2017; and 'Healthcare before the Welfare State' in Prague, March 2018. Thank you also to Dr Pete Smith for his kind permission to reproduce a graphic representing the 'symptom iceberg'. And, finally, I would like to thank the Wellcome Trust for their support (grant no. WT 092782).

1 Roy Porter, 'The Patient's View: Doing Medical History from Below', *Theory and Society* 14:2 (1985), 175–98, 194.

2  Anne McAteer, Alison Elliott and Philip Hannaford, 'Ascertaining the Size of the Symptom Iceberg in a UK-Wide Community-Based Survey', *British Journal of General Practice* 61 (2011), 1–11.
3  Percy Stocks, *Sickness in the Population of England and Wales* (London: HMSO, 1949); John Horder and Elizabeth Horder, 'Illness in General Practice', *Practitioner* 173 (1954), 177–87.
4  Karen Dunnell and Ann Cartwright, *Medicine Takers, Prescribers and Hoarders* (London: Routledge & Kegan Paul, 1972).
5  There was review article published in 1981 which called for more research. Kathryn Dean, 'Self-Care Responses to Illness: A Selected Review', *Social Science Medicine* 15A (1981), 673–87.
6  Anne McAteer, Alison Elliott and Philip Hannaford, 'Revisiting the Symptom Iceberg in Today's Primary Care: Results from a UK Population Survey', *BMC Family Practice* 12 (2011), 1–11. The sample was from thirty GPs in the Grampian region of Scotland. There was a mix of urban and rural practices. Although Grampian has one of the lowest population densities in the United Kingdom, its population is concentrated in towns and cities, particularly Aberdeen, and GP services are strong.
7  Ibid., 3.
8  One interesting dissenter, though not a historian, would be David G. Green, who has controversially argued that self-help, friendly societies and philanthropy provided a denser, more consumer/patient responsive service than the NHS did after 1948. See David G. Green, *Working-Class Patients and the Medical Establishment: Self-Help in Britain from the Mid-Nineteenth Century to 1948* (London: St Martin's Press, 1985).
9  Pam Schweitzer (ed.), *Can We Afford the Doctor?* (London: Age Exchange, 1985).
10  See Lloyd (Meadhbh) Houston and Anne Hanley's chapters in this collection. Michael Worboys, 'Unsexing Gonorrhoea: Bacteriologists, Gynaecologists, and Suffragists in Britain, 1860–1920', *Social History of Medicine* 17:1 (2004), 41–59.
11  Self Care Forum, 'What We Do We Mean by Self-Care and Why It Is Good for You', www.selfcareforum.org/about-us/what-do-we-mean-by-self-care-and-why-is-good-for-people (accessed 14 July 2020). Also see: BMA, 'Self-Care: Question & Answer', Online publication, November 2019, www.bma.org.uk/media/1936/bma-plg-selfcare-nov-19.pdf (accessed 16 July 2020).
12  William G. Rothstein, *Public Health and the Risk Factor: A History of an Uneven Medical Revolution* (Rochester: Rochester University Press, 2003); Jeremy Greene, *Prescribing by Numbers: Drugs and the Definition of Disease* (Baltimore: Johns Hopkins University Press, 2007).

13 Roberta Bivins, Hilary Marland and Nancy Tomes, 'Medicine in the Household: Recovering Practice and "Reception"', *Social History of Medicine* 29:4 (2016), 669–75.
14 Alex Mold, *Making the Patient-Consumer: Patient Organisations and Health Consumerism in Britain* (Manchester: Manchester University Press, 2016).
15 Nancy Tomes, *Remaking the American Patient: How Madison Avenue and Modern Medicine Turned Patients into Consumers* (Chapel Hill: University of North Carolina Press, 2016).
16 Michael Sigsworth and Michael Worboys, 'The Public's View of Public Health in mid-Victorian Britain', *Urban History*, 21:4 (1994), 237–50.
17 Neil Pemberton, and Michael Worboys, *Mad Dogs and Englishmen: Rabies in Britain, 1830–2000* (Houndmills: Palgrave Macmillan, 2007). Revised and reprinted as *Rabies in Britain: Dogs, Disease and Culture, 1830–2000* (London: Palgrave, 2012).
18 Aya Homei and Michael Worboys, *Fungal Disease in Britain and the United States: Mycoses and Modernity* (Basingstoke: Palgrave, 2013), 55–6.
19 Rachael Russell, 'Nausea and Vomiting: A History of Signs, Symptoms and Sickness in Nineteenth-Century Britain' (unpublished PhD Thesis, University of Manchester, 2012).
20 Charles E. Rosenberg, 'The Therapeutic Revolution: Medicine, Meaning, and Social Change in Nineteenth-Century America', *Perspectives in Biology and Medicine*, 20:4 (1977), 485–506.
21 Tearfund – Prayer Survey (January 2018), www.comresglobal.com/polls/tearfund-prayer-survey (accessed 15 January 2019).
22 The percentage figures for the main religious groups were: Christian 42 per cent; Muslim 39 per cent; Hindu 31 per cent; Jewish 47 per cent; Sikh 55 per cent; Buddhist 25 per cent; Other religion 45 per cent; No religion 34 per cent.
23 Joanna Bourke, *The Story of Pain: From Prayers to Painkillers* (Oxford: Oxford University Press, 2014). Similarly, Charles E. Rosenberg argued that in cholera outbreaks between the 1830s and 1860s there was a shift: 'the gospels of Snow and Chadwick, not those of Mark and John promised deliverance from cholera'. Charles E. Rosenberg, *The Cholera Years: The United States in 1832, 1849, and 1866* (Chicago: University of Chicago Press, 1987), 213.
24 Philip Williamson, 'State Prayers, Fasts and Thanksgivings: Public Worship in Britain 1830–1897', *Past & Present* 200:1 (2008), 121–74.
25 Alasdair Raffe, 'Nature's Scourges: The Natural World and Special Prayers, Fasts and Thanksgivings, 1541–1866', *Studies in Church History* 46 (2010), 237–47. See also John V. Pickstone, 'Establishment and Dissent in Nineteenth-Century Medicine: An Exploration of

Some Correspondence and Connections Between Religious and Medical Belief-Systems in Early Industrial England', *Studies in Church History* 19 (1982), 165–89.
26 Frank M. Turner, 'Rainfall, Plagues, and the Prince of Wales: A Chapter in the Conflict of Religion and Science', *Journal of British Studies*, 13:2 (1974), 46–65. See also Gordon Huelin, 'The Church's Response to the Cholera Outbreak of 1866', *Studies in Church History* 6 (1970), 137–48.
27 Turner, 'Rainfall', 60.
28 Ibid. See also 'The National Thanksgiving: The State Ceremony at St. Paul's Cathedral', *Manchester Guardian* (28 February 1872), 4–5.
29 Report, 'The Prince of Wales', *Lancet* 1 (1872), 123.
30 Rosenberg, 'Therapeutic Revolution', 493.
31 Francis Galton, 'Statistical Inquiries into the Efficacy of Prayer', *Fortnightly Review* 12 (1872), 125–35. For a modern discussion of the issues, see Richard P. Sloan and Rajasekhar Ramakrishnan, 'Science, Medicine, and Intercessory Prayer', *Perspectives on Biology and Medicine* 49:4 (2006), 504–14.
32 For example, see Antony Fletcher, 'The Death of Charlotte Bloomfield in 1828: Family Roles in an Evangelical Household', *Studies in Church History* 50 (2014), 354–65.
33 George Reid, 'The National Thanksgiving', *Lancet* 1 (1872), 169.
34 Leading Article, 'Gratuitous Medical Services', *British Medical Journal* 2 (1860), 843–4; Editorial, 'Naval Medical Officers', *British Medical Journal* 1 (1869), 499.
35 Guenther B. Risse, Ronald L. Numbers and Judith W. Leavitt (eds), *Medicine Without Doctors: Home Health Care in American History* (New York: Science History Publications, 1977).
36 Roy Porter (ed.), *The Popularization of Medicine* (London: Routledge, 1992); Roger Cooter (ed.), *Studies in the History of Alternative Medicine* (London: Macmillan, 1988).
37 James Harvey Young, 'Patient Medicines and the Self-Help Syndrome', in Guenther B. Risse, Ronald L. Numbers and Judith W. Leavitt (eds), *Medicine Without Doctors: Home Health Care in American History* (New York: Science History Publications, 1977), 95–116, 112. James Harvey Young wrote many books on patent medicines and health quackery in the United States. Victoria A. Harden, 'James Harvey Young (1915–2006)', *Perspectives on History* 45:2 (2007), www.historians.org/publications-and-directories/perspectives-on-history/february-2007/in-memoriam-james-harvey-young (accessed 20 April 2020).
38 Georgia McWhinney shows how, in the particular circumstances of the trenches of the First World War, fellow soldiers, as new friends, were resources for ideas and actions with wounds and disease. See McWhinney's chapter in this collection.

39  Risse, Numbers and Leavitt (eds), *Medicine Without Doctors*, 4. James Cassedy's chapter, promisingly sub-titled 'Alone with their Disease', only considered quacks, itinerants and alternative healers. James H. Cassedy, 'Alone with their Disease', in Guenther B. Risse, Ronald L. Numbers and Judith W. Leavitt (eds), *Medicine Without Doctors: Home Health Care in American History* (New York: Science History Publications, 1977), 31–47.
40  Keith Bakx, 'The "Eclipse" of Folk Medicine in Western Society', *Sociology of Health and Illness* 13:1 (1991), 20–38, 21.
41  There is a literature on the subject by folklorists for the United States. The most comprehensive studies are by Wayland D. Hand: Wayland D. Hand, *American Folk Medicine: A Symposium* (Berkeley: University of California Press, 1976); Wayland D. Hand, *Magical Medicine: The Folkloric Component of Medicine in the Folk Belief Custom and Ritual of the Peoples of Europe and America* (Berkeley: University of California Press, 1980).
42  Dunnell and Cartwright, *Medicine Takers*, 120.
43  Cecil G. Helman, '"Feed a Cold, Starve a Fever": Folk Models of Infection in an English Suburban Community, and their Relation to Medical Treatment', *Culture, Medicine and Psychiatry* 2 (1978), 107–37.
44  Charles Leslie, 'Medical Pluralism in World Perspective', *Social Science and Medicine. Part B. Medical Anthropology* 14:4 (1980), 191–5 and other articles in the special issue of the journal.
45  Helman, '"Feed a Cold"', 125.
46  Dunnell and Cartwright, *Medicine Takers*, 26–9, 107–9.
47  Helman, '"Feed a Cold"', 129. Also see E. Wilkes, 'The Treatment of Cough in General Practice', *Prescribers Journal* 14 (1974), 98–103.
48  Samuel X. Radbill, 'Whooping Cough in Fact and Fancy', *Bulletin of the History of Medicine* 13:1 (1943), 33–53; Isaac A. Abt, 'Treatment of Whooping Cough: A Study in the History of Therapeutics', *American Journal of the Diseases of Childhood* 48:3 (1934), 617–29
49  Radbill, 'Whooping Cough in Fact and Fancy', 41–3.
50  James F. Goodhart, *The Disease of Children* (London: J. & A. Churchill, 1893), 239–40.
51  Hand, *Magical Medicine*, 276. See also Michael Worboys, *Spreading Germs: Disease Theories and Medical Practice in Britain, 1865–1900* (Cambridge: Cambridge University Press, 2000).
52  Sigsworth and Worboys, 'The Public's View', 244; Helen Bynum, 'Riding the Waves: Optimism and Realism in the Treatment of Tuberculosis', *Lancet* 380 (2012), 1465–6.
53  'The Whooping Cough Cure', *Gippsland Times* (7 January, 1926), http://slightlywashedoutgoth.blogspot.com/2015/05/the-gasworks-cure-for-whooping-cough.html (accessed 11 October 2019).

54  Ibid.
55  Ibid.
56  Ibid.
57  Peter G. Homan, Briony Hudson and Ray C. Rowe, *Popular Medicines: An Illustrated History* (London: Pharmaceuticals Press, 2008).
58  Ibid., 74–83.
59  British Medical Association, *Secret Remedies: What They Cost and What They Contain Based on Analyses Made for the British Medical Association* (London: BMA, 1909); British Medical Association, *More Secret Remedies: What They Cost and What They Contain Based on Analyses Made for the British Medical Association* (London: BMA, 1912). Stuart Anderson, *Making Medicines: A Brief History of Pharmacy and Pharmaceuticals* (London: Pharmaceutical Press, 2005), 223–42; Lori Loeb, 'British Patent Medicines: Injurious Rubbish?', *Nineteenth Century Studies* 13 (1999), vi–21.
60  Harvey Young, 'Patient Medicines', 95–116.
61  Stuart C. Anderson and Peter G. Homan, 'Best for Me, Best for You: A History of Beecham's Pills, 1842–1998', *Pharmaceutical Journal* 269 (2002), 921–4.
62  'The Most Reliable Friend', *Star* (7 December 1869), 1.
63  'Holloway's Pills: Dismiss Your Doubts', *Bell's Life in London* (20 June 1874), 5, emphasis added.
64  Nick Hubble, *Mass Observation and Everyday Life: Culture, History, Theory* (Basingstoke: Palgrave, 2005); James Hinton, *The Mass Observers: A History, 1937–1949* (Oxford: Oxford University Press, 2013).
65  Jack N.P. Davies, 'Self-Medication and Patent Medicines', *British Medical Journal* 2 (1944), 87–9; Jack Davies worked in Uganda in the 1950s and did pioneering work on kwashiorkor and Burkitt's lymphoma. He returned to England to work at the Hammersmith Hospital, before moving to Albany Medical College where he developed a career as a forensic pathologist. Michael Hutt, 'Jack Neville Phillips Davies', *British Medical Journal* 317 (1998), 1662.
66  Davies, 'Self-Medication', 88.
67  Ibid., 89.
68  Emma Griffin, 'Diets, Hunger and Living Standards During the British Industrial Revolution', *Past & Present* 239:1 (2018), 71–111.
69  John Burnett, David Vincent and David Mayall (eds), *The Autobiography of the Working Class: An Annotated, Critical Bibliography 1790–1945* (Brighton: Harvester, 1984, 1987, 1989).
70  See 'May Jones', in John Burnett, David Vincent and David Mayall (eds), *The Autobiography of the Working Class: An Annotated, Critical Bibliography 1790–1945* (Brighton: Harvester, 1984), 23–4

71 Eli O. Anders, 'Between Hospital and Home: English Convalescent Care from Nightingale to the National Health Service' (unpublished PhD Thesis, Johns Hopkins University, 2017), http://jhir.library.jhu.edu/handle/1774.2/60858 (accessed 28 October 2019).
72 Amelia Bonea, Jennifer Wallis, Melissa Dickson and Sally Shuttleworth, *Anxious Times: Medicine and Modernity in Nineteenth-Century Britain* (Pittsburgh: University of Pittsburgh Pres, 2019).
73 University of Sussex Special Collections, Mass Observation Archive, *Report on Taking Medicines in Wartime* (May 1943), 1–10 SxMOA1/1/8/5/20; Daniel Ussishkin, *Morale: A Modern British History* (Oxford: Oxford University Press, 2017).
74 *Report on Taking Medicines in Wartime*, 5; oral vaccines for the common cold were available, but the general medical opinion is that they offered no protection. Anon., 'Oral Vaccine for "Colds"', *British Medical Journal* 2 (1944), 424.
75 'Colds and Influenza', *Daily Mail* (30 January 1939), 4.
76 'What the Consumer Thinks of Self-Medication', *Manufacturing Chemist and Manufacturing Perfumer* (August 1943), 236–7, www.massobservation.amdigital.co.uk/Documents/Images/FileReport-1889/45 (accessed 28 October 2019).
77 'The Drugs Trade's Case Has Not Been Heard', *Manufacturing Chemist and Manufacturing Perfumer* (August 1943), 238, www.massobservation.amdigital.co.uk/Documents/Images/FileReport-1889/47 (accessed 28 October 2019).
78 Ibid.
79 Laura Robson-Mainwaring, 'Branding, Packaging and Trade Marks in the Medical Marketplace, 1870–1920' (unpublished PhD Thesis, University of Leicester, 2019), https://ethos.bl.uk/OrderDetails.do?uin=uk.bl.ethos.784766 (accessed 28 October 2019).
80 Matthew Thompson and Fiona Walter, 'Increases in General Practice Workload in England', *Lancet* 238 (2016), 2270–2.
81 '"3 before GP": New RCGP Mantra to Help Combat Winter Pressures in General Practice', Royal College of General Practitioners (29 December 2017), www.rcgp.org.uk/about-us/news/2017/december/3-before-gp-new-rcgp-mantra-to-help-combat-winter-pressures-in-general-practice.aspx (accessed 20 April 2020).
82 RCGP Learning, 'Helping Patients to Help Themselves: Self Care for Minor Ailments' (2018).
83 Self Care Forum, 'What Do We Mean by Self-Care?'.
84 *NHS Long Term Plan*, London (January 2019), www.longtermplan.nhs.uk (accessed 20 June 2019).

# 2

# Family not to be informed? The ethical use of historical medical documentation*

*Jessica Meyer and Alexia Moncrieff*

Public interest in war service, particularly in the global conflicts of the twentieth century, has led to increasingly open archival practices. The attestation papers of Australians who served in the First World War have all been digitised and are free to access online. Meanwhile, work to open up Australian post-war repatriation files is on-going. In Canada, the pension files of the roughly 200,000 disabled veterans who returned from the First World War are currently being digitised. In Britain, service records are available through genealogy websites and digital catalogues. A search of The National Archives' (TNA) records will garner the researcher information about the name, rank, regiment and pensionable disability of individuals who made claims for British post-First World War disability pensions, while the Imperial War Museum's online catalogue of manuscripts contains a range of details about donors and their families. The Wellcome Library has digitised the Royal Army Medical Corps Muniments Collection, previously held by the Army Medical Services Museum, making many previously unpublished memoirs and diaries, of both medical service personnel and their patients, freely available online. The centenary of the First World War, meanwhile, has been used by organisations ranging from community research projects to the Red Cross and the BBC both to make records more accessible via online platforms and to solicit material for such projects in the name of memory, commemoration and education.

While the increased accessibility of this range of records is of huge benefit to historians not only of the war but related historical fields, it also raises questions about the ethical use of the information being made available. Many of these archives contain comparatively unproblematic details about individuals, which form the building blocks of much social and cultural history. Some of the content, however, has the potential to reveal sensitive information about the lives of the men and their families. This has implications not only for historians who make use of personal narratives as central primary sources, but also those whose work contextualises specific, sometimes marginalised or even stigmatised, perspectives, such as historians of medicine and disability. It is the implications of accessing, analysing and disseminating sensitive material generated by the patient voice that this chapter considers. In doing so, it contextualises and complicates the analysis in other chapters in this collection, particularly those of Houston and Hanley, in its consideration of the archival afterlife of stigma and its effect on how patients are heard by historians. Creative approaches not only enable access to historic patient experience but suggest ways in which patients and their agency are understood as historical actors beyond the archival records of their conditions. Set within the context of ethical considerations and the requirements of disciplinary norms such as complete referencing, the effectiveness and utility of such approaches can be more fully understood.

Within the context of the wider collection, therefore, this chapter considers the implications of accessing and using patient voice for the policies that govern historical research, such as those relating to consent, referencing and anonymisation. Yet, as with all the chapters in this collection, this analysis also has contemporary relevance due to its focus on the case study of pension files. The sorts of sensitive medical and social material in such files continue to be collected by government departments charged with administering welfare. The collection of such information exposes the systems of state surveillance which underpin such administration. Consideration of the ethics of accessing and analysing such material highlights the role not only of the historian in perpetuating such surveillance practices, but also archivists and those engaged with policies around the digitisation of historic materials. As governments and institutions across the globe turn increasingly to digital practices to preserve data and disseminate historical material, the question of the ethics of such preservation becomes ever more important.[1]

## The ethical use of historical medical documentation 63

In exploring these questions of ethical approach and their policy implications, this chapter uses as its starting point a case study of the British soldiers' pension files created during and after the First World War. The paperwork generated by the bureaucratic processes associated with the First World War, including enlistment and conscription, service and demobilisation, were collected in these files. All have the potential to reveal intensely personal details of men's bodies and lives, including as they do everything from vital statistics to marital and employment status and religious affiliation. After the end of the war, the process for applying for a pension created paper trails with the power to expose the personal experiences of disabled ex-servicemen, sometimes in intimate detail. Take, for example, the case of a British man who had been stationed in India, whose wife bore two illegitimate children while he was away at war before he succumbed to oesophageal cancer, leaving his legitimate daughter in the care of an orphanage in Kodaikanal.[2] Then there is the case of the ex-serviceman, with stricture of the anus and subsequent incontinence, who abandoned his wife and three children when he migrated to America and subsequently to Canada. The Ministry of Pensions paid his pension, in full, to his estranged wife and marked his file 'Man not to be informed' after the Ministry discovered his indiscretions. This was despite attempts by the man to get the pension commuted to a lump sum and paid directly to himself.[3] These two examples are taken from the 22,829 British Ministry of Pensions files that form the PIN 26 series at TNA. As well as publicly accessible information such as name, rank, regiment, date of birth and theatres of service, this series contains sensitive details of medical conditions and diagnoses, as well as material concerning stigmatising social circumstances, including domestic violence, prostitution, illegitimacy and even potentially criminal activity.

The potential of this archive as a resource for historians of medicine, disability and twentieth-century British society is immense, as is demonstrated by the range of scholars who have used it in their research.[4] The Men, Women and Care project at the University of Leeds, which is utilising this archive to examine the care provided to disabled ex-servicemen of the First World War in relation to religious charities, social stigma, distance and disability, is the first project to attempt a comprehensive analysis of this archive. Moreover, it is the first actively to consider the ethical implications of using such material in historical analysis. Through the process of creating a database of the demographic information in and metadata of the individual pension award records, the project is identifying a variety of information produced by both individuals and institutional bureaucracies held by these files. Analysis of this material, when read alongside related institutional and other archival records, is demonstrating the ways in which the treatment of war attributable disability shaped government policy, charitable practice and family life in Britain in the years after the First World War. Such analysis has the potential fundamentally to shape our understanding of British society at all levels, from the domestic to the global. It is built, however, on the stories of individual men, their families and associates, whose data has been captured by a historic bureaucracy.

The database we have developed, which is designed to be publicly accessible and searchable, contains a range of demographic and non-medical information to enable researchers to use the archives more effectively to explore relevant topics in social, cultural and medical history of Britain in the interwar period, including quantitative analysis of the sample as a whole. Men, Women and Care is not, however, a digitisation project. In part, this is a reflection of the project as one of historical analysis rather than archive preservation and curation, with all project participants undertaking significant social history research using the PIN 26 material.[5] The database will, however, enrich TNA's Discovery catalogue through its recording of details beyond name, rank, unit and pensionable disability. An equally important limit to the methodology of data circulation employed by the project, and its consequent output, has been the ethical considerations which emerged early on as a significant question about the project's methodology as a whole. These are the ethical questions we want to consider in this chapter, suggesting some strategies for tackling them but also leaving much open for further discussion as to the responsibility of historians using this material to gain a better understanding of periods and people still within living memory. In doing so, we aim to demonstrate how conscious considerations of historical practice can shape our work as historians, particularly in relation to use of the patient voice as a historical source with clear contemporary resonances.

Using material drawn from PIN 26 and the process of creating and populating the database, this chapter asks what use historians

## The ethical use of historical medical documentation 65

can and should make of the sort of information contained in government-generated files which record intimate medical and social information about individuals. It considers how such archives can be made more available as part of the impact agenda while adhering to ethical considerations about medical confidentiality. These questions are of relevance not only to historians of medicine and disability, but also those concerned with memory and commemoration in a field where family histories and personal narratives have formed the basis of both historiographic debates and government policy.[6] They also resonate with debates among current medical practitioners in the NHS about government mandated requirements for patients to be given online access to their medical records, debates which raise issues of resource, comprehension and state intervention in clinical practice.[7] In considering key questions of ethical and scholarly practices of research and dissemination, including informed consent and referencing requirements, this chapter demonstrates the practical issues that this sort of material raises for historical researchers in particular. It goes on to discuss the theoretical significance of historical practice in relation to these files, highlighting tensions both in the social definition of modernity (with increased government data collection leading to increased demands for personal privacy) and in the modern public sphere (through the evidence they present of individual and community agency in relation to the nascent welfare state). Finally, it considers what steps the historical community might take to articulate a code of ethics around practice that is sensitive both to family feeling and academic enquiry, and which may speak to wider questions of the digitisation of medical information.

### PIN 26: First World War pensions award files

The 22,829 files that make up the PIN 26 series are described by TNA as a 2 per cent representative sample of all pension files created.[8] The files themselves contain a wealth of material, much of it medical. Even the shortest file includes service and discharge records, complete with medical histories, as well as details of the claim for the pensionable disability. The more complex files contain hospital records, doctors' notes, correspondence, receipts, reports, appeals, hospital admissions records and medical reports. Some include x-rays (almost all badly damaged due to poor preservation), while some have detailed anatomical sketches to illustrate an injury or physical complaint. While much of this material is associated with the bureaucratic processes of enlistment, discharge and pensioning in the context of a modernising military engaged in and after mass warfare, the files have the power to expose intimate details of the personal lives of their individual subjects. As such, the files form a vital record for understanding the social history of twentieth-century Britain. However, the dissemination of this material, whether through developing practices in digital humanities or through more traditional forms of historical analysis, raises a number of ethical issues.

In many cases, the details contained in the PIN 26 files are not only specific but potentially embarrassing to the descendants of these men who, although all dead themselves, may have relatives who knew them intimately while still alive. The research undertaken by the team thus far has uncovered medical histories of incontinence, venereal disease, images of facial disfigurement and reports of suspected malingering, fraud and infidelity. That such records might be perceived as shaming if made public is evident from the files themselves, which include correspondence such as that of the ex-serviceman who begged the Ministry not to alert his employer to the fact that he was in receipt of a pension for neurasthenia because 'they are not aware that I am a pensioner, if they knew my job would not be secure'.[9] Indeed, Eilis Boyle's PhD research for the project directly addresses the question of how facial disfigurement and psychological trauma, as stigmatising conditions, shaped the care and treatment of men who suffered from them, including their treatment in the workplace.[10] At the same time, the existence of personal correspondence within government generated records provides evidence of the need pensioners had to lay claim to agency in relation to their impairments. As Helen Bettinson notes in her history of the Ministry of Pensions as an institution, 'the challenge [faced by the Ministry] was to make pensions conform to the needs and expectations of the pensioner, rather than vice versa'.[11]

While our primary consideration in this chapter is around protecting the privacy of the patient while still enabling the patient's voice to have agency in the creation and analysis of the historical record, it is important to note that it is not only their voices present in the archive. Letters of advocacy from family members formed part of the process of applying for pensions. These included parents, siblings, in-laws and wives, with letters often discussing dependent children, some of whom may still be alive. Indeed, in Canada in 2016, there were still fifty-four First World War widows in receipt of Canadian pensions.[12] With men claiming First World War pensions into the 1980s, it is likely that some, either current or former, medical practitioners who authored the case notes and correspondence that appear in the files are still alive. This was raised as a possibility when one of us discovered her childhood GP had responsibility for the medical care of one man whose file is in the 'Overseas' subsection of PIN 26. The pensioner had migrated to Adelaide and accessed medical care there into the 1970s. The doctor in question, who wrote to the Ministry of Pensions on behalf of the pensioner as well as writing medical case notes contained in the file, died as recently as 2015. The people who appear in these files are not located in the distant past.[13]

While the detailed and explicit medical nature of these files would seem to imply that their access should be curtailed by considerations of medical confidentiality, as part of TNA these records are classified as open public records which can be viewed by anyone on request. In this they differ from Ministry of Health files from the Second World War which still remain classified, although researchers believe these files contain entirely administrative, rather than personal, material.[14] In addition, much of the medical and personal data contained in PIN 26 was generated or collected by government bodies or contractors on behalf of a government ministry and is thus covered by Crown Copyright, so can be disseminated without additional requests for permission to use from either those who are the direct subjects or their descendants. There are also powerful reasons why knowledge of the existence of these files and the material they contain should be made more accessible. The material in the files speaks to contemporary debates over the allocation and administration of state support for disabled people, the gendering of mental illness and social and medical care for veterans.[15] Additionally, the centenary of the First World War, and the investment made in its commemoration in Britain, has led to increased interest in the war from both educational institutions and individuals.[16] While the culmination of the centenary in November 2018 has led to less formal investment in community and commemorative practice around the war, the material in PIN 26 and other sections of the Ministry of Pensions archives continues to offer opportunities to foster public interest in and education about the history of not only the war years but the longer legacies of the war for British and indeed global society. How these files can be used ethically as such a tool is thus a significant and timely question, demanding that we consider the material they contain not only in terms of their utility for scholars but also as memorial and memory for their descendants. More broadly, understanding the utility of historical medical data for historians and historical understanding may be useful for the collection and preservation of such data by state actors such as the NHS today.

## The ethics of consent

The dual roles of personal medical records collected by the state lies at the heart of the ethical issues around their use as a source of patient voice. The Ministry of Pensions records have formed an important source for historians exploring the social and cultural impact and legacy of the First World War over the past twenty-five years, particularly in relation to disability, gender and the body.[17] To date they have tended to be under-utilised by social and medical historians as the format of TNA's catalogues tends to prioritise information pertinent to family historians, making it more difficult to address broader historical queries as effectively. One of the goals of the Men, Women and Care database is to make it easier for historians of the First World War, disability and twentieth-century Britain to identify relevant files across the sample. Yet we must approach the method of making this information available with some care. As April Hathcock has suggested in relation to the records of vulnerable or marginalised communities, the uncritical use of such files, let alone making them readily available online through digitisation, might be construed as 'an act of aggression and oppression'.[18] Hathcock's argument centres on the issue of digitisation of historical records more widely, pointing out that digitisation projects which are made accessible via forms of Creative Commons licensing may be interpreted by those who produced the original material as 'a form of cultural and informational colonialism, taking the works of the marginalised – such as the feminists, dissident GIs, campus radicals, Native Americans, anti-war activists, Black Power advocates, Latinos, gays, lesbians and more [...] and forcing it into (uncompensated) availability without their express consent'.[19] Those whose information is contained in historical medical records are generally the subject rather than the creators of the archive. As such, the use of these sources might be perceived as a form of 'informational colonialism' through the forced access to physical and psychological information that, in other contexts, would be deemed confidential. Certainly, the use of historical medical material (although not specifically historical medical records) for research purposes has been shown to be oppressive to individuals, as in the case of the HeLa cell line taken without consent from Henrietta Lacks.[20]

The subjects of the PIN 26 files are made vulnerable by their mortality, rather than their race, gender, sexuality or class. Their deaths leave them unable to provide informed, un-coerced consent. And although the dead feel no shame, their still-living descendants can. The exposure of intimate medical details of men who survived the war with impaired bodies is particularly sensitive in the context of British memorial culture which, in the words of Alex King, 'canonised the common people' through memorial narratives of both physical and moral courage.[21] Originally invoked in relation to those who died during the war, over the past century this narrative of commemorative canonisation has expanded to cover all those who fought in it or, in extreme instances, lived through it.[22] Combined with the narrative of family connection that underpins memorial practice in Britain and elsewhere, historians who discuss intimate and embarrassing details of the physical and psychological aftermath of the war for men, in ways that are often deeply unheroic, risk angering and alienating the descendants of these men. Is deepening our historic understanding of a particular period or social concept through open discussion of such material sufficient justification for the infliction of pain or discomfort on these descendants? This is very much an open question, as illustrated most recently by the debates around the outing as gay of Robert Wyndham Ketton-Cremer, the last squire of Fellbrigg Hall, by the National Trust as part of its Prejudice and Pride programme.[23]

Ethical concerns raised over the failure to gain consent from vulnerable groups for the use of sensitive personal material would seem to suggest that historians should avoid using such material. But there are equally important arguments supporting the identification of vulnerable actors within the historical narrative. Hathcock's concern relates to the particular types of Creative Commons license used for digitised archives that allow for their manipulation; the simple dissemination of the material has the power to bring these groups visibility that would otherwise be denied them. In the case of those who died in war, the practice of naming as a way of making visible has, since the mass casualties of the First World War, become a central element of commemorative practice. This was evident in Britain where state policy to not repatriate the war dead meant that the naming of the dead became a primary site of mourning.[24] Similar policies enacted in Australia were compounded by the great distances between families and the graves of their loved ones.[25] The importance of this naming practice – of making the dead visible as historic actors – can be seen in the proliferation of lists of names on war memorials around the world. In the United States, the practice arguably reached its apotheosis in Maya Lin's Vietnam War Memorial where 'the names act as surrogates for the bodies of the Vietnam War dead'.[26] As Jay Winter points out, the memorial 'brought the American dead of the Vietnam war back into American history'.[27] The inclusion of names and stories in historical analysis can potentially play a similar role in memorialising individuals by making them historically visible.[28]

Additionally, the academic analysis of personal information and material relating to medical conditions has the potential not only to cause pain and discomfort but also to nuance understandings of particular conditions in ways that challenge historical understandings of stigma. This is particularly relevant to histories of facial injury, where the detailed medical records kept by pioneering surgeons such as Harold Gillies and Archibald McIndoe have enabled a range of significant studies into the importance of their work for their patients.[29] This in turn has led to work such as Boyle's which has supplemented the medical record with personal narratives to show that facially disfigured men such as Reg Evans were not necessarily isolated in post-war Britain but rather were able successfully to reintegrate into their local communities as active members.[30] To show how men were able to negotiate social challenges, such analysis requires discussion of potentially uncomfortable details, such as the embarrassment Evans faced when eating in company as his impairment made chewing difficult. These examples suggest that there is value to be gained, not from unrestricted dissemination, but from the study and thoughtful broadcast of historical medical material. Scholars, society and even family members stand to gain a more nuanced picture.

As we have already indicated, the Men, Women and Care project is attempting to address the question of sensitive public dissemination by harvesting almost exclusively demographic and archival information only for inclusion in the database. We are opening up the files to researchers through improved metadata rather than through the dissemination of their content. The only reference to medical information that will be available will be the recorded pensionable disability, an indication of whether the pensioner received hospital treatment as part of his care and a general indication as to whether files contain medical records without details of what, precisely, those records consist. Researchers will be able to use this information to identify files that they wish to explore in more detail and make their own (informed) decisions on how they disseminate the material they find. In this way, we aim to make the men whose lives are captured, at least in part, in these files, more visible without wantonly exposing them to a public scrutiny to which they are unable to consent. However, there is an analytic element to the project, which goes beyond capturing data and metadata. Using material from selected files, we are exploring questions of how the care provided to these men was gendered. This raises additional important issues about how we undertake our historical analysis and what our professional responsibilities as historians are when it comes to using this material. In our work, this question has crystallised around the anonymisation of subjects and professional norms of referencing in our subject area.

## The professional paraphernalia of history

To the hapless undergraduate, finishing essays at the last minute and frantically sorting out their referencing, their tutors' obsession with style and footnotes can be a source of frustration. Yet proper referencing is not only an important tool of scholarship that supports reproducibility and the development of argument and analysis, but also a moral act. In his 2016 meditation on the craft of history, Tom Griffiths describes the moral contract historians have with the past. Griffiths writes: 'Footnotes are not defensive displays of pedantry; they are honest expressions of vulnerability, generous signposts to anyone who wants to retrace the path and test the insights, acknowledgements of the collective enterprise that is history.'[31] He portrays this collective enterprise as a conversation both between historians and between the historian and the past, asking where our responsibility lies. Griffiths continues,

> Historians feed off the power of the past, exploiting its potency [...] but historians also constantly discuss the ethics of doing that. To whom are we responsible – to the people in our stories, to our sources, to our informants, to our readers and audiences, to the integrity of the past itself? How do we pay our respects, allow for dissent, accommodate complexity, distinguish between our voice and those of our characters? The professional paraphernalia of history has grown out of these ethical questions.[32]

Historians, then, must hold in tension these sometimes conflicting responsibilities. When publishing our research based on the PIN 26 files, how do we respect the people whose stories we are telling while also enabling our readers to follow our footsteps in the archive?

As we work through the files in PIN 26 and enter them into the database, we are giving each of the men an individual anonymisation code. This code consists of their first and last initials and a randomly generated number. Anonymisation is a standard tool of social studies research, with its own set of methodological practices.[33] Yet, in the case of the pensions archives, as we use these codes to discuss the details of files and the personal experiences of disabled ex-servicemen, we are confronted with the problem that the men are still identifiable because of how their records have been archived. In this chapter, and in previous historians' use of PIN 26, references have included the file number listed in TNA's Discovery catalogue (e.g. PIN 26/18).[34] Yet, if we reference in this way, all a reader needs to do to discover the identity of the pensioner is to search for that number in TNA's catalogue. The search will return the soldier's name and pensionable disability. A recent Friends of The National Archives project to enhance the catalogue record as part of TNA's range of projects commemorating the centenary of the war means that there is now more information useful to family historians readily available through the catalogue system, compounding this problem for academic historians. At present, we have no answers for how we might address this particular challenge.[35] The Men, Women and Care project currently has an agreement with our funding body that any publications will be scrutinised by our faculty's research ethics committee to assess the suitability of our referencing practice, a compromise which has a number of practical drawbacks, principally the additional time and burden of labour that this will add to the publication and dissemination process.

The problem of anonymity is not confined to British records and is particularly problematic if using the digitised and openly accessible Australian Imperial Force attestation papers at the National Archives of Australia (NAA). The archival reference for these files is the name of the man who served (e.g. B2455/Schramm Cyril Charles), making it difficult simultaneously to preserve anonymity and maintain professional standards of referencing.[36] While, in theory, these files do not contain medical information, they do contain details of when and for what reason a man transferred between different units, including when and why he was admitted to a medical unit.

Previous histories that have made use of these files have used pseudonyms when discussing sensitive details of individual's lives, thus concealing their identity but also preventing the sources from being traced in the archive.[37] This practice reflects wider treatment of sensitive archival material within the history of medicine, particularly the treatment of asylum records by historians of psychiatry and mental health. The choice of whether the privacy of individuals or disciplinary referencing standards are prioritised is dependent on the researcher's interpretation of the sensitivity of the information in the files, as well as the practice prescribed by the particular archive, which can vary enormously. While researchers working within institutions can be guided by the recommendations of ethics committees in instances such as these, independent and enthusiast researchers, who author a large proportion of the publications in military history and war studies, do not necessarily have equivalent resources to turn to. When adherence to copyright law is the sole or primary standard required for publication, as is increasingly

2.1 Cyril Charles Schramm Casualty Form – Active Service

the case, the deeply personal medical histories of servicemen (as well as other groups under state care) can make their way into the public realm. Indeed, this has happened already with the uncritical publication of lists of Australian First World War soldiers who had contracted various venereal diseases (VD) in the early stages of the war.[38] The men listed sought medical care for VD prior to the Australian Army Medical Corps changing its policy on recording the names of men who were infected. The policy was changed after publicity and shame were identified as significant factors preventing men from becoming active agents in the maintenance of their sexual health.[39] The identification of VD as a stigmatising condition was not sufficient to prevent the publication of the men's names while their immediate descendants are still alive. These variations in policy towards recording and disseminating identifying information across time highlights the complexity of responses to stigmatising conditions explored by Lloyd (Meadhbh) Houston and Anne Hanley in this collection. The case also highlights the potential contemporary relevance that the treatment of such records has well beyond their import for historical understanding.

The vast quantities of evidence created by various countries' wartime bureaucracies and now made easily accessible may yet cause difficulties for the descendants of pensioners, beyond concerns of shame. Given that these records contain information about all types of ailments that become apparent during military service, including heritable conditions and not just those incurred on the battlefield, further protections are needed to prevent the unethical use of this information. As a result of the 'Code on Genetic Testing and Insurance', an agreement between the British government and the Association of British Insurers, insurance companies are prevented from making underwriting decisions based on predictive (as opposed to diagnostic) genetic test results and customers are not required to disclose predictive results.[40] Originally signed in 2014 as the 'Concordat and Moratorium on Genetics and Insurance', the 2018 Code recognises that 'a minority of patients might be deterred from taking predictive genetic tests, if they are unaware that the Concordat protects their fair rights of access to insurance'.[41] Historical medical documentation, like that in the PIN 26 files, is not covered by this agreement and it is doubtful that all countries with accessible medical documentation have protections. Should this type of information be released in subsequent years for later wars, individuals with traditions of military service (or potentially state care) in their family could be at a distinct disadvantage if they also had a heritable condition in their family's medical history. As historians increasingly seek to engage with the public and to mobilise history to intervene in discussions over public policy, it is worth considering how our practice may have unintended as well as intended effects on both individuals and society.

## Bureaucracy and personal privacy: tensions in the First World War archive

These questions are not only significant because of the methodological implications for historians working in this space. From a more analytical perspective, the systematisation of this post-war provision and the development of new processes and procedures provide evidence for the increasing bureaucratisation of the modern state and the development of what would become the welfare state. These developments have important implications for our understanding of the concept of privacy, an idea of particular significance to historians of medicine and one that, as Margaret Pelling has noted, is multi-layered and historically contingent.[42] The questions raised by the pension records relate both to definitions of modernity as a process of bureaucratisation and debates over the nature of the modern public sphere and the way it can be shaped by the mobilisation of the private body.[43] The ways in which patients used their voices in reaction to these processes serves to blur the line between public and private, with implications for the role of the historian in using them.

Roger Cooter and Steve Sturdy, in their discussion of the relationship between war, medicine and modernity, centre their arguments on Max Weber's definition of modernity, which they define as the crystallisation of 'a constellation of social processes', most notably in the era of the First World War.[44] These processes, symptomatic of the shift from a 'traditional' society to a 'rational' one, included 'the growth, differentiation and integration of bureaucracy and other organisational and managerial systems; the standardisation and routinisation of administrative action; and the employment of experts to define and order such systems'.[45] The relationship between medicine and bureaucracy, standardisation and expertise in the First World War is well documented.[46] What is less clear is how these expressions of modernity translated into the interwar period. It is here that pension files, including the medical information they contain, can play a key role in our developing understanding. Cooter and Sturdy suggest that the processes of medical modernisation during the First World War resulted in the emergence of new ways of thinking about how best to harness resources, especially manpower, for the national effort. From this point on, they argue, war was perceived as:

> a process of technical, strategic and social innovation that tested the vigour and adaptability, not just of the military, but of the social organism as a whole. In this context, medicine in both its military and civilian aspects was increasingly seen to fulfil a vital function in the organisation, mobilisation and management of entire societies.[47]

The First World War as a total war, then, resulted in the blurring of boundaries between civilian and military concerns in the decisions to allocate resources.[48]

In the early twentieth century, the emergence of the health of its people as integral to the economic and military success of an industrialised society resulted in the application of modern processes of organisation and bureaucratisation to welfare provision. As a result, 'the welfare and the warfare state increasingly become indistinguishable from one another'.[49] The British Ministry of Pensions, established during the war to address the problems with the previous system of pensions that were created by conscription, functioned at the intersection of welfare and warfare.[50] Thus the PIN 26 files provide the source material to enable an analysis of a new government department as it transferred bureaucratic management methods from the military in wartime to the administration of demobilised men during and after war. Mark Harrison has called for further research into whether attitudes learnt in military service had a lasting effect on medical practice after the war.[51] Because the Ministry of Pensions relied on the expertise of demobilised medical personnel, the PIN 26 files also provide evidence for the influence of military service on the development of the nascent welfare state.

While the PIN 26 files provide substantial evidence of bureaucratisation, they also enable analysis of opposing facets of the social definition of modernity. Jay Winter has noted that the bureaucratisation of medical care led, in turn, to demands for personal privacy. Ana Carden-Coyne argues this period also saw increasing discussion of patient rights,[52] while Mark Harrison suggests that in the First World War medical care was an important facet of the relationship between soldier and the state, forming an unwritten social contract or covenant supported by the humanitarian ideals and political will of British society.[53] All these arguments draw on the state's records of men's bodies and bodily health as part of their evidence base.

The historian's analysis thus has the power to intervene in debates about the bodily autonomy of the soldier, both historic and contemporary. With the act of enlistment – a process that entailed at some level the soldier signing over his body to the state – an individual person made his health a matter of government concern. As such, it became part of the public record, to be archived and preserved in line with state policy rather than the personal wish of the individual. Those records are now available *because* a man either enlisted or was conscripted into military service.[54] Indeed, conscription serves to highlight the limits of consent around bodily autonomy in relation to military service during the war. As Lois Bibbings has demonstrated, the body became the site of protest by conscientious objectors to forced military service through their refusal to attend medical inspections or to wear military uniform. In response, the state mobilised shame and punishment to coerce consent.[55] The existence of such protests raises questions about the consent of all conscripts to having their bodies inspected and their data recorded, creating yet another ethically grey space of research and analysis.

For the disabled ex-serviceman, his service may have lasted five years but, if he sought financial assistance for illness or injury associated with the war, his body continued to be inspected by the state and subject to government decision-making until either the end of his pension or his death. The state has subsequently made information that might otherwise have been considered private or for a limited audience available publicly, including (potentially) to people who knew him intimately. By making such material the subject of analysis, the historian plays a part in exposing the soldier's body to further scrutiny, well beyond the time limits of his military service. The practice of this form of history is thus implicated in the ethics of state data collection and storage practices, much of which occurs without the permission of the subjects of such analysis. While the lack of informed consent could be said to apply to all subjects of historical analysis, the practice of naming the war dead arguably places them in a public space within historical memory that they may or may not have themselves consented to occupy. The narrative of family-centred commemorations which have grown up in the centenary period, particularly in Britain, exerts a countervailing pull towards the rights of descendants to retain control over the memories and family narratives of their ancestors. Thus, tensions persist over who has the right to use and interpret the voice of an individual captured and preserved by a public body. It behoves us, therefore, to question the ethics of our practice, whoever the subject of our research may be.

While the use of the PIN 26 files forces us to question the ethics of our historical practice, it also demonstrates the ways in which the work of social historians of medicine which uses patient voice contributes to formative debates in and on civil society. As the contributors to Steve Sturdy's 2002 collection on *Medicine, Health and the Public Sphere in Britain, 1600–2000* consistently demonstrate across the period, medical history approaches provide a useful methodology for challenging the pessimistic view of the modern public sphere and its relation to the welfare state taken by Jürgen Habermas in *The Structural Transformation of the Public Sphere* (1962).[56] They also, Sturdy argues, demonstrate the ways in which 'concerns about configuring the private were central to many areas of public activity, and might even be regarded as one of the primary purposes of public association'.[57] Medical institutions, and the political bodies designed to regulate them, developed and now function at the boundaries between the private body and the public good, the individual and the collective, the intimate and the mass.

Sturdy suggests that historical critiques and analyses of the Habermasian public sphere have tended 'to neglect the extent to which institutions of various kinds were implicated in the structuration of the public sphere itself'.[58] But institutions are themselves made up of individuals whose identities become implicated in the public discourse. In medico-political institutions, these identities are related to the private body and private life. The PIN 26 archives allow insight into the variety of ways individuals attempted to engage with the state to shape its provision of care for themselves and for others. These strategies could include the detailing of physical incapacity, domestic breakdown and failure to achieve social norms. CE1, for example, laid bare his failures to fulfil the male breadwinner norm, writing: 'I am now living on my wife's people, being unable to follow employment, and having no means to carry on. [...] [T]he public would make a great outcry if the facts of my case were made known to them. And I shall feel compelled, unless something definite is done *this week*, to obtain help in a way which may cause publicity.'[59] Here, CE1 placed his private domestic circumstances within the public discourse as a way of gaining leverage in relation to the bureaucratic state. While such interventions do not necessarily correlate with Habermas's definition of the authentic bourgeois public sphere as collective discussion among individuals emancipated from identification with the state, they do provide evidence of a sense of agency among recipients of state care and their advocates.

Within such agency can be found articulations of how pensioners and their families defined their own sense of privacy in relation to their conditions. Whether demanding that the Ministry not make the details of a man's pension available to his employers or threatening public exposure of perceived ill treatment in the press, pensioners' own relationship to their impaired bodies complicated the status of those bodies as either public or private. In mobilising their bodies and domestic lives as part of public discourse aimed at shaping state policy, pensioners may be said to have entered the public sphere, laying claim to agency in relation to the nascent welfare state in the process. For historians, to refrain from critically examining such interventions because of concerns over privacy is potentially to deny these men the very agency over their subjective understandings of their disability that they sought in writing to the Ministry. As Jennifer Wallis has noted in relation to medical images: 'by presenting the face and body of a patient to public view [without identifying information] we also run the risk of reducing the patient to an abstract representation of a disease'.[60] If those whose lives are recorded in PIN 26 have anything to tell us, it is that their identities were defined by far more than their pensionable illness or injury. Thus, if we should respect the right to privacy of the historical subject, we should also respect the right of the subject to be heard. What they have to tell us may have significant implications for our understanding of the power of the public sphere to shape state practice both historically and in the present. Fostering such understanding through respecting the right of historical actors to be heard also forms part of our duty of care as historians to the individuals whose lives and views are the subject of our research.

## Conclusions: towards a code of ethical practice

What this chapter points to is the number of tensions that exist when it comes to the ethics of accessing and analysing patient voice as captured by state bureaucracies. On the one hand, patients may fall into the category of vulnerable subjects, particularly when speaking about their illness. Consent, therefore, forms an important criterion for considering using their stories in historical analysis. Yet historical subjects cannot give consent from beyond the grave. Not to use such voices in our work because they cannot consent, however, may deny visibility to marginalised groups whose histories deserve to be told and to those who actively sought to locate

## The ethical use of historical medical documentation 81

themselves and their personal histories within the public sphere. While anonymisation offers one option for using patient voice ethically, archiving practices, particularly those associated with official government records, create forms of traceability when referencing conventions are fully applied. These tensions between concern for the subject and rigorous historical practice have implications not only for the holders of records and the writers of history, but also the families of the patients involved, whose sense of personal history, both narrative and genetic, may be exposed and challenged. The use of official records as a source for patient voice also implicates the historian in the bureaucratic processes of bodily and mental assessment and surveillance, giving them an often-unwitting role in the continuation of these practices long after the individual patient's death. Such a role may serve an important purpose in shaping our understanding of the past in ways which resonate with contemporary concerns over the recording and accessing of medical data. It remains important to acknowledge this aspect of the historian's work, along with its role in constructing historical actors *as* patients.

While this article does not seek to provide concrete answers as to how to resolve these tensions, the questions they raise are important ones for scholars in the field. One avenue for discussion that is relevant to these issues is the development of a code of ethical practice for historians. Indeed, in his 2008 book *Responsible History*, Antoon De Baets sets out a 'proposed code of ethics for historians', drawing on the UNESCO Recommendation Concerning the Status of Higher-Education Teaching Personnel (1997) and the Constitution of the International Committee of Historical Sciences (2005).[61] The Royal Historical Society has also produced a Statement of Ethics, originally published in 2004 and republished in 2015. Unfortunately, even with this update, neither document directly deals with the challenges posed by digitisation to the dignity to be accorded to the historical subject and their descendants or to the historian's role in scholarly analysis and dissemination. Indeed, the Royal Historical Society explicitly states that the maintenance of professional ethical standards involves 'observing the ethical and legal requirements of the repositories and collections they use' without any reflection on the ethical implications attached to extracting the data from the archives for analysis.[62] Similarly De Baets, while on the one hand arguing that 'aware of the universal rights of the living and the universal duties to the dead, historians shall respect the dignity of the living and the dead they study', also suggests 'that maximal, free, and equal access to information is the rule and that restrictions are exceptional and only for purposes prescribed by law and necessary in a democratic society'.[63] At present, the laws governing the digitisation of archives and access to information contained therein are such as to ensure the latter condition, but in ways, we would suggest, that contravene the former.

This is not to say that a code of ethics relating to the digitisation of historical archives and historians' use of such material would not be useful, simply that it has not yet been written. This, to some extent, reflects wider debates around the open internet and its emerging use as a repository, including those among current medical practitioners and politicians. As the examples given already indicate, the process of digitisation has enabled the work of non-professional historians, who may not view themselves as bound by a professional code of ethics even if it did exist. It also has the power to make previously hidden historic actors publicly visible in ways that positively affirm their identities, experiences and social and cultural significance. Nonetheless, if the transformation of the historical record into a digital resource is a genie that cannot be returned to its bottle, for those of us who do engage with history as professionals, these are questions that demand our attention. As we gather and analyse data, we must think about the tools that we utilise for the purposes of preservation, just as we must think about our citation practice and the work of surveillance that our analysis may do, however unintentionally. Doing so with care is a duty that we, as historians, owe to the living and the dead.

## Notes

* We would like to thank the European Research Council who funded this research (Starting Grant no. 638694), the members of the University of Leeds School of History Health, Medicine and Society Research Cluster for feedback and Jessamy Carlson for advice and literature recommendations.
1 Sam Trendall, 'How the National Archive Is Digitizing 1,000 Years of History', PublicTechnology.net (5 October 2017), www.publictechnology.net/articles/features/how-national-archives-digitising-1000-years-history

(accessed 25 March 2020); David Underdown, Alex Green, Sonia Ranade and Alec Mullinder, 'A Bayesian Model of Preservation Risk', The National Archives (TNA), www.nationalarchives.gov.uk/documents/digital-projects-at-the-national-archives.pdf (accessed 25 March 2020); Warwick Cathro and Susan Collier, 'Developing *Trove*: The Policy and Technical Challenges', VALA2010 Conference, www.vala.org.au/vala2010/papers2010/VALA2010_127_Cathro_Final.pdf (accessed 25 March 2020).
2 PIN 26/20328, TNA, London.
3 PIN 26/20384, TNA, London.
4 See, for example, Helen Bettinson, '"Lost Souls in the House of Restoration?" British Ex-Servicemen and War Disability Pensions, 1914–1930' (unpublished PhD Thesis, University of East Anglia, 2002); Deborah Cohen, *The War Come Home: Disabled Veterans in Britain and Germany, 1914–1939* (Berkley: University of California Press, 2001); Marjorie Levine-Clark, *Unemployment, Welfare, and Masculine Citizenship: 'So Much Honest Poverty' in Britain, 1870–1930* (Basingstoke: Palgrave, 2015), chapter 6.
5 The four projects being undertaken are: Jessica Meyer, exploring the gendering of care provision in domestic and community spaces; Alexia Moncrieff, exploring the effects of distance and dislocation in the lives of men living outside of Britain; Eilis Boyle, 'Gender and Care in Interwar Britain: An Examination of the Care Provision and Experiences of Care for Facially Wounded and War-Neurotic Ex-Servicemen'; Bethany Rowley, 'Christianity and Charitable Care-Giving for Disabled Ex-Servicemen in Inter-War Britain'.
6 Helen McCartney, 'The First World War Soldier and His Contemporary Image in Britain', *International Affairs* 90:2 (2014), 299–315.
7 Valeria Fiore, 'GPs Must Give Patients Online Access to Past Medical Records from 2020', *Pulse* (4 February 2019), www.pulsetoday.co.uk/news/gp-topics/it/gps-must-give-patients-online-access-to-past-medical-records-from-2020/20038203.article (accessed 27 July 2020).
8 'Catalogue Description: Ministry of Pensions and Successors: Selected First World War Pensions Awards Files', TNA, http://discovery.nationalarchives.gov.uk/details/r/C11539 (accessed 18 January 2019).
9 CA3, Letter to the Ministry of Pensions (13 May 1932) PIN 26/21097, TNA, London.
10 Eilis Boyle, 'Gender and Care in Interwar Britain: An Examination of the Care Provision and Experiences of Care for Facially Wounded and War-Neurotic Ex-Servicemen' (unpublished PhD Thesis, University of Leeds, 2020).
11 Bettinson, 'Lost Souls in the House of Restoration?', 6.

12 Patrick Cain, 'Dozens of Canadian First World War Veterans' Widows Still Get Pensions' (8 September 2016), https://globalnews.ca/news/2923384/dozens-of-canadian-first-world-war-veterans-widows-still-get-pensions (accessed 12 February 2019).
13 For discussion of the some of the ethical implications for historians working on social and cultural history of the more distant past, see Laura Sangha, 'The Living, the Dead and the Very, Very Dead', Storying the Past (22 May 2018), https://storyingthepast.wordpress.com/2018/05/22/the-living-the-dead-and-the-very-very-dead-ethics-for-historians-by-laura-sangha (accessed 12 February 2019).
14 Dr Linsey Shaw Cobden, correspondence with Jessica Meyer (15 August 2017).
15 Jessica Meyer and Eilis Boyle, Evidence to the Women's and Equalities Committee Mental Health of Men and Boys Enquiry (22 May 2019), http://data.parliament.uk/writtenevidence/committeeevidence.svc/evidencedocument/women-and-equalities-committee/mental-health-of-men-and-boys/written/96646.html (accessed 9 March 2020).
16 Catriona Pennell, 'Taught to Remember? British Youth and First World War Centenary Battlefield Tours', *Cultural Trends* 27:2 (2018), 83–98; Helen McCartney, 'Commemorating the Centenary of the Battle of the Somme in Britain', *War and Society* 36:4 (2017), 289–303.
17 See for example, Joanna Bourke, *Dismembering the Male: Men's Bodies, Britain and the Great War* (London: Reaktion Books, 1996); Jessica Meyer, *Men of War: Masculinity and the First World War in Britain* (Basingstoke: Palgrave, 2011).
18 April Hathcock, 'Creative Commons Requires Consent', At the Intersection (20 March 2016), https://aprilhathcock.wordpress.com/2016/03/20/creative-commons-requires-consent (accessed 12 February 2019).
19 Ibid.
20 Rebecca Skloot, *The Immortal Life of Henrietta Lacks* (New York: Random House, 2010).
21 Alex King, *Memorials of the Great War in Britain: The Symbolism and Politics of Remembrance* (London: Bloomsbury Academic, 1998), chapter 7.
22 McCartney, 'The First World War Soldier and His Contemporary Image in Britain', 301–4.
23 'National Trust Criticised for "Outing" Country Squire', *The Telegraph* (29 July 2017), www.telegraph.co.uk/news/2017/07/28/national-trust-criticised-outing-country-squire (accessed 18 January 2019); Catherine Bennett, 'Is Outing People Really the Remit of the National Trust?', *The Observer* (13 August 2017), www.theguardian.com/commentisfree/2017/aug/12/is-outing-people-remit-of-national-trust (accessed 18 January 2019).

24 Jay Winter, *Sites of Memory, Sites of Mourning: The Great War in European Cultural History* (Cambridge: Cambridge University Press, 1995), 104–5, 113–15.
25 Bart Ziino, *A Distant Grief: Australians, War Graves and the Great War* (Perth: University of Western Australia Press, 2007); Kenneth S. Inglis assisted by Jan Brazier, *Sacred Places: War Memorials in the Australian Landscape*, 3rd edition (Melbourne: Melbourne University Press, 2008), 171–80.
26 Marita Sturken, *Tangled Memories: The Vietnam War, the AIDS Epidemic, and the Politics of Remembering* (Berkeley: University of California Press, 1997), 60.
27 Winter, *Sites of Memory*, 104.
28 For some of the ambiguities of this process, see Bette London, 'The Names of the Dead: "Shot at Dawn" and the Politics of Remembrance', in Kellen Kurchinski, Steve Marti, Alicia Robinet, Matt Symes and Jonathan F. Vance (eds), *The Great War: From Memory to History* (Ontario: Wilfred Laurier University Press, 2015), 171–92.
29 Andrew Bamji, *Faces from the Front: Harold Gillies, The Queen's Hospital, Sidcup and the Origins of Modern Plastic Surgery* (Solihull: Helion & Co. Ltd., 2017); Emily Mayhew, *The Reconstruction of Warriors: Archibald McIndoe, the Royal Air Force and the Guinea Pig Club* (London: Greenhill Books, 2004); Kerry Neale, '"Without the Faces of Men": Facially Disfigured Great War Soldiers of Britain and the Dominions' (unpublished PhD Thesis, University of New South Wales, 2015).
30 Eilis Boyle, 'The Social and Psychological Impact of Facial Injuries During and After the First World War' (unpublished MRes. Thesis, University of Leeds, 2016).
31 Tom Griffiths, *The Art of Time Travel: Historians and Their Craft* (Melbourne: Black Inc., 2016), 131.
32 Ibid.
33 Jennifer Wallis, *Investigating the Body in the Victorian Asylum: Doctors, Patients and Practices* (Basingstoke: Palgrave, 2017), 34; Andrew Clark, 'Anonymising Research Data', NCRM Working Paper Series 7/06 (Manchester: ESRC National Centre for Research Methods, 2006), http://eprints.ncrm.ac.uk/480/1/0706_anonymising_research_data.pdf (accessed 4 March 2020). For a discussion of ethical issues around methodological practices, see Jane C. Richardson and Barry S. Godfrey, 'Towards Ethical Practice in the Use of Archived Transcripted Interviews', *International Journal of Social Research Methodology* 6:4 (2003), 347–55.
34 Bourke, *Dismembering the Male*; Meyer, *Men of War*.
35 We consider the methodological implications of these challenges further in Jessica Meyer and Alexia Moncrieff, 'Glimpsing the Lives of First

World War Veterans: Working in a Fragmentary Archive', *Archives & Manuscripts* (forthcoming).
36 Used with the permission of Cyril Schramm's surviving son.
37 Marina Larsson, *Shattered Anzacs: Living with the Scars of War* (Sydney: University of New South Wales Press, 2009), 11.
38 Raden Dunbar, *The Secrets of the Anzacs: The Untold Story of Venereal Disease in the Australian Army, 1914–1919* (Melbourne: Scribe, 2014).
39 George Raffan, 'Suggested Reform in the Management of the Venereal Disease Problem' (3 October 1916). Australian War Memorial (AWM): AWM15 14379/7.
40 HM Government and Association of British Insurers, 'Concordat and Moratorium on Genetics and Insurance' (2014), www.abi.org.uk/globalassets/sitecore/files/documents/publications/public/2014/genetics/concordat-and-moratorium-on-genetics-and-insurance.pdf (accessed 12 February 2019).
41 Ibid., 2.
42 Margaret Pelling, 'Public and Private Dilemmas: The College of Physicians in Early Modern London', in Steve Sturdy (ed.), *Medicine, Health and the Public Sphere in Britain, 1600–2000* (London: Routledge, 2002), 28–9.
43 Tony and Dagmar Waters, *Weber's Rationalism and Modern Society: New Translations on Politics, Bureaucracy, and Social Stratification* (Basingstoke: Palgrave, 2015), 73–127; Jürgen Habermas, *The Structural Transformation of the Public Sphere: An Inquiry into a Category of Bourgeois Society*, trans. by Thomas Burger and Frederick Lawrence (Cambridge: Polity Press, 1989).
44 Roger Cooter and Steve Sturdy, 'Of War, Medicine and Modernity: Introduction', in Roger Cooter, Mark Harrison and Steve Sturdy (eds), *War, Medicine and Modernity* (Stroud: Sutton, 1999), 1–21, 1.
45 Ibid., 1.
46 See, for example, Kate Blackmore, *The Dark Pocket of Time: War, Medicine and the Australian State, 1914–1935* (Adelaide: Lythrum Press, 2008); Bourke, *Dismembering the Male*; Ana Carden-Coyne, *The Politics of Wounds: Military Patients and Medical Power in the First World War* (Oxford: Oxford University Press, 2014); Mark Harrison, 'Medicine and the Management of Modern Warfare: An Introduction', in Roger Cooter, Mark Harrison and Steve Sturdy (eds), *Medicine and Modern Warfare* (Atlanta: Editions Rodopi B.V., 2004), 1–27; Mark Harrison, *The Medical War: British Military Medicine in the First World War* (Oxford: Oxford University Press, 2010); Alexia Moncrieff, *Expertise, Authority and Control: The Australian Army Medical Corps in the First World War* (Cambridge: Cambridge University Press, 2020).
47 Cooter and Sturdy, 'Of War, Medicine and Modernity', 15.

48 J.M. (Jay) Winter, *The Great War and the British People*, 2nd edition (Basingstoke: Palgrave, 2003), 25.
49 Cooter and Sturdy, 'Of War, Medicine and Modernity', 4.
50 Meyer, *Men of War*, 100.
51 Harrison, 'Medicine and the Management of Modern Warfare', 12.
52 Carden-Coyne, *The Politics of Wounds*, 12.
53 Harrison, *The Medical War*, 11–12.
54 A similar process of (involuntary) recording of the body by the state can be seen in relation to the Poor Law patients discussed by Paul Carter and Steve King. See Carter and King's chapter in this collection.
55 Lois Bibbings, *Telling Tales About Men: Conceptions of Conscientious Objectors to Military Service during the First World War* (Manchester: Manchester University Press, 2011).
56 Steve Sturdy, 'Introduction: Medicine, Health and the Private Sphere', in Steve Sturdy (ed.), *Medicine, Health and the Public Sphere in Britain, 1600–2000* (London: Routledge, 2002), 1–4.
57 Ibid., 5.
58 Ibid., 4.
59 CE1, Letter to the Ministry of Pension (9 April 1920), PIN 26/21580, TNA, London.
60 Wallis, *Investigating the Body in the Victorian Asylum*, 34.
61 Antoon De Baets, *Responsible History* (New York: Berghahn Books, 2008), chapter 6.
62 *RHS Statement on* Ethics, 12 January 2015 (originally published December 2004), https://royalhistsoc.org/rhs-statement-ethics (accessed 12 February 2019).
63 De Baets, *Responsible History*, 192–3.

# II

## Voices from the institution

# 3

# Lunatics' rights activism in Britain and the German Empire, 1870–1920: a European perspective*

*Burkhart Brückner*

Participation and empowerment are core issues in contemporary mental health policy. Involving (ex-)users as 'experts by experience' has become an internationally accepted guiding principle for civil society health promotion, especially in the wake of the 2006 *UN Convention on the Rights of Persons with Disabilities*. However, this 'mainstream user involvement' also meets with scepticism from user self-advocacy initiatives and organisations.[1] This can, for example, be seen in the words of Diana Rose, a 'user/survivor academic' at London's King's College, who, while criticising the austerity policy in the British healthcare system, emphasises the significance of local, 'hidden' and often radical grassroots groups:

> This activism is barely visible socially because 'the mad organising' is an oxymoron and there are material conditions for not being persistently open. It is hidden, it is suspicious and it is angry but with a righteous anger.[2]

This quote addresses key topics of today's 'consumer/survivor/ex-patient' (c/s/x) movement: structural disadvantaging, emotionalised protest, mobilisation capacity and media (in-)visibility; in short, the chances and contradictions of (ex-)users' political 'struggles for recognition'.[3]

The history of this movement, however, has not yet been fully explored. Historical discussions are usually limited to the second half of the twentieth century; moreover, comparative studies are missing so far. The main objective of this chapter, therefore, is to investigate the lunatics' rights activism between 1870 and 1920, both in bilateral comparison and in the European context. A historical comparison of this kind allows us not only to reconstruct the scale of this early activism as a precursor of today's c/s/x movements but also to more closely examine the strategies and patterns of self-advocacy, mobilisation and political lobbying. Actually, in Europe around 1900, the criticism of psychiatry and the associated activism were not 'hidden' but rather on everybody's lips.

The first (ex-)patient organisations emerged in the mid-nineteenth century in England in reaction to a number of asylum scandals, such as the arbitrary internment of the writer Rosina Bulwer Lytton (1802–82) in a private madhouse at the instigation of her husband Edward Bulwer Lytton (1803–78). This event caused a considerable stir in 1858, and the scheme against Lady Lytton was condemned by several commentators, among them John Stuart Mill (1806–73), Karl Marx (1818–83) and the lunatics' rights activist John Thomas Perceval (1803–76).[4] This and other scandals during the years 1858/59 intensified the Victorian public's scepticism towards the lunacy law reform of 1845.[5] The Alleged Lunatics' Friend Society (ALFS), an early self-advocacy organisation of former patients co-founded by John Perceval in 1845, achieved a parliamentary inquiry in 1859 – but their most important demand, a timely judicial review of committals, was only met in 1890 with the passing of the Lunacy Act of that year.[6] This 'triumph of legalism', as this liberal law has been labelled, thus was the result of decade-long debates over the 'lunacy question' in England.[7] Such debates were not restricted to Britain: they occurred in the whole of Western Europe, and the people involved included physicians, jurists and politicians, as well as former patients. This critical discourse by ex-inmates and their allies has repeatedly been investigated for France, Britain, Germany and Switzerland, and traces can be found across the continent.

Against this backdrop, this chapter will point out the prerequisites for the emergence of lunatics' rights activism as well as its chances for political success by discussing two key figures, the British spiritualist Louisa Lowe (1820–1901) and the German merchant Adolf Glöklen (1861–c.1935), former patients who initiated influential self-advocacy organisations. Drawing on their examples, I explore the intersections between expert and lay discourse, medical science and the judiciary, social structure and individual fate. How did

Lowe and Glöklen become such prominent critics of psychiatry? What were their experiences and motives, their preferred alliances and political strategies? And can the campaigns that they initiated be considered social movements in the proper sense?

To answer these questions, I interpret the history of psychiatry around 1900 from the perspective of a social history of (user) experience.[8] Using the activists' self-narratives as a starting point, I draw on concepts developed in disability history and the political sociology of social movements and use the term 'self-advocacy' as a key concept.[9] Roy Porter has been discussing self-narratives of (ex-)inmates since the 1980s, referring to them as 'communications in their own right' and as expressions of a specific subculture.[10] In 2010, Aude Fauvel argued along the same lines by questioning Michel Foucault's propositions regarding the 'absence of madness' in modernity:

> Parallel to a history of exclusion, there is thus another history: that of the ways through which the insane have tried to re-inhabit the public scene – a history of the 'return of the repressed', as it were, which should seek to explore the impact of the patient's expressions both on a national *and* a transnational perspective.[11]

This historical trajectory begins in eighteenth-century Britain with early polemics on the 'trade in lunacy'.[12] Like the women's movement, the first wave of Europe-wide criticism of psychiatry emerging in the late nineteenth century can be seen as a predecessor to the second wave that occurred between 1960 and 1990. This, in turn, resulted in user involvement policies and the consumer/survivor/ex-patient movement in the twenty-first century.

## Lunacy panic all over Europe

What were the themes and trends, and who were the people shaping lunatics' rights activism in Western Europe between 1870 and 1920? In Britain, even novelists seized the topic.[13] Small but media-savvy ex-patient organisations formed when new asylum scandals came to light after 1870. In France, calls for a reform of the 1838 *Loi des aliénes* first emerged during the 1860s.[14] An even stronger wave of criticism arose in the 1870s. Several ex-inmates were involved in these campaigns, like Léon Sandon (1823–72), Hersilie Rouy (1814–81) or Raymond Seillière (1845–1911), but no evidence is available of any self-advocacy association.[15]

Although several other European countries had also passed lunacy laws between the 1830s and 1880s, non-specific administrative and civil law provisions or local regulations largely prevailed. In the German Empire of the late 1880s, numerous ex-patients, alongside several politicians, called for the creation of a uniform lunacy law. Ex-patient organisations emerged from 1907 onwards.[16] In Switzerland, the press started covering cases of allegedly wrongful confinement in the late 1870s.[17] In 1897, anti-vivisectionist Ludwig Fliegel (1865–1947) founded the Zurich-based Irrenrechts-Reformverein [Association for Lunacy Law Reform], active until 1904. In the Austro-Hungarian Empire, conflicts intensified around 1890.[18] Heated debates arose over actress Helene Odilon's (1865–1939) quest to have her husband assessed by alienists and the six-year-long confinement of Princess Louise of Saxe-Coburg (1858–1924) between 1898 and 1904. In Belgium, two patients died at Maison de Santé d'Evere in Brussels in 1871. Consequently, the institution was closed and legislation was reviewed in 1873.[19] In the Netherlands, Johanna Stuten-te Gempt (1829–98) exposed the malpractice experienced during her treatment at Slijkeinde in The Hague in 1889/90. Directors and staff were dismissed and the 1884 law was reviewed.[20] In northern Europe, public distrust of asylums first emerged in the Grand Duchy of Finland, then part of the Russian Empire, during the 1870s.[21] In Denmark, scandals around psychiatrist Knud Pontoppidan (1853–1916) lead to his resignation as head of the psychiatric department at Copenhagen Municipal Hospital in 1898.[22] And in Sweden, press coverage started in 1890 and significant controversies arose in 1907 and 1913.[23] Similar conflicts emerged in the US and Japan. Only few traces, however, can be found in eastern or southern Europe, for instance in Spain and Portugal.[24]

Around 1890 at the latest, European psychiatry's reputational problems accumulated. Hundreds of polemics by former inmates, escape stories, stories of clinic directors resigning, investigative reports and collective appeals filled the papers, while at the same time sharp increases in patient numbers – alongside growing doubts in brain psychiatry, diverging classification systems and deficits in legislation – presented psychiatry with fundamental reform challenges. The years after 1900 saw transformations such as a growing focus on outpatient services and the standardisation of classifications of mental disorder. In Britain, the criticism abated with the 1890 Lunacy Act; in Germany, it intensified well into the 1920s.

Materials from twelve European countries clearly indicate that lunatics' rights activism had its geographical hotspots in Central and Western Europe, in other words, in countries that already had relatively modern systems of psychiatric care. But the international dissemination of political activism organised by (ex-)patients and their allies has received little scholarly attention so far. According to Alexandra Bacopoulous-Viau and Aude Fauvel, a 'history of collective "mad" cultures' is missing for two reasons: first, because 'medical history from below' in the tradition of Porter is preoccupied with the personal accounts of allegedly insane patients; second, because the writings of Foucault suggest a lack of relevant sources.[25] But a history-of-experience perspective, as applied in this study, can reveal the historical continuities in ex-inmates' political struggles for recognition as stakeholders in modern psychiatry, which started in the nineteenth century.

Considering the conditions in psychiatric institutions in Britain and Germany around 1900, we can assume that procedural irregularities had become more likely due to overcrowding, low release rates, poor staffing and the prevalence of hereditarianist theories. The bilateral comparison of activists' biographies, motives and social environments brings to light structural similarities in their protest practices, media presence and networking as well as intersections with other categories of social history, like 'class', 'gender' and 'body'. This shall first be shown with regard to Britain.

## Louisa Lowe: 'I have a right to my liberty'

The history of experience explores how individuals deal with and interpret social practice. In 1883, the spiritualist Louisa Lowe (1820–1901) published *The Bastilles of England; or, the Lunacy Laws at Work* (Figure 3.1), a book that became iconic of lunatics' rights activism in Britain.[26] Very little is, however, known about her life prior to 1870/71 when her husband had her treated in three private asylums. What we do have are three personal accounts from

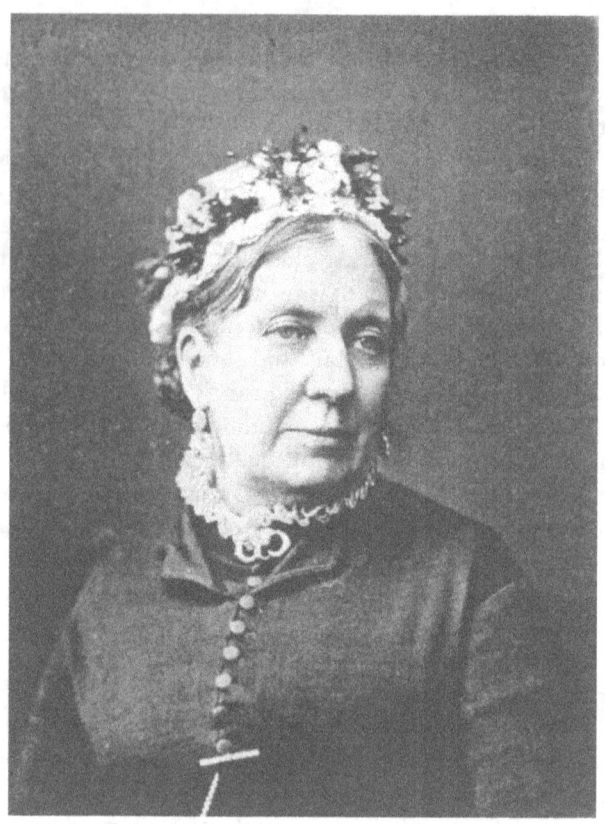

3.1 Portrait Louisa Lowe (1820–1901)

1872/73, parliamentary proceedings from 1877, Lowe's newly discovered memoirs from 1888, and several essays and press reports.[27] The medical files from the asylums and her own notes taken there have survived only in fragments or gone missing altogether. These absent sources – classified reports, intercepted letters and occult messages – have fuelled the disputed discourses of knowledge on Lowe's case ever since. Given the limited sources, going beyond the established paths in telling her story is no easy task, which is yet another argument in favour of a comparative analysis.

Louisa Lowe, nee Crookenden, was the youngest daughter of Thomas Crookenden (1761–1842), a landowner from Suffolk.[28] On 1 September 1842, shortly after her father's death, she married the

Anglican vicar George Lowe (1813–85) from Upottery, Devonshire. She raised six children, but her marriage turned out to be unhappy. Around 1850, she began suffering from 'increasing nervousness', was treated by John Conolly (1794–1866) for some days and, in 1855, survived severe opium intoxication, most likely an attempted suicide.[29] What is clear, however, is that the marital conflicts intensified in the summer of 1869 due to her new commitment to spiritualism, a Franco-American movement that fascinated Victorian audiences.[30] Having attended a séance together with her sister Emily Chamier, Lowe was convinced she possessed medial powers and engaged in the 'passive notation' of supposed messages from deceased persons.[31]

After a marital row in early September of 1870, Lowe fled to nearby Exeter where she complained to her family physician, Dr Thomas Shapter (1809–1902), about her husband's 'infidelity' and 'impotence'. Shapter later testified that she had attributed these allegations to 'mesmeric influences'.[32] Shortly after this encounter, she received an unsolicited visit from Dr Kempe, a surgeon. Using the certificates from these two doctors, George Lowe signed the formal order for his wife's committal to an asylum on 23 September. Two days later, she was forcefully taken to Brislington House, an exclusive private sanatorium near Bristol. Accommodated on the ward for 'violent maniacs', she deemed her barred cell 'utterly unfit for a gentlewoman's occupation'.[33] Her urgent request for legal counsel was denied by the institution's director, Superintendent Charles Henry Fox (1837–1915). This was in fact in line with the 1845 Lunacy Act, which revoked an inmate's right to immediate judicial review under *habeas corpus*, as had been stipulated in the Madhouse Act of 1774.[34] Committals like that of Lowe required no more than an order signed by a relative and certificates from two 'qualified and independent' doctors. Reviewing committals for procedural correctness was now exclusively the task of the eleven-member Lunacy Commission, then chaired by Lord Shaftesbury (1801–85).[35]

In mid-October 1870, two Commissioners, surgeon James Wilkes (1811–94) and barrister Robert Wilfred Skeffington Lutwidge (1802–73), visited Lowe. She complained about serious procedural irregularities, the poor quality of her food and the harassment directed at her by other inmates. The Commissioners, however, deemed the confinement formally legitimate. One of the certificates stated 'various delusions about her husband, &c, &c, &c.', while Fox diagnosed 'sub-acute mania', 'utterance without coherence' and 'perversion of the moral sentiments'.[36] Apparently, Lowe learned neither about her husband's order claiming that she had been 'in treatment for 20 years' nor about the fact that 'for hysteria' had been added on 1 October without the Commission's approval.[37] What she did know was that her release could only be initiated by her husband or the Commission.[38]

Over the next months, Lowe wrote upwards of eighty letters asking friends, clerics and politicians for help. Fox confiscated almost all letters and handed them to her husband, which was against the law.[39] On 19 and 20 January 1871, Reverend Lowe and the Commissioners recommended that she be discharged, but according to Fox, her sister Emily raised objections.[40] On 14 February 1871, Lowe was transferred to Lawn House, Henry Maudsley's (1835–1918) small and expensive private asylum in Hanwell. There she continued her spiritualist practices – which may have proved her doom in four more meetings with the Commissioners. 'All spiritualists are mad,' Lutwidge and Wilkes reportedly stated on one occasion.[41] On 25 September, she was transferred to Otto House in Hammersmith where George Fielding Blandford (1829–1911) declared her 'recovered' and 'legally competent' at the end of December 1871. She was released on trial to an apartment on London's Russell Square and into the supervision of a 'legal adviser'. In March, Bethlem Hospital physician William Rhys Williams (1837–93) confirmed that she was mentally healthy, whereupon she regained her full civil rights in April 1872, eighteen months after the initial committal.[42]

Lowe was free but feared the 'foul madhouse reek' and 'isolation' as a 'recovered lunatic'. To escape the stigma, she politicised the problem, as we can read in her 1888 memoirs: 'To rehabilitate myself, if possible, and at any rate to make my past agonies minister to the public in future became the main object of my life'.[43] Her first action was to fight off her husband's attempts to get hold of her assets; then she sued the Commissioners.[44] In November 1872, at the Court of Queen's Bench, she emphasised the innocuousness of her spiritualism, regretted accusing her husband of unfaithfulness, admitted to having been over-excited in September 1869 and claimed, 'I have a right to my liberty'.[45] Not finding any 'intentional' mistakes in the Commissioners' handling of the matter, the Court dismissed the case, whereupon Lowe started interpreting her fate as a 'test' for the medico-legal system, as she called it in 1888.[46]

Lowe's founding of the Lunacy Law Reform Association (LLRA) in June 1873 was followed by several reports and calls for action. The organisation also provided support in a number of individual cases. In 1876, the Lunacy Law Amendment Association (LLAA) seceded from the LLRA. Its secretary, James Billington, claimed that Lowe's business methods and 'spiritualistic views' had proved detrimental to their political cause.[47] The LLAA was dominated by men and initially had no ex-inmates among its members. Both associations remained fairly small but the activists managed to stage efficient campaigns and Lowe became the most prominent figure within a few years.[48]

In the spring of 1877, increasing public attention led to establishing a House of Commons Select Committee chaired by the Welsh liberal politician Lewis L. Dillwyn (1814–92). Conservative alienists like Lyttelton Stewart Forbes Winslow (1844–1913) declared the inquiry to be based on 'imaginary grievances, morbid fancies, actual delusions, and in the hostility and antipathies of those who had been subjected to asylum restraint'.[49] A report for the British Medico-Psychological Association was more objective in tone but similarly critical of the ex-patients' claims.[50] Other doctors, however, supported them. Joseph Mortimer Granville (1833–1900) denounced overcrowded institutions, the 'cruelty of attendants', the misery of pauper lunatics, rashly issued 'emergency certificates' and the use of 'chemical restraint', while the Scottish physician Lockhart Robertson (1825–97) claimed that one third of the inmates in private asylums were able to be released.[51]

Testifying before the Committee on 3 and 8 May 1877, Lowe argued that her husband's 'order' and the medical certificates had been 'perfectly false' as she had been 'perfectly sane'.[52] Maudsley, the leading alienist of his generation, tried to point out the difference between 'genuine spiritualistic ideas' and her allegedly delusional 'direct communications with the Almighty'.[53] This disagreement occurred within the historical context of increasing debates over 'psychical research' and the pathologisation of spiritualism, normative medical constructs like 'moral insanity' or 'hysteria' and unreliable cross-sectional diagnoses. Lowe declared:

if a patient protests his sanity [...] he is adjudged an excitable, troublesome subject, and is punished; if he takes things quietly, and makes the best of it, which was my course, he is adjudged morbidly apathetic.[54]

When asked about her demands, she argued that committals should be subject to prior examination by a court, a justice of the peace would only suffice in urgent cases of 'acute mania'. She explained:

the first thing would be to define clearly what is, and what is not coercible lunacy. The second thing, I think, is to render prosecution for breaches of the lunacy laws as easy as for any other misdemeanour, to throw open the power of prosecution to the public.[55]

The Committee eventually found the Commissioners of Lunacy not guilty of any misdemeanour and that the certificates from Drs Shapter and Kempe cleared the asylum doctors of blame. What seemed more problematic though was the lucrative months-long prolongation of Lowe's confinement.

In its 1878 final report, the Committee stated that the system was 'not free from risks' but 'allegations of *mala fides* or of serious abuses were not substantiated'.[56] It recommended a closer examination of medical certificates, shorter stays, the protection of patient mail and the gradual closure of private asylums. However, these measures were only implemented in 1889; for the time being, Lowe's initiative had failed.[57] This may explain the harsh rhetoric that marked her main work, *The Bastilles of England* (1883). Comparing the medical certificates to the *lettres de cachet* of French despotism, she presented over a dozen cases to substantiate her criticism of 'cruelties and malpractices in asylums', the 'moral death' suffered by the inmates, and the 'autocratic' Commission in Lunacy.[58] On 31 January 1887, her complaint against Fox reached the House of Lords but was finally dismissed.

In their respective studies, Nicholas Hervey labels the LLRA as 'highly polemical' and Michael Clark attributes its 'militant and uncompromising tone' to Lowe's 'personality, experiences and prejudices'.[59] Alex Owen describes Louisa Lowe as 'radical and unorthodox' and Helen Nicholson refers to her as a 'not always easy woman'.[60] Sarah Wise highlights Lowe's fierce conflicts with other members of the British National Association of Spiritualists around 1880, with former allies as well as with two of her children.[61] But despite these problems, Lowe managed to initiate effective networks, foster debates among experts and create a media presence.

The decisive case came in 1878. On 14 April, the singer and spiritualist Georgina Weldon (1837–1914) fled to Lowe's house to escape the order issued by her husband and from two doctors who had secretly tried to assess her mental state.[62] Weldon published her story, *How I Escaped the Mad-Doctors*, in 1879, successfully filed a suit for damages under the 1882 Married Women's Property Act and, with the LLAA's support, initiated legal proceedings in at least seventeen instances, all of which generated tremendous media attention.[63] The London-based activists operated within networks of women's rights campaigners, spiritualists, anti-vivisectionists and anti-vaccinationists. One of their vital allies was the National Association for the Defence of Personal Rights, founded in 1871 in the fight against the Contagious Diseases Acts. This association advocated a libertarian, anti-statist and anti-interventionist stance and also promoted women's rights.[64] As a political player, however, these networks proved too weak. Yet, Clive Unsworth argues that the British establishment of the 1880s sought to defend its position in society against the increasingly influential workers' movement by promoting modern legalistic concepts ('the rule of law').[65] Lunacy legislation seemed a suitable case. That was why, after the Select Committee's recommendations, the inquiry report published by the *Lancet* and increasing press coverage, powerful liberal and conservative politicians and jurists like Lord Selborne (1812–95) and Lord Chancellor Halsbury (1823–1921) supported a series of draft laws between 1880 and 1889.[66] The Medico-Psychological Association, which advocated early interventions, found itself put on the defensive, and the controversies over medical monopolies and specialist decision-making ended with the Royal Assent to the Lunacy Act on 29 March 1890.

The consolidating Act met some of the LLRA and LLAA's demands. Committals to private madhouses now required a 'legal certificate' (or 'reception order') issued by a justice of the peace, a county court judge or a magistrate, and patients were given the right to appeal. Committals of pauper lunatics also required both judicial and medical approval ('summary reception order').[67] This was the first modern legalistic lunacy legislation and shaped the British system up to the Mental Health Act of 1959.[68] The Act further stipulated that the licensing of private asylums be stopped. Of the 101 facilities existing in 1876, only 55 were still in operation in 1926, catering for around 3,500 patients.[69] The closure of asylums also meant that most of their medical records got lost – as in the case of Louisa Lowe. Both the LLRA and LLAA ended their activities around 1900; effective successor organisations, like the National Council for Lunacy Reform (1920–23) and the National Society for Lunacy Reform (1923–32), formed only after the First World War.[70] The doctors then tapped other sources of income: 'consultant psychiatry', 'voluntary admissions' or 'early intervention programmes'.[71]

Endowed with upper middle-class privileges and assets, Louisa Lowe became an effective 'expert by experience'. Her radical criticism contributed to shaping the political opportunity structure for democratising lunacy legislation in Britain. This contribution too is part of the history that led to the founding of the National Health Service in 1948 and the 'deinstitutionalisation' of psychiatry in the 1960s. Can we find similar dynamics when looking at lunatics' rights activism in the German Empire around 1900?

### Adolf Glöklen: 'I was of a sound mind'

Criticism of the asylum system in the German Empire ballooned after 1880. Until around 1925, more than 250 books, pamphlets and brochures appeared, denouncing allegedly false confinements, legal incapacitations and abuses in asylums. Most prominent were the juridical writings of Austrian right-wing socialist Eduard August Schroeder (1852–1928) and a call, initiated by the Protestant theologist and antisemitic politician Adolf Stoecker (1835–1909), for a 'tighter control of asylums' signed by 111 members of the high nobility and military that was published in the ultra-conservative *Neue Preußische Zeitung* in 1892.[72] In 1894/95, reports about practices similar to what would today be called water-boarding at an asylum run by the Alexian Brothers in Mariaberg near Aachen shocked the public.[73] Alienists defended their profession against the clerical rivals and endorsed calls for nation-wide regulations and better training of staff but denied almost all incriminated cases, speaking of 'querulous individuals'. From 1897 onwards, the national parliament repeatedly supported demands for a uniform lunacy law and a supervisory body.⁷⁴ A bill failed in 1902 but a new wave of criticism began to surface in 1907.

In that year, the ex-patient Georg Wetzer (1878–1914) founded the (albeit short-lived) Zentrale für die Reform des Irrenwesens [Centre for Lunatic Care Reform] in the Bavarian city of Hersbruck.⁷⁵ In 1908, the Deutsche Verein für Psychiatrie [German Psychiatric Association] established a press commission to monitor campaigns. In 1909, the Bund für Irrenrechts-Reform und Irrenfürsorge (BIRIF) [Association for Lunacy Law Reform and Lunatics' Welfare] was initiated by the Heidelberg merchant Adolf Glöklen (Figure 3.2), who soon became a key figure among German reformers. Glöklen described his asylum experience in the brochure *Zustände in der Heidelberger Universitäts-Irren-Klinik oder 5 Tage lebendig begraben* [Conditions at Heidelberg University's Lunatics' Clinic, or Five Days Buried Alive], published in 1908.⁷⁶ Unlike Louisa Lowe, Adolf Glöklen, along with his essays, is almost forgotten today. But in his case, the medical files have been preserved and will serve here to illustrate the mutual relationship between the perspective 'from below' and the clinical gaze 'from above'.⁷⁷

Glöklen's account of his treatment at Heidelberg University Clinic between 13 and 17 June 1907 highlighted the 'other side' of this well-renowned research clinic that had to provide mental healthcare for three counties.⁷⁸ Initially a cigar manufacturer, Glöklen went

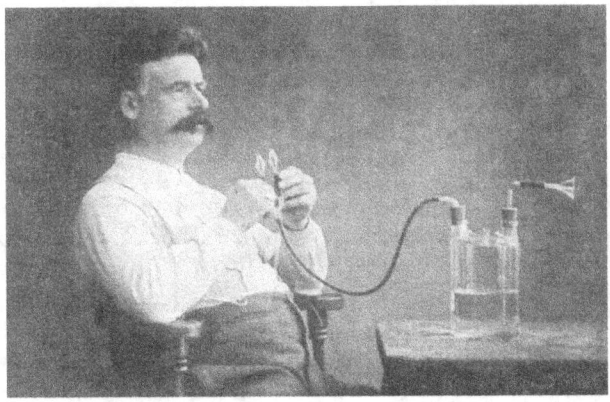

3.2 Presumably Adolf Glöklen (1861–c.1935), demonstrating his healing device for breathing therapy

bankrupt in 1904 and became a travelling salesman. On 3 April 1907, his nineteen-year-old daughter committed suicide after her fiancé broke their engagement. The young man took his own life three weeks later. Shattered by these events, Glöklen applied for health resort treatment, especially since he had also lost his employment.[79] Following his family doctor's advice, Glöklen went to the Heidelberg Clinic on 13 June to get a certificate for his health insurance. At the clinic, Dr Karl Wilmanns (1873–1945) first examined him and then had a one-to-one conversation with Glöklen's wife, Berta. Glöklen himself recalled being taken to a 'locked corridor' shortly thereafter. Berta Glöklen signed the admission form, apparently without being aware of the document's purpose: she later claimed that she thought it had been about cost coverage.[80]

The clinic doctors noted that Berta Glöklen had informed them about her husband having 'repeatedly' expressed 'suicidal thoughts'. They considered his 'current fit' to be 'curable' but were nonetheless convinced that he posed 'a threat to himself and others'.[81] While Glöklen was given a bath, two attendants searched his clothes and then assigned him to a bed on a surveillance ward in the second- and third-class unit with about forty patients.[82] His questions regarding the expected examination were dismissed. The place seemed frightening:

> My ward is where all the sick are first taken for observation. On this ward, one is never for a moment safe, day or night, from being attacked by a patient whose condition is still unknown even to the doctors themselves. This feeling was not beneficial to my ailing nerves and my ailing mind! The rooms were that overcrowded that patients had to be placed in the corridor.[83]

Glöklen learned that the clinic's surveillance ward also held forensic cases and that the observation period could take up to six weeks:

> Defenceless, like a child, I was lying there, had to be guided and commanded by the juvenile attendants like a child. I was treated like a mute, bereaved of reason, since I was declared mad and put among madmen. My words were not believed! When I kept calm and quiet, I was considered lugubrious, when I wanted to move around, I was considered agitated, when I gave explanations, I had idées fixes, when I wrote letters, I had a writing mania, but yet, I was of a sound mind just like any other person.[84]

Apart from this argument, which was also brought forward by Louisa Lowe,[85] Glöklen complained about dirty toiletries, mail delays, 'prison food' and 'harshly' ordered bed rest. He was initially unaware of the fact that the obligatory 'certificate of urgency' from the district medical officer was only issued on 18 June – one day after Glöklen's release.[86] On the other hand, he soon learned what the alienists thought about him. After a fierce dispute with the head attendant on 15 June, ward doctor Otto Ranke (1880–1917) reportedly confronted him with his file in the presence of the clinic's director, Franz Nissl (1860–1919), pointing out entries alleging 'litigiousness' and a family history of 'melancholic and mental disorder'.[87] Glöklen angrily rejected any reading of his reactions as symptoms.

After four days at the clinic, his wife and son came to visit and arranged for his transfer to a private institution in nearby Neckargmünd, against medical advice. On 17 June Glöklen left the clinic, which he described as 'pretty' like a 'small castle or villa', so that 'nobody would suspect the kind of torture chambers to which these corridors lead'.[88] This sarcastic comment may also have referred to the diagnostics applied. Ranke actually based his discharge diagnosis of 'cyclothymia' on hereditarianist assessment, as Glöklen's medical file reveals: it includes the case sheet of a 'feeble-minded' aunt, his mother and grandmother were referred to as 'lugubrious', and two brothers bore the label 'cyclothymic'. Glöklen admitted that he had 'always suffered mood swings' but referred to them as 'non-pathological' nervousness.[89] While 'nervous disease' seemed still respectable, 'cyclothymia' was the epitome of bourgeois death: hereditary madness, possibly incurable. Similar to Lowe, Glöklen sought to fight against this stigma. He nonetheless experienced the ensuing compulsory four-week stay at a private sanatorium in Neckargmünd as utterly relaxing.[90] Afterwards, he first went into 'family care', then spent some weeks with a 'curative educator' in Bonn where he started writing his protest 'brochure', published in 1908. The ninety-five-page pamphlet documents his background, treatment, conclusions and correspondence, including some self-composed poems. Glöklen repeatedly asked his Heidelberg doctors for compensation but his claim was dismissed by the state court in 1911.[91]

In 1909, Glöklen started giving lectures on his asylum experience, turned to naturopathy, and founded the publishing company Jünger & Co. That same year, he initiated the BIRIF and became the editor of its journal *Die Irrenrechts-Reform* [The Lunacy Law Reform]. He also developed breathing exercises, marketed 'medical healing devices', opened his own psychology practice, and wrote an article on suggestion therapy.[92] Like Lowe, Glöklen created for himself a new social identity and became an 'expert by experience'.

His BIRIF merged with its Swiss counterpart during the First World War and presented itself as the mouthpiece of the 'psychiatric group' within the Allgemeiner Deutscher Kulturbund [General German Cultural Association], then run by the radical *völkisch*-nationalist publisher Johannes Lehmann-Hohenberg (1851–1925).[93] This right-wing political strategy can most likely be attributed to Glöklen himself. The BIRIF is believed to have had several hundred members, both in and beyond Germany. Among its supporters were freethinkers, naturopaths, monists, life reformers, anti-vivisectionists and anti-vaccinationists, as had been the case in England. Bernhard Beyer (1879–1966), a doctor from Bayreuth, spoke of an 'anti-psychiatry movement' for the first time as early as in 1909.[94] The BIRIF journal *Die Irrenrechts-Reform* appeared bimonthly, with a reputed circulation of up to 10,000 copies. Constantly ridiculing and mocking the mad-doctors, it featured calls, petitions, 'provable reports of maltreatment', legal essays and readers' contributions. In 1908, Glöklen had only demanded that admissions should require 'advice and assessment by a lay commission' and that asylum staff should be competent and adequately paid.[95] Ten years later, the BIRIF listed twelve demands, above all the introduction of 'monitoring commissions', with a law stipulating provisions for their proper implementation, as well as the sanctioning of abuses, the monitoring of private asylums, the establishment of separate institutions for alcoholics and the introduction of 'social welfare'.[96] In 1914, these calls for reform were also supported by social democrats like Karl Liebknecht (1871–1919).[97]

After the 1918 revolution, the BIRIF managed to float its ideas within the Prussian Ministry of People's Welfare. The official in charge, the Social Democrat physician Alfred Beyer (1885–1961), consulted with BIRIF representatives to prepare a draft bill. Well aware of these negotiations, the National Minister of the Interior ordered the drafting of a national bill: *Grundzüge zu einem Schutzgesetz für Geisteskranke (Irrenschutzgesetz)* [Basic Features of a Law for the Protection of the Mentally Diseased (Lunatics' Protection Law)]. It built on legalistic principles and was officially presented in July 1923. Committals were to be restricted to patients 'who constitute a danger to the public' and would require a court order and patients were to be given the right to appeal.[98] The draft was rejected both by psychiatrists' associations and the German states and was eventually withdrawn in the spring of 1924. Efforts to create a revised Prussian state law or a 'custodial' lunatics' welfare law, as advocated by the expert associations, also petered out.[99] The last issue of *Die Irrenrechts-Reform* appeared in 1922, shortly before the onset of the hyperinflation crisis of 1923. Reports on abuses in mental institutions continued well up to the end of the Weimar Republic.[100]

Adolf Glöklen returned to private life. The final document in his medical file, added by the young Walter von Baeyer (1904–87), who visited him at his home in 1931, states that seventy-year-old Glöklen was healthy, leading a bourgeois life and had remarried in 1920. He reportedly complained about his low income but enthusiastically spoke of his work as a 'psychotherapist', as he knew from his time at the clinic 'what the mentally ill need and what they miss'.[101]

Scholars vary in their assessment of German lunatics' rights activism. While Cornelia Brink associates the heterogeneous scene of activists with the 'Wilhelminian reformist milieu', Ann Goldberg identifies the BIRIF's affiliations with 'anti-liberal' bourgeois populism and Hans-Walter Schmuhl depicts the campaigners as civil-society actors in opposition to medical 'claims to omnipotence' and attempts of 'social engineering' in the modernising Empire.[102] The failure to implement a nationwide lunacy law during the years of the Weimar Republic resonates to this day, as present-day Germany still has no uniform legislation. Laws and regulations governing compulsory hospitalisation differ between the federal states, the Bundesländer, in some they are part of public order laws, in others part of social welfare laws.

## Patterns of self-advocacy

The following comparative analysis of the presented cases draws on concepts developed in disability studies and in the political sociology of social movements. The model of 'self-advocacy', as defined by Sian Anderson and Christine Bigby in 2017, provides a suitable *tertium comparationis*: 'The dominant narrative about self-advocacy has been about speaking out, having a say and developing skills in empowerment.'[103] These three elements structure the analysis to highlight the similarities between Lowe's and Glöklen's careers at both the individual and collective level. This analysis reveals the chances and contradictions of user self-advocacy – some of which matter still today – as well as some typical problems associated with their historical reconstruction.

## Speaking out

Louisa Lowe and Adolf Glöklen described similar experiences and structural problems. Both complained about deceitful admission practices, a lack of doctors' attention, harassment by fellow patients, low hygiene, mail censorship, substandard food, and the harsh and sometimes violent treatment by attendants and alienists alike.[104] They dealt with these experiences by developing an 'injustice frame' that focused on humiliation and the deprivation of rights.[105] 'Speaking out' was meant to convey this message. Lowe did so in third person: 'say that which she does know, and testify to that she has seen'.[106] 'Speaking out' transcends the status of the patient as objects of medical treatment and creates a self-determined narrative.[107]

Both activists communicated their biographical disruption in a radical and scandalising tone. Glöklen saw himself as having been 'assassinated' at the clinic, while Lowe bemoaned her 'lingering death in life, this moral torture of incarceration among maniacs'.[108] The polemical rhetoric was typical of this kind of protest literature. The radical perspective created a collective politics of identity but, at the same time, impeded alliances with liberal doctors or politically moderate patients. Moreover, this perspective largely ignored the working conditions of asylum staff as well as the possibility that some of the activists' relatives – like Glöklen's wife and Lowe's sister – may have actively contributed to their institutionalisation.[109] However, neither of the two ever demanded the wholesale abolition of psychiatry. Lowe asked for a 'just and safe Lunacy System' and Glöklen hoped 'that the reputation of capable doctors and decent institutions is not being undermined and that the sick no longer have to be afraid of going to an asylum'.[110]

Lowe's and Glöklen's personal justifications contested medical indications to rid themselves of stigma. They drew a different line between being healthy or being in need of treatment, and insisted on the normality of 'nervous' conditions and denied ever having posed a threat to either themselves or others.[111] This may explain why both distanced themselves from their fellow patients while at the asylum and why Cornelia Brink concludes that the German protesters were 'more concerned with securing their own status as healthy individuals than with those who actually lived at the asylums'.[112]

## Having a say

When social movements emerge, the public response attests to the political relevance of the chosen interpretive framework. The ensuing years of networking are documented in Lowe's *The Bastilles of England* and in the journal *Die Irrenrechts-Reform*. The key strategy was to uncover new cases of allegedly wrongful confinement. This created a counter-public sphere where the voices of Lowe and Glöklen mattered. The 'new journalism' around 1900 facilitated political agitation. The press created a critical public, albeit with the danger of opportunistic coverage.[113] Alienists in particular feared that the latter would be the case, among them British psychoanalyst Ernest Jones (1879–1958), who wrote in his 1910 review of Clifford Beers' (1876–1943) *A Mind That Found Itself*:

> America has now a great opportunity to repudiate the 'yellow press' methods of asylum reform indulged in by German agitators, and to show the world how a sober but enthusiastic campaign against avoidable evils should be carried on.[114]

In Britain, the campaigns were affiliated with conservative liberalism and individualism. The legal settlement thus entailed serious political trade-offs. The 1890 Lunacy Act expanded the Commissioners' authority and, in accordance with the Medico-Psychological Association's demands, exempted doctors from liability if they had acted in 'good faith'.[115] The German alliances, in contrast, seem more unstable and give an overall impression of political opportunism. Ann Goldberg interprets the fact that the BIRIF's 'radical-democratic' and 'emancipatory' populism managed to integrate right-wing nationalist and antisemitic positions as an expression of radicalising bourgeois politics on Germany's 'Sonderweg' towards Nazism.[116] The BIRIF's libertarian rhetoric of freedom could thus easily be exploited for nationalist ends. The organisation was, however, striving for a non-partisan image and their reform proposals repeatedly gained support from left-liberal and Marxist politicians too. In the years after 1920, this created opportunities entirely different from those in Victorian Britain, a post-revolutionary alliance with social democratic health policy-makers.

## Empowerment skills

Lowe's and Glöklen's professionalisation as 'experts by experience' is a vivid example of their empowerment strategies. Their asylum experiences served to substantiate their organisations' demands in 1885 and 1919 for the implementation of independent supervisory bodies and judicial reviews as well as sanctions for violations and abuses committed by staff.[117] To gain influence, their associations offered legal advice and assistance. In Britain, the links with the early women's movement are evident, although the stereotype of the 'locked-away Victorian wife' has now become obsolete.[118] The German organisations, in contrast, were dominated by men and notions of masculine honour.[119]

In terms of public relations, self-labelling is an important means of empowerment. We know that in Britain James Billington spoke of a 'movement' in 1877, while Lowe used the term 'lunacy law reformers' in 1883.[120] In a 1911 issue of *Die Irrenrechts-Reform*, psychiatry-experienced visitors to an expert conference labelled themselves as 'well-experienced' and 'self-trained laypersons'; one year later, there was talk of a 'lunacy law reform movement', and in 1917 the wording was 'modern lunatics' rights reformers'. On top of this, we also find the self-labelling expression 'anti-psychiatry movement' in a 1914 book published by the jurist and editor of *Die Irrenrechts-Reform*, Paul Elmer.[121] Despite being introduced in the expert discourse by the German psychiatrists Bernhard Beyer and Georg Lornmer (1877–1957) in 1909 in order to discredit critics once and for all, the term 'anti-psychiatry' may then have already been in use within the movement, or they may have reappropriated the initially derogatory catchword for their own purposes soon thereafter. Regardless of its two historical predecessors – the designations 'Anti-Insane Asylum Society' (1868) in the US and 'Anti-Aliéniste' in France (1893) – this specific self-label cannot be traced in the writings examined here, except in Elmer.[122] The term 'antipsychiatry' is thus not suitable for historicising the entire criticism of psychiatry at that time, but is likely to have been used only by a particular wing of the reform movement, just as it is today.

## Conclusions

The sources examined here support Eric J. Engstrom's argument that the 'history of the criticism of psychiatry' does not begin in the 1960s and that we need a 'broad perspective' spanning from 'the single patient's subjectivity to the larger political and social contexts'.[123] It has become clearer now that concepts like 'self-advocacy', 'speaking out', 'empowerment' and 'rights-based legalism' had specific predecessors around 1900. This particularly holds for the positive claims to legal protection, democratisation and de-stigmatisation but also for the problematic aspects, like populist rhetoric, libertarian postulates of freedom and particularistic politics of identity. The careers of Louisa Lowe and Adolf Glöklen reveal similarities in both individual and collective patterns of argumentation, action and organisation. Both described their asylum experience and, at the same time, developed from laypersons to experts by analysing this experience. 'Ex-patients' or 'post-patients' thus deserve group-specific historiographical attention, similar to what Michael Worboys argues with respect to 'non-patients' and 'pre-patients'.[124] As a result, their early and partly 'catalytic' contribution to the development of psychiatry becomes visible and open to scholarly debate. In this sense, the present study sheds light on the historical background and the politics of today's consumer/survivor/ex-patient movement.

In the imperialist era around 1900, marked by the urbanisation, industrialisation and medialisation of society, lunatics' rights discourses were influenced by gender, class and corporeality. It is clear that both Lowe and Glöklen represented gender-specific voices. Glöklen's attitudes and his association were bound to the male-dominated zeitgeist of Imperial Germany and Lowe's activities were linked to the early British women's movement. Moreover, traditional social historiography of psychiatry has highlighted the connection between the rise of asylums and poor relief in the nineteenth century as well as the dramatic increase in patient numbers in the context of industrialisation, capitalist economy and the 'social question'.[125] The divide between public asylums and workhouses for the majority of penniless patients and exclusive private facilities – as a sign of class distinction – also influenced Lowe's and Glöklen's narratives. In this sense, we can speak of a 'bourgeois protest' in both countries. Paul Carter and Steve King have, however, shown that we can systematically reconstruct calls for legal counsel from first-person accounts by inmates of Britain's nineteenth-century poor- and workhouses, too.[126] According to Peter Bartlett, the 1890 Lunacy Act actually changed neither the social gradient in public asylums nor the revolving-door effect of the workhouse system.[127] This is why the Act has often been considered a custodial and paternalistic compromise, especially since it failed to prevent further asylum scandals.[128] The German draft law of 1923 would have restricted coercive measures to the coincidence of 'insanity' and 'constituting a public danger', but with the effect of segregating those patients within the institutions. The structural problems reflected the limits of expert knowledge. Treated by leading doctors of their time, both Lowe and Glöklen rejected hereditarian models of disorder and, by doing so, addressed yet another structure of social inequality, one that directly targeted their bodily disposition.

Can we now speak of social movements in the proper sense? Organisations like the LLRA or the BIRIF do not by themselves constitute a social movement. Social movements can be defined as 'networks' of individuals who share a 'collective identity' and seek to foster 'social change' through 'public protest'.[129] This, indeed, applies to both countries' lunatics' rights activists. A comparison with their US counterparts might help to gain a clearer picture; the same holds for the French movement. We know that French, Austrian and Swiss campaigns had an impact on the German movement, whereas British activists apparently had no international connections prior to 1900. Except for a German translation of one of Lowe's essays in the context of 'psychical research', there is also no further evidence of British–German exchange.[130]

British historians have recently suggested placing more emphasis on 'the experience of all service users' and the 'interaction between officials and expert and lay networks in shaping policy and legislation' in the twentieth century.[131] Indeed, very little is known about lunatics' rights discourses between 1920 and 1960. In the case of Britain, this would mean including campaigns by the National Society for Lunacy Reform from 1923 onwards and the National Council for Civil Liberties around 1950. German lunatics' rights campaigns fell silent after 1933 and it was not until the late 1960s that patient organisations started re-emerging in West Germany.[132]

All things considered, the activists and organisations presented in this chapter can, without any doubt, be regarded as historical predecessors of today's consumer/survivor/ex-patient movement. The analysis brings to light typical structures and contradictions: legal certainty, political participation and the protection against violence and discrimination are still on the agenda of contemporary self-advocacy organisations. In historical retrospect, the bilateral comparison reveals similar motives for and means of activism in Britain and Germany but different chances of political realisation. In this respect, the sources describe the crisis of modernisation in European psychiatry around 1900 from the perspective of individuals with asylum experience. Dirk Blasius identified the significance of this type of sources with regard to the social history of German-speaking psychiatry already in 1980; in the English-speaking world, Dale Peterson's 1982 work *A Mad People's History of Madness* was followed by Roy Porter's studies.[133] So we know by now that Louisa Lowe's and Adolf Glöklen's writings document the classic pattern of madhouse literature as it has been known for 350 years, as a personal confession, an account of treatment and recovery, a polemic on health policy and a testimony of resistance.

## Notes

* The author would like to thank the editors of this collection for their support and Jacques Hochmann, Rafael Huertas, Bernhard Leitner, Benoît Majerus, Bob Peel, Doris Noell-Rumpeltes, Annika Söderland and Sarah Wise for their advice on sources for this study, as well as Andrea Tönjes for the translation.
1 Cf. Linda Morrison, *Talking Back to Psychiatry: The Psychiatric Consumer/Survivor/Ex-patient Movement* (London: Routledge, 2013); Nancy Tomes, 'From Outsiders to Insiders: The Consumer-Survivor Movement and its Impact on U.S. Mental Health Policy', in Beatrix Hoffman, Nancy Tomes, Rachel Grob and Mark Schlesinger (eds), *Patients as Policy Actors* (New Brunswick: Rutgers, 2011), 111–31;

Nick Crossley, *Contesting Psychiatry: Social Movements in Mental Health* (London, New York: Routledge, 2006).
2 Diana Rose, 'A Hidden Activism and its Changing Contemporary Forms: Mental Health Service Users/Survivors Mobilising', *Journal of Social and Political Psychology* 6 (2018), 728–44, 738.
3 Cf. Mohammed Abouelleil Rashed, *Madness and the Demand for Recognition* (Oxford: Oxford University Press, 2019).
4 John Stuart Mill, 'The Law of Lunacy', *Daily News* (31 July 1858), 4; Correspondent of the *New York Tribune* [Karl Marx], 'Imprisonment of Lady Bulwer Lytton', *New York Daily Tribune* (4 August 1858), 6; John Thomas Perceval, 'To the Editor of The Morning Advertiser', *Morning Advertiser* (12 August 1858), 4.
5 Sarah Wise, *Inconvenient People: Lunacy, Liberty and the Mad-Doctors in Victorian England* (London: Bodley Head, 2012), 252–90; Dan Degerman, '"Am I Mad?" The Windham Case and Victorian Resistance to Psychiatry', *History of Psychiatry* 30:4 (2019), 1–12; Rebecca Wynter, '"Horrible Dens of Deception": Thomas Bakewell, Thomas Mulock and Anti-Asylum Sentiments, 1815–58', in Thomas Knowles and Serena Towbridge, (eds), *Insanity and the Lunatic Asylum in the Nineteenth Century* (London: Pickering & Chatto, 2015), 27–44.
6 Wise, *Inconvenient People*, 65–93; Nicholas Hervey, 'Advocacy or Folly: The Alleged Lunatics' Friend Society, 1845–63', *Medical History* 30:3 (1986), 245–75; House of Commons, *An Act to Consolidate Certain of the Enactments Respecting Lunatics* (London: Her Majesty's Stationery Office, 1890). The ALFS emerged from the Society for the Protection of Alleged Lunatics founded by Thomas Mulock in 1840.
7 Kathleen Jones, *Mental Health and Social Policy, 1845–1959* (London: Routledge and Kegan, 1960), 7–42. On the significance of legalist concepts, see Penny Weller (ed.), *Rethinking Rights-based Mental Health Laws* (Oxford: Bloomsbury, 2010).
8 Burkhart Brückner, Thomas Röske, Maike Rotzoll and Thomas Müller, 'Geschichte der Psychiatrie "von unten". Entwicklung und Stand der deutschsprachigen Forschung', *Medizinhistorisches Journal* 54 (2019), 347–76.
9 Anne Waldschmidt, Anemari Karačić, Andreas Sturm and Timo Dins, '"Nothing About Us Without Us": Disability Rights Activism in European Countries. A Comparative Analysis', *Moving the Social* 53 (2015), 103–37, 110; James M. Jasper, *The Art of Moral Protest: Culture, Biography, and Creativity in Social Movements* (Chicago, London: University of Chicago Press, 1997).

10  Roy Porter, *Social History of Madness: The World Through the Eyes of the Insane* (New York: Weidenfeld & Nicolson, 1987), 2, 5; Geoffrey Reaume, 'From the Perspective of Mad People', in Greg Eghigian (ed.), *The Routledge History of Madness and Mental Health* (London: Routledge, 2017), 277–96.

11  Aude Fauvel, 'A World-Famous Lunatic: The "Seillière Affair" (1887–1889) and the Circulation of Anti-Alienists' Views in the Nineteenth Century', in Waltraud Ernst and Thomas Müller (eds), *Transnational Psychiatries: Social and Cultural Histories of Psychiatry in Comparative Perspective, 1800–2000* (Newcastle: Cambridge Scholars Publishing, 2010), 200–28, 228; Michel Foucault, *Folie et déraison: Histoire de la folie à l'âge classique* (Paris: Plon, 1961).

12  Dana Gliserman-Kopans, 'One Cannot Be Too Secure: Wrongful Confinement, or, the Pathologies of the Domestic Economy', in Chris Mounsey (ed.), *The Idea of Disability in the Eighteenth Century* (Lewisburg: Bucknell University Press, 2014), 130–57.

13  See, for example, Charles Reade, *Hard Cash: A Matter-of-Fact Romance* (London: Ward, 1863).

14  Ian Dowbiggin, *Inheriting Madness: Professionalization and Psychiatric Knowledge in Nineteenth-Century France* (Berkeley: University of California Press, 1991), 93–115.

15  Aude Fauvel, 'Cerveaux fous et sexes faibles (Grande-Bretagne, 1860–1900)', *Clio: Femmes, Genre Histoire* 37 (2013), 41–64, 54; Jacques Hochmann, *Les Antipsychiatries: Une histoire* (Paris: Odile Jacob, 2015).

16  Cornelia Brink, *Grenzen der Anstalt: Psychiatrie und Gesellschaft in Deutschland 1860–1980* (Göttingen: Wallstein 2010), 36–56, 145–92; Ann Goldberg, *Honor, Politics and the Law in Imperial Germany, 1871–1914* (Cambridge: Cambridge University Press, 2010), 168–91; Burkhart Brückner, *Delirium und Wahn: Geschichte, Selbstzeugnisse und Theorien von der Antike bis 1900*, Vol. II, *Das 19. Jahrhundert – Deutschland* (Hürtgenwald: Pressler, 2007), 161–77.

17  Brigitta Bernet, *Schizophrenie. Entstehung und Entwicklung eines psychiatrischen Krankheitsbildes um 1900* (Zurich: Chronos, 2013), 89–102.

18  Leslie Topp, *Freedom and the Cage: Modern Architecture and Psychiatry in Central Europe, 1890–1914* (University Park: Penn State University Press, 2007), 16–23.

19  Godart Gauthier, *L'Asile en procès: Le scandale d'Evere (1871–1872) et la prise en charge de la folie en Belgique* (Louvain-la-Neuve: Presses Universitaires de Louvain, 2019).

20 Joost Vijselaar, 'Egodocumenten van psychiatrische patienten uit de negentiende eeuw', *Amsterdams Sociologisch Tijdschrift* 14 (1988), 645–61.
21 Kirsi Tuohela, 'Hospitalised: Patients' Voices in Nineteenth-Century Finnish Newspapers', in Tuomas Laine-Frigren, Jari Eilola and Markku Hokkanen (eds), *Encountering Crises of the Mind: Madness, Culture and Society, 1200s–1900s* (Leiden: Brill, 2018), 115–38. On Russian-governed Latvia, see Parcival Baron Lieven, 'Die soziale Stellung des Psychiaters', *Rigaische Zeitung* (20 August 1912), 1.
22 Niels Reisby, 'An Anti-psychiatry Debate of the 1890's', *Acta Psychiatrica Scandinavica* 52 (1975), 15–20.
23 Patrik Möller, *Hemligheternas värld. Bror Gadelius och psykiatrins genombrott i det tidiga 1900-talets Sverige* (unpublished PhD Thesis, University of Gothenburg, 2017), 59–98.
24 On the US, see Jeffrey Geller, 'Advocacy: The Push and Pull of Psychiatrists', in Hunter L. McQuistion, Wesley E. Sowers, Jules M. Ranz and Jacqueline Maus Feldman (eds), *Handbook of Community Psychiatry* (New York: Springer, 2012), 61–78; Mary De Young, *Madness: An American History of Mental Illness and Its Treatment* (Jefferson: McFarland, 2010), 90–170. On Japan, see Susan L. Burns, 'Constructing the National Body: Public Health and the Nation in Nineteenth-Century Japan', in Timothy Brook and Andre Schmid (eds), *Nation Work: Asian Elites and National Identities* (Michigan: The University of Michigan Press, 2000), 17–49. On Spain and Portugal, see Rafael Huertas and Enric J. Novella, 'L'Aliénisme français et l'institutionalisation du savoir psychiatrique en Espagne: L'affaire Sagrera (1863–1864)', *L'Évolution Psychiatrique* 76 (2011), 537–47; Manuela Gonzaga, *Maria Adelaide Coelho da Cunha: doida não e não! Um escándalo em Portugal no início do século XX* (Lisboa: Bertrand, 2009).
25 Alexandra Bacopoulous-Viau and Aude Fauvel, 'The Patient's Turn: Roy Porter and Psychiatry's Tales, Thirty Years On', *Medical History* 60:1 (2016), 1–18, 3.
26 Louisa Lowe, *The Bastilles of England; or, the Lunacy Laws at Work* (London: Crookenden, 1883).
27 Wise, *Inconvenient People*, 291–324; Helen Nicholson, 'Women, Madness and Spiritualism: Introduction to the Writings of Louisa Lowe', in Bridget Bennett, Helen Nicholson and Roy Porter (eds), *Women, Madness and Spiritualism* Vol. I (New York: Routledge, 2003), 139–53; Alex Owen, *The Darkened Room: Women, Power and Spiritualism in Late Victorian England* (Chicago: University of Chicago Press, 1989), 168–201; Charlotte MacKenzie, *Psychiatry for the Rich: A History of Ticehurst Private Asylum, 1792–1917* (London:

Routledge, 1992), 107–13. Lowe's twelve-part retrospective, hitherto unnoticed by scholars, appeared in 1888. See Louisa Lowe, 'Fifteen Months in Lunatic Houses: I', *Evening News* (23 March 1888), 2.
28 TNA, London, Will of Thomas Crookenden of Rushford or Rushford Lodge, PROB 11/1963/326, fol. 3.
29 Louisa Lowe, 'No 1: Report of a Case Heard in Queen's Bench', *Quis Custodiet Ipsos Custodes?* (London: Burns, 1872/73), 7–10, 17; House of Commons, *Report from the Select Committee on Lunacy Law; Together with the Proceedings on the Committee, Minutes of Evidence and Appendix* (London: Her Majesty's Stationery Office, 1877), q. 7308.
30 Lowe, 'No 1: Report', 6, 22.
31 Louisa Lowe, 'No 3: How an Old Woman Obtained Passive Writing and the Outcome Thereof', *Quis Custodiet Ipsos Custodes?* (London: Burns, 1873); Anthony Enns, 'The Undead Author: Spiritualism, Technology and Authorship', in Tatiana Kontou and Sarah Willburn (eds), *The Ashgate Research Companion to Nineteenth-Century Spiritualism and the Occult* (London: Routledge, 2012), 55–78.
32 *Select Committee on Lunacy Law* (1877), qq. 7192–235.
33 Lowe, 'Fifteen Months: I', 2.
34 House of Commons, *An Act for Regulating Mad-Houses* (London, 1774).
35 House of Commons, *Act for the Regulation of the Care and Treatment of Lunatics* (London: Her Majesty's Stationery Office, 1845), 45, 99.
36 *Select Committee on Lunacy Law* (1877), q. 5316. Both certificates had to include the finding 'lunatic' or 'insane person' or 'idiot' or 'person of unsound mind'; *Act for the Regulation of the Care and Treatment of Lunatics*, 46, Appendix: Schedule B; Carol Berkenkotter and Cristina Hanganu-Bresch, 'Occult Genres and the Certification of Madness in a 19th-Century Lunatic Asylum', *Written Communication* 28:2 (2011), 228–32.
37 *Select Committee on Lunacy Law* (1877), qq. 5307, 5499; Lowe, 'No 1: Report', 8. On alterations to the order, see J.M. Moorsom, 'Louisa Lowe, Appellant and Charles Henry Fox, Respondent', in A.P. Stone (ed.), *The Law Reports* (London: Clowes and Sons, 1887), 206–17.
38 *Act for the Regulation of the Care and Treatment of Lunatics*, 72–7.
39 Patients' mail was to be forwarded unopened and the fine for non-compliance was £20. See House of Commons, *Lunacy Acts Amendment Act* (London: Her Majesty's Stationery Office, 1862), 40.
40 *Select Committee on Lunacy Law* (1877), qq. 7636, 7644, 7676.
41 *Ibid.*, q. 5423; Louisa Lowe, 'Lunacy Law Reform', *The Spiritualist* (1878), 239.

42 Lowe, 'Fifteen Months in Lunatic Houses: VI', *Evening News* (29 March, 1888), 2.
43 Ibid.; *Select Committee on Lunacy Law* (1877), q. 1540.
44 *Select Committee on Lunacy Law* (1877), qq. 7366, 7378, 7468. Lowe, 'No 1: Report', 4, 14, 20–3.
45 Lowe, 'No 1: Report', 18, 21.
46 Lowe, 'Fifteen Months in Lunatic Houses: XII', *Evening News* (7 April 1888), 2.
47 *Select Committee on Lunacy Law* (1877), qq. 6902–11.
48 On the size of these organisations, see Lunacy Law Reform Association (ed.), *The First Report of the Lunacy Law Reform Association* (London, 1874); *Select Committee on Lunacy Law* (1877), q. 7162; Lowe, *Lunacy Law Reform*, 239; Michael J. Clark, 'Does a Certificate of Lunacy Affect a Patient's Ethical Status? Psychiatric Paternalism and its Critics in Victorian England', in Andrew Wear, Johanna Geyer-Kordesch and Roger French (eds), *Doctors and Ethics: The Earlier Historical Setting of Professional Ethics* (Amsterdam: Rodopi, 1993), 274–93, 283; Clive Unsworth, *The Politics of Mental Health Legislation* (Oxford: Clarendon Press, 1987), 93–6.
49 Stewart Lyttleton Forbes Winslow, 'The Dillwyn Committee', *Journal of Psychological Medicine and Mental Pathology* 3:2 (1877), 311–25, 311.
50 Thomas S. Clouston, 'The Evidence Given Before the Select Committee of the House of Commons on Lunacy Law, 1877', *Journal of Mental Science* 23:104 (1878), 457–525, 496.
51 *Select Committee on Lunacy Law* (1877), qq. 892, 8896, 8902–11, 8967.
52 *Ibid.*, qq. 4403–552, 5296–639. The Committee also heard from ex-patients Walter Marshall (b. 1837) and Reverend J.W. Thomas.
53 *Select Committee on Lunacy Law* (1877), qq. 7277–9. Maudsley claimed that nobody had succeeded in correcting Lowe, that she had no longer been able to care for her children, declared herself a 'female Christ' and believed that her husband entered the sanatorium via the chimney to haunt her.
54 Louisa Lowe, 'Dr. Forbes Winslow's Pamphlet', *The Spiritualist* (1876), 201; *Select Committee on Lunacy Law* (1877), qq. 5309, 5554. On psychical research, moral insanity and spiritualism, see Owen, *The Darkened Room*, 139–67.
55 *Select Committee on Lunacy Law* (1877), q. 5630.
56 House of Commons, *Report from the Select Committee on Lunacy Law with the proceedings of the Committee* (London: Her Majesty's Stationery Office, 1878), iii; *Select Committee on Lunacy Law* (1877), qq. 1771, 7443.

57 House of Commons, *Lunacy Acts Amendment Act* (London: Her Majesty's Stationery Office, 1889).
58 Lowe, *The Bastilles of England*, 63, 1, 56.
59 Hervey, 'Advocacy or Folly', 245; Clark, 'Does a Certificate of Lunacy Affect a Patient's Ethical Status?', 283.
60 Owen, *The Darkened Room*, 200; Nicholson, 'Women, Madness and Spiritualism', 150.
61 Wise, *Inconvenient People*, 319–22.
62 Ibid., 325–73; Roy Porter, 'Introduction: Georgina Weldon and the Mad Doctors', in Bridget Bennett, Helen Nicholson and Roy Porter (eds), *Women, Madness and Spiritualism* Vol. I (New York: Routledge, 2003), 3–27.
63 Georgina Weldon, *How I Escaped the Mad-Doctors* (London, 1879).
64 Maureen Wright, '"The Perfect Equality of All Persons before the Law": The Personal Rights Association and the Discourse of Civil Rights in Britain, 1871–1885', *Women's History Review* 24:1 (2015), 72–95.
65 Unsworth, *The Politics of Mental Health Legislation*, 80–111; Jones, *Mental Health and Social Policy*, 29–42, 80–110; Peter McCandless, 'Dangerous to Themselves and Others: The Victorian Debate over the Prevention of Wrongful Confinement', *Journal of British Studies* 23:1 (1983), 84–104.
66 Joseph Mortimer Granville, *The Care and Cure of the Insane: Being the Reports of the Lancet Commission on Lunatic Asylums, 1875–6-7* Vols I and II (London: Hardwicke and Bould, 1877).
67 House of Commons, *An Act to Consolidate Certain of the Enactments Respecting Lunatics* (1890), I, 9, 15. The Act included changes to the *Lunacy Law Amendment Act* (1889).
68 House of Commons, *Mental Health Act* (London: Her Majesty's Stationery Office, 1959), 72.
69 *Select Committee on Lunacy Law* (1877), q. 578, Appendix 5; William L. Parry-Jones, *The Trade in Lunacy: A Study of Private Madhouses in England in the Eighteenth and Nineteenth Centuries* (London: Routledge & Kegan Paul, 1972), 27.
70 Phil Fennell, *Treatment Without Consent: Law, Psychiatry and the Treatment of Mentally Disordered People since 1845* (London: Routledge, 1996), 104–16; Hervey, 'Advocacy or Folly', 345; Rachel Grant-Smith [Rachel Godde-Smith], *The Experiences of an Asylum Patient* (London: Allen & Unwin, 1922), 30.
71 Akinobu Takabayashi, 'Surviving the Lunacy Act of 1890: English Psychiatrists and Professional Development during the Early Twentieth Century', *Medical History* 61:2 (2017), 246–69; Jones, *Mental Health and Social Policy*, 29–42.

72 Rebecca Schwoch, 'Eduard August Schröder – ein Protagonist der Psychiatriekritik um 1900', *Schriftenreihe der Deutschen Gesellschaft für Geschichte der Nervenheilkunde* 13 (2007), 208–32; Eric J. Engstrom, 'Pastoral Psychiatry and *"Irrenseelsorge"*: Religious Aspects of the Anti-Psychiatry Debates in Germany in the 1890s', in Lutz Greisiger, Sebastian Schüler and Alexander van der Haven (eds), *Religion und Wahnsinn um 1900. Zwischen Pathologisierung und Selbstermächtigung* (Würzburg: Ergon, 2017), 289–99.

73 Ann Goldberg, 'The Mellage Trial and the Politics of Insane Asylums in Wilhelmine Germany', *Journal of Modern History* 74:1 (2002), 1–32; Arthur von Kirchenheim and Heinrich Reinartz, *Zur Reform des Irrenrechts: Elf Leitsätze zur Besserung der Irrenfürsorge und Beseitigung des Entmündigungsunfugs* (Wiemann: Barmen 1894).

74 Ernst Rittershaus, *Die Irrengesetzgebung in Deutschland: Nebst einer vergleichenden Darstellung des Irrenwesens in Europa* (Berlin, Leipzig: de Gruyter, 1927), 12–15; Sandra Kuban, *Das Recht der Verwahrung und Unterbringung am Beispiel der 'Irrengesetzgebung' zwischen 1794 und 1945* (Frankfurt am Main: Lang, 1997), 47–70; Lenzmann, '[Rede] 1 February 1902', *Stenographische Berichte über die Verhandlungen des Reichstags* (Berlin: Norddeutsche Verlags-Anstalt, 1901/1902), 5, 3838–42.

75 Bernd Ottermann and Ulrich Meyer, 'Der Irren-Reformer Georg Wetzer aus Herbruck. Ein Beitrag zur Geschichte der antipsychiatrischen Bewegung des beginnenden 20. Jahrhunderts', *Würzburger medizinhistorische Mitteilungen* 5 (1987), 311–21; Bernhard Beyer, *Die Bestrebungen zur Reform des Irrenwesens: Material zu einem Reichsirrengesetze* (Halle: Marhold, 1912), 611–20.

76 Adolf Glöklen, *Zustände in der Heidelberger Universitäts-Irren-Klinik oder 5 Tage lebendig begraben* (Heidelberg: Jünger, 1908). Glöklen presumably published a second part under a pseudonym: D. Jusmann, *Ein Kampf um Wahrheit, Recht und Existenz! Nachklänge der Broschüre: Zustände in der Heidelberger Universitätsirrenklinik* (Heidelberg: Jünger, 1910); Goldberg, *Honor, Politics and the Law*, 172–3; Beyer, *Die Bestrebungen zur Reform des Irrenwesens*, 11, 396.

77 Universitätsarchiv Heidelberg, Sig. L-III-1907/159 (University Clinic; henceforth: UAH 07/159) and Historisches Archiv der Psychiatrischen Universitätsklinik Heidelberg (Neckargmünd; henceforth: HAP-Glök).

78 Werner Janzarik, '100 Jahre Heidelberger Psychiatrie', *Heidelberger Jahrbücher* 22 (1978), 93–113; Eric J. Engstrom, *Clinical Psychiatry in Imperial Germany. A History of Psychiatric Practice* (Ithaca and London: Cornell University Press, 2003), 121–40, 177–86.

79 Glöklen, *Zustände*, 25.

80 UAH 07/159, *Abschrift Gr. Landgericht Heidelberg, 29.9.1910, Glöklen gegen Fiskus*, 11.
81 UAH 07/159, *Krankengeschichte*, 13.VI.07.
82 Glöklen, *Zustände*, 26.
83 Ibid., 31.
84 Ibid., 44; Engstrom, *Clinical Psychiatry*, 132–5.
85 Lowe, 'Dr. Forbes Winslow's Pamphlet', 201.
86 UAH 07/159, *Krankengeschichte*, 7. Regulations applying to Glöklen's case included *Landesherrliche Verordnung: Das Verfahren der Aufnahme von Geisteskranken und Geistesschwachen in öffentlichen Irrenanstalten betreffend vom 3. Oktober 1895* (GVBl 29, 367–327), with § 4, sec. 1 stipulating that 'urgent' and 'immediate, caring admission' be allowed on examination by a clinic's superintendent, and the *Statut für die Irrenklinik Heidelberg* from 12 October 1878 in the version of 23 March 1887 (GVBl 8, 87–88). The committal was to be 'immediately approved' by the district medical officer in charge.
87 Glöklen, *Zustände*, 46.
88 Ibid., 51.
89 UAH 07/159, *Krankengeschichte, 15.VI.07*; Christopher Baethge, Paola Salvatore and Ross J. Baldessarini, 'Cyclothymia, a Circular Mood Disorder by Ewald Hecker, Introduction', *History of Psychiatry* 14:3 (2003), 377–89.
90 HAP-Glök, *Krankengeschichte, 18.6.1907*; Glöklen, *Zustände*, 55–9.
91 UAH 07/159, *Abschrift Gr. Landgericht Heidelberg Civilkammer I, Nr. 2739, 11. März 1911, Urteil*.
92 Knieper, 'Bemerkungen zu einer Broschüre und einem Vortrag "Zustände in der Heidelberger Universitäts-Irren-Klinik"', *Psychiatrisch-Neurologische Wochenschrift* 5 (1909), 42–4; Adolf Glöklen, *Meine Atmungs-Methode: Nebst Anwendung des gesetzlich geschützten Lungenkräftigungs- und Inhalations-Apparates 'Glia'* (Heidelberg: Jünger, 1913); Adolf Glöklen, 'Hypnotismus im Dienste des Gewerbes und der Krankenbehandlung', *Akademische Mitteilungen für die Studierenden der Ruprecht-Karls-Universität zu Heidelberg* 19 (1914), 3–5.
93 Rupert Gaderer, 'Johannes G. Lehmann-Hohenberg – Wahnsinn, Presse und Recht im Deutschen Kaiserreich', in Heinz-Peter Schmiedebach (ed.), *Entgrenzungen des Wahnsinns – Psychopathie und Psychopathologisierung in urbanen und provinziellen öffentlichen Räumen um 1900* (Berlin and Boston: De Gruyter, 2016), 225–40.
94 Bernhard Beyer, 'Antipsychiatrische Skizze', *Psychiatrisch-Neurologische Wochenschrift* 11 (1909), 275–8, 278.
95 Glöklen, *Zustände*, 77–9.
96 Bund für Irrenrechts-Reform, 'Unsere Forderungen', *Die Irrenrechts-Reform* (1919), 195–6. The BIRIF chairmanship was assumed by

Wilhelm Winsch (1863–1945), a naturopath and anti-vaccinationist, around 1918.
97 Karl Liebknecht, '[Rede] 14 February 1914', *Stenographische Berichte über die Verhandlungen des Preußischen Hauses der Abgeordneten* (Berlin: Preußische Verlagsanstalt, 1914/15), 21, 2195–200.
98 Geheimes Staatsarchiv Preußischer Kulturbesitz Berlin, Sig. I. HA, Rep. 84a, Nr. 1013 (henceforth GeStA 1013), Rudolf Oeser, *An sämtliche Landesregierungen*, 17 July 1923, *Grundzüge zu einem Schutzgesetz für Geisteskranke*. This draft bill is printed in Rittershaus, *Irrengesetzgebung*, 130–8. On the negotiations, see Brink, *Grenzen der Anstalt*, 162–4; Kuban, *Das Recht der Verwahrung*, 86–8; Rittershaus, *Irrengesetzgebung*, 26–31, 116–62.
99 GeStA 1013, circulars by Adolf Gottstein of 3 December 1923 and 15 February 1924.
100 Paul Elmer, 'Um die Reform des Irrenrechts. Antwort an Professor Rittershaus', *Dortmunder General-Anzeiger* (20 August 1931), sheet 2.
101 UAH 07/159, *Besuch bei Adolf Glöklen, 'Heilpsychologe'*, 27.6.1931. V. Baeyer was the director of the Heidelberg clinic from 1955 to 1972.
102 Brink, *Grenzen der Anstalt*, 149, 151; Goldberg, *Honor, Politics and the Law*, 188 f.; Hans-Walter Schmuhl, 'Experten in eigener Sache. Der Beitrag psychiatrischer Patienten zur "Irrenrechtsreform" im 19. und frühen 20. Jahrhundert', *Sozialpsychiatrische Informationen* 39 (2009), 7–9.
103 Sian Anderson and Christine Bigby, 'Self-Advocacy as a Means to Positive Identities for People with Intellectual Disability: "We just help them, be them really"', *Journal of Applied Research in Intellectual Disabilities* 30:1 (2017), 109–20, 110. On applying the 'disability' concept to the field of psychiatry, see Helen Spandler, Jill Anderson and Bob Sapey (eds), *Madness, Distress and the Politics of Disablement* (Bristol: Policy Press, 2015).
104 *Select Committee on Lunacy Law* (1877), q. 5297; Lowe, 'No 1: Report', 3–20; Glöklen, *Zustände*, 26, 35, 42, 44, 61, 67; Louisa Lowe, 'No 2: Gagging in Madhouses, as Practiced by Government Servants, in a Letter to the People', *Quis Custodiet Ipsos Custodes?* (London: Burns, 1873), 5.
105 Jasper, *The Art of Moral Protest*, 12–29, 78–80.
106 Lowe, *The Bastilles of England*, 3.
107 Michele L. Crossley and Nick Crossley, '"Patient" Voices, Social Movements and the Habitus: How Psychiatric Survivors "Speak Out"', *Social Science and Medicine* 52 (2001), 1477–89.
108 Glöklen, *Zustände*, 27, 47; Lowe, 'No 1: Report', 15, 17; Lowe, *The Bastilles of England*, 3, 120, 123–4.

109 UAH 07/159, *Landgericht 29.10.1910, Zeugin Frau Glöklen*; Glöklen, *Zustände*, 62; *Select Committee on Lunacy Law* (1877), qq. 7238–54.
110 Lowe, *The Bastilles of England*, 127; Adolf Glöklen, '[untitled]', *Volkstümliche Zeitschrift des Bundes für Irrenrechts-Reform und Irrenfürsorge* (1910), 1.
111 Lowe, 'No 1: Report', 8, 14; Lowe, 'Fifteen Months in Lunatic Houses: XI', *Evening News* (April 6 1888), 2; UAH 07/159, *Krankengeschichte, 15.VI.07*; UAH 07/159, *Dr. R. Fürst, Fiskalanwalt, 11.1.1910*.
112 Brink, *Grenzen der Anstalt*, 149.
113 Marion T. Marzolf, 'American "New Journalism" Takes Root in Europe at End of Nineteenth Century', *Journalism Quarterly* 61:3 (1984), 529–691.
114 Ernest Jones, 'A Mind That Found Itself: An Autobiography', *The Journal of Abnormal Psychology* (1910), 42.
115 House of Commons, *An Act to Consolidate Certain of the Enactments Respecting Lunatics* (1890), 315, 330.
116 Goldberg, *Honor, Politics and the Law*, 168–91.
117 Lowe, *The Bastilles of England*, 129–33; Bund für Irrenrechts-Reform, 'Unsere Forderungen'.
118 Wise, *Inconvenient People*, xvii. Marilyn J. Kurata, 'Wrongful Confinement: The Betrayal of Women by Men, Medicine and Law', in Kristine Ottesen Garrigan (ed.), *Victorian Scandals: Representations of Gender and Class* (Athens: University of Ohio Press, 1992), 43–68.
119 Goldberg, *Honor, Politics and the Law*, 168–91.
120 *Select Committee on Lunacy Law* (1877), q. 7135; Lowe, *The Bastilles of England*, 3.
121 Anon., 'Unser Bund auf dem Kongreß der Irrenärzte', *Die Irrenrechts-Reform* (1911), 140–4, 142; Paul Elmer, 'Praktische Vorschläge zur Irrenrechtsreform', *Die Irrenrechts-Reform* (1911), 169; Anon., 'Hochadel, Wissenschaft, Parlamente und Presse gegen die Irrenrechtswillkür', *Die Irrenrechts-Reform* (1917), 74–9, 76; Paul Elmer, 'Ist ein Zusammenarbeiten des Bundes und der Psychiatrie zum Zwecke der Irrenrechtsreform möglich?', *Die Irrenrechts-Reform* (1912), 220–2, 220; Paul Elmer, *Geld und Irrenhaus* (Berlin: Rosenthal & Co. 1914), 8.
122 Elizabeth P.W. Packard, *The Prisoners' Hidden Life, Or Insane Asylums Unveiled* (Chicago: The Author, 1868), 144; Tanka Gagné Tremblay, 'Le débat anti-aliéniste français au XIXe siècle: une campagne de presse', *L'Évolution Psychiatrique* 80 (2015), 600–24.
123 Eric J. Engstrom, 'Zur Geschichte der Psychiatriekritik im 19. Jahrhundert', *Themenportal Europäische Geschichte* (2011), www.europa.clio-online.de/2011/Article=507 (accessed 21 August 2020).
124 See Michael Worboys's chapter in this collection.

125 Andrew Scull, *The Most Solitary of Afflictions: Madness and Society in Britain, 1700–1900* (New Haven, London: Yale University Press, 1993); Klaus Dörner, *Bürger und Irre: Zur Sozialgeschichte und Wissenschaftssoziologie der Psychiatrie* (Frankfurt am Main: EVA, 1969).
126 See Paul Carter and Steve King's chapter in this collection.
127 Peter Bartlett, *The Poor Law of Insanity: The Administration of Pauper Lunatics in Mid-Nineteenth Century England* (London: Leicester University Press, 1999), 12.
128 Allan Beveridge, 'Britain's Siberia: Mary Coutts's Account of the Asylum System', *The Journal of the Royal College of Physicians of Edinburgh* 35 (2005), 175–81; Marcia Hamilcar, *Legally Dead: Experiences During Seventeen Weeks' Detention in a Private Madhouse* (London: Ouseley, 1910).
129 Dieter Rucht, 'Leadership in Social and Political Movements. A Comparative Exploration', in L. Helms (ed.), *Comparative Political Leadership* (Houndmills: Palgrave Macmillan, 2012), 99–118, 104.
130 Anon. [Gregor Constantin Wittig], 'Dr. Forbes Winslow über wahnsinnige Spiritualisten', *Psychische Studien* (1877), 77–9.
131 John Turner, Rhodri Hayward, Katherine Angel, Bill Fulford, John Hall, Chris Millard and Mathew Thomson, 'The History of Mental Health Services in Modern England: Practitioner Memories and the Direction of Future Research', *Medical History* 59:4 (2015), 599–624, 622.
132 Burkhart Brückner, '"Nichts über uns ohne uns!" Psychiatrieerfahrene im Prozess der deutschen Psychiatriereform, 1970–1990', in Jürgen Armbruster, Anja Dieterich, Daphne Hahn and Katharina Ratzke (eds), *40 Jahre Psychiatrie Enquete—Blick zurück nach vorn* (Cologne: Psychiatrie-Verlag, 2015), 138–47.
133 Dirk Blasius, *Der verwaltete Wahnsinn: Eine Sozialgeschichte des Irrenhauses* (Frankfurt am Main: Suhrkamp, 1980); Dale Peterson (ed.), *A Mad People's History of Madness* (Pittsburgh: University of Pittsburgh Press, 1982).

# 4

# Narrating and navigating patient experiences of farm work in English psychiatric institutions, 1845–1914*

*Sarah Holland*

Asylum and hospital farms, the agricultural land managed by psychiatric institutions and on which some patients worked, represented transitional spaces between the institution and the wider community, and are pivotal to understanding the experience of patients who worked the land. Patients' experiences of work undertaken while in a psychiatric institution were typically narrated by medical superintendents, and thus mediated through an institutional lens. Arguably the voice of these patients has been silenced as a result. Yet even in the absence of personal testimonies, patients 'narrated' and 'navigated' their experiences through their actions and reactions. Patient records, particularly case notes, can provide valuable insights into the treatment and experiences of patients.[1] Maintaining casebooks became mandatory after the 1845 Lunacy Act, although some institutions already kept detailed case notes before this date. The notes performed medical, bureaucratic and legal roles, and entries became increasingly detailed.[2] The relationship between patients and farm work was not narrated consistently, even within the case notes for one asylum. Frustratingly, references are often fleeting in nature and inconsistent in content. Some, however, do provide more information, and even allude to the way in which a patient responded to work.

Jonathan Andrews acknowledges that case notes present challenges for the historian interested in patients, as they more often reflected the preoccupations of the asylum than a complete patient history.[3] Constructed within the wider context of institutional goals, case notes could be censored to assert expertise in treating the insane.[4] This is apparent in some references to farm work discussed later in this chapter, where the case notes are positioned within the context of the institutional rhetoric concerning the value of outdoor work in the treatment and management of patients. Similarly, Brendan D. Kelly comments that case notes rely on official records written by medical superintendents rather than direct patient accounts, and as such could be consciously or unconsciously manipulated.[5] This is in contrast to the patient advocacy discussed by Burkhart Brückner in Chapter 3, which was a response to the lack of a patient voice. Nevertheless, although casebooks had a very specific function, both Andrews and Kelly demonstrate how it is still possible on occasions to access the patient voice, albeit in a mediated form.[6] Case notes reflect patient behaviour and how medical authorities interpreted it, and as such present 'a unique and crucial account of the patient's experience'.[7] Hazel Morrison highlights the role of the patient in case notes, directly or indirectly narrating their own stories. She argues that case notes were the product of 'construction and reconstruction' at different levels including by the patients and psychiatrists.[8] Similarly, although focusing specifically on voluntary boarders in psychiatric institutions, Sarah Chaney argues that 'representations of madness were the product of a two-way process of negotiation between alienist and patient', with patients participating in 'the construction and circulation of medical notions by serving as active intermediaries between medical and lay perceptions of madness'.[9] Chaney demonstrates that a more nuanced understanding can be gained by looking in depth at how positive and negative experiences were depicted in case notes.[10] By revisiting case notes, this chapter extrapolates aspects of the patient experience and, in some instances, the 'patient voice' relating to farm work. To simply interpret casebook entries as mediated assessments of treatment and recovery undermines the patient as a person and the active role they played in making sense of work and the wider institutional environment.

Evidence of patient experiences of farm work is drawn from case notes, which, although written by medical superintendents, were the process of co-narration incorporating the patient 'voice'. However, the process by which patients could 'narrate' their experiences of farm work necessitates looking beyond merely what patients said, and undertaking a close analysis of the case notes to understand how actions, reactions and behavioural traits, coupled with occupational identities, could allude to their role in negotiating and curating their experience. Lynn M. Thomas reminds us that 'agency should not be the endpoint of our analyses' but it can be an important concept that enables us to explore why people do things.[11] This approach can be applied to the lives of patients undertaking farm work in psychiatric institutions by 'drawing attention to individual choices, motivations and intentions'.[12] This is crucial in providing a nuanced insight into how different patients reacted to and experienced farm work, which suggests that at least for some patients their understanding of institutional space and the use of work shaped their experiences.

The experience or 'voice' and identity of the patients who worked on the farm are at the heart of this chapter, so it is important to reflect on how they are referred to throughout. As Jennifer Wallis argues, 'there is something particularly dehumanising about taking away the patient's real name and replacing it with a pseudonym'.[13] Patients are therefore referred to by their first name and the initial of their surname. This offers some anonymity without rendering the person void of any identity beyond that of a patient. The exception is where patients are only referred to by their initials or a number in the documentary evidence. Similarly, where information about patients before their admission to the asylum is discussed, it is included not as a means of identifying patients but rather in recognition of their lives beforehand and how this might have shaped their experiences while in the institution.

The importance of psychiatric spaces in shaping patient experiences has been demonstrated in *Madness, Architecture and the Built Environment: Psychiatric Spaces in Historical Context*.[14] In the introduction, James Moran and Leslie Topp acknowledge how spatial separation was a common response to madness and, as such, these spaces warrant detailed exploration including consideration of how spaces were created, used, exploited and related to the space beyond their boundaries.[15] Other chapters in the volume examine how spaces were 'constructed' and what they meant to patients. Barry Edginton, in his appraisal of the York Retreat and its influence on asylum design, highlights the connections made between body and mind as part of moral treatment and the fundamental role that the environment could play in this.[16] Chris Philo explores the ideal of the ruralised asylum and the role of nature's perceived capacity to 'elevate the mind of the distressed lunatic'.[17] Farms are, however, only briefly discussed.

The farms managed by psychiatric institutions were transitional spaces, which are pivotal to understanding patient experiences of work. This was a place in which multiple identities came to the fore and where the experience of work could be shaped by the patients' understanding and use of institutional space. Identity and experience were further determined by the spatial demarcation of living arrangements, with some patients accommodated in the farm house rather than the main institution. The economy of the institution and the moral treatment of patients may have converged on the farm, but for those patients who worked outside on the land it provided opportunities to 'navigate' institutional space and 'narrate' their own experiences, making the farms invaluable spaces for the study of patient experiences.

By considering the ways in which patients 'navigated' institutional spaces, this chapter explores how space could be reconfigured to express new identities and experiences and yet also be a tool of authority, and adds a spatial perspective to our understanding of farm work within a psychiatric setting. Records documenting institutional spaces, such as maps, plans and building records, together with case notes, are used to provide insight into how the farm was 'constructed' as an institutional space and how patients who undertook farm work understood and 'navigated' this space and the effect it had on their identity. Maps, for example, visualise the spatial relationship between institution and farm, and how specific institutional geographies affected this relationship. Correspondence between architects, institutions and the Commissioners in Lunacy regarding the construction or conversion of buildings to accommodate patients working on the farm, are used in conjunction with architectural plans, memoranda and minutes of meetings pertaining to these decisions at an institutional level. Case notes, minutes and annual reports for psychiatric institutions contain evidence of how patients used, perceived and negotiated space, including the multiple identities forged and the opportunities for escape.

This chapter uncovers the nuanced experiences of farm work in public psychiatric institutions in England during the nineteenth and early twentieth centuries, and assesses the extent to which these patients had the opportunity to express themselves and whether the patient 'voice' is ever present. By exploring the relationship between how work was represented at institutional level and experienced by individuals, and the role of the patient in 'narrating' and 'navigating' this process, the chapter has parallels with the work of Brückner (Chapter 3) and Paul Carter and Steve King (Chapter 5) in this volume, both of which foreground the experience of the patient or pauper within an institutional and/or hierarchical context. Further, by considering how patients experienced welfare policy in practice, it exposes the structural factors which shaped their lives within institutions. This has contemporary resonance in terms of the processes by which experiences of mental healthcare continue to be recorded. As we will see, the absence of the personal 'voice' continues to be articulated by patients in a twenty-first-century context.

The chapter is divided into three sections. Section one positions these institutional farms within the wider context of Victorian and Edwardian welfare policies, and examines the rationale for advocating farm work for psychiatric patients. This provides an insight into the institutional lenses through which patient records were constructed. Section two reassesses what we can learn about patient experiences of farm work using case note methodologies, and argues that the patient voice can be found in requests to work on the farm as well as in strong behavioural or emotional reactions. Actions, reactions and other behavioural indicators were ways in which patients could 'narrate' their experience, injecting their personality and identity. Section three focuses on the farm as a crucial space in which the patient experience was shaped both by its location and transitional nature, and through the actions and reactions of patients while on the farm, which enabled them to navigate institutional spaces.

## Work, therapy, economy and the farm

Work became 'a major cornerstone of treatment' of the 'insane' from the early nineteenth century.[18] It was part of what was referred to as 'moral treatment' or 'moral therapy', which represented a move away from mechanical restraint and sought to restore rational thought and prepare patients for their return to society.[19] Key ideas, principles, and language of moral treatment recognised the link between mind and body, and the value of occupation 'in diverting the mind from itself towards muscular action'.[20] Significantly, this was not an Anglo-centric phenomenon, with studies of America, Canada and Europe also evidencing the way in which physical, outdoor work was thought to restore rational habits.[21] While not the purpose of this chapter, the comparative perspective, advocated by Brückner in Chapter 3 and by Waltraud Ernst in her edited book on *Work, Psychiatry and Society*, offers great potential for further understanding the use and experience of farm work within institutional settings in different countries. Although 'moral treatment' remained an ideal in England through the mid- to late nineteenth century, the gap between theory and practice widened within the context of large-scale public pauper asylums with an increased focus on 'managing' the burgeoning asylum population.

The continued centrality of work was closely interlinked with Victorian and Edwardian welfare policies that increasingly segregated the poor and the ill and saw the rise of institutionalisation in the form of workhouses and asylums.[22] Whereas the 1808 Asylums Act permitted the construction of and containment of 'pauper lunatics' within specially designated premises, the 1845 legislation provided for compulsion, although the classification of patients remained complex and contested.[23] Welfare policies, as Anne Borsay reminds us, were neither linearly progressive nor singular in nature. Indeed, the experience of patient work could be both aligned to and in conflict with official narratives of institutional treatment.[24] Rationales for patient work, which aligned to welfare policies, focused on the economic, management and therapeutic aspects, albeit to differing extents. Asylums were, in essence, Poor Law institutions, and as such were considered to have a responsibility to ratepayers.[25] They were expensive institutions, and the employment of patients in productive work was recognised often as lowering the cost per patient, so an increasing emphasis was therefore placed on institutional profits. The Lunacy Commission (LC), a public body established by the 1845 Lunacy Act to oversee asylums and the welfare of patients, remained committed to the principles of moral treatment and stressed that patients should only be employed where it was in their own interests rather than those of the institution.[26] However, the LC praised those asylums where patients undertook profitable work and saved the institution money, recognising the aforementioned responsibilities and thus the economic imperative of work in this context.[27] Social control has also been considered another dimension of patient work, although the extent to which Michel Foucault emphasised the repressive nature of occupation within an institutional context has been repeatedly challenged.[28] Others have retained a focus on the therapeutic nature of work and highlighted the important role work played in both recovery and life beyond the asylum.[29] Work could be of benefit from both a therapeutic and financial perspective, and medical, moral and economic motivations were often intertwined in providing a rationale for patient labour.[30]

This focus on the principles and application of policy, however, positions the patient as passive. By moving beyond this, and examining the ways in which patients experienced policy in practice, we can begin to understand the nuanced experiences which underpin 'work' within institutional contexts. Indeed, to understand the use and experience of work, and particularly the active role patients could perform in this process, we should pay attention to the interplay of structural factors, which according to Borsay shaped experiences of exclusion.[31] Gender was particularly influential in shaping experiences of work within psychiatric institutions, with female patients generally allocated work in the laundry or kitchen and male patients assigned to the workshops or outdoor labour.[32] In addition, mental state and occupational identities could affect how individual patients responded to and experienced 'work'.

It was within this context that farms became such a prominent feature of nineteenth-century psychiatric institutions. They provided a space for the outdoor occupation of patients and an opportunity to reduce the cost per patient by producing food for consumption within the institution. Farm work, alongside other forms of physical outdoor labour, was often advocated as part of moral treatment. William Tuke, who established the York Retreat, was a pioneer in the use of space, place and design as methods of treatment, and this included the farm.[33] Tuke's influence can be seen elsewhere, including in the work of John Conolly.[34] Conolly wrote at length on the employment of patients in *On the Construction and Government of Lunatic Asylums*. He argued that work was a crucial means of 'relieving patients from the monotony of an asylum', 'preserving bodily health', 'improving the condition of the mind' and 'promoting recovery'.[35] Work should, however, according to Conolly, always be carefully managed and in the interests of the patients, noting that for some patients work or certain types of work could be detrimental, as could forcing patients to work against their will.[36] Conolly paid particular attention to farm work, asserting that 'more men recover who work in the gardens and on the farm than in the tailors' or the shoemakers' shops' as such work was 'not only more active, but more various, and therefore more remedial'.[37]

The dual motivation of therapy and economy for employing patients on farms is widely acknowledged by historians of psychiatric institutions.[38] Few studies, however, have looked specifically at the patients who undertook this work. Jennifer Laws asserts that therapeutic work had rarely been the subject of historical analysis, and began to readdress this in her detailed and nuanced investigation.[39] Ernst also argues patient work has 'not received any in-depth, systematic assessment' with the exception of a few case studies.[40] This in part is no doubt interconnected with the wider absence of patient narratives that Roy Porter highlighted in the 1980s.[41] Although historians of psychiatry responded to Porter's call for patient orientated histories, there are still gaps where patients are 'curiously underwritten'.[42] In Chapter 5, Carter and King highlight that patient voices are often still not foregrounded despite being crucial to understanding experiences of lunacy. As the 2016 'Voices of Madness' conference at the University of Huddersfield highlighted, this is still a fertile field for research. Sarah Ann Pinto, in her work on lunatic asylums in colonial Bombay, positions patient voices as 'an important part of the asylum soundscape', emphasising that despite being manipulated, interpreted and managed these voices performed a significant role.[43] While *Work, Psychiatry and Society*, edited by Ernst, offers an international perspective on work and psychiatry, and emphasises the importance of the patients who worked as well as the work they undertook, patients undertaking farm work receive only brief mention.

The absence of these experiences in scholarly accounts is perhaps not surprising owing to the types of sources that record the work undertaken. The voices of 'experts' were most frequently recorded, including the work of John Conolly, medical textbooks and individual medical superintendents. All advocated the role of work in the treatment of patients in psychiatric institutions. Annual reports and the minutes of Visiting Committees provide further evidence of the desirability of farm work, the extent to which this was realised, and any challenges encountered. The patient voice is far removed from such documents and yet these accounts can, as discussed in the introduction, facilitate an understanding of how patient narratives were constructed. This chapter therefore contributes to a new understanding of work within psychiatric institutions by focusing on *patients' experiences* of farm work.[44] If asylums were, as Borsay argues, embodiments of the social values and social relations attached to mental impairment, then the farms run by these institutions created complex spatial dynamics which conflated values embodied within and outside the institution but also enabled unique ones based on occupational identities and the patient's understanding of institutional space to come to the fore.[45]

## Recovering the patient experience from mediated case notes

To recover the patients' experience of farm work, and in some instances their 'voice', it is first necessary to contextualise the production of case notes and address the *silencing* of the patient voice. References to work in patient records were underpinned by institutional priorities. Asylum rule books reveal the importance placed on farm work. At Hull Borough Asylum, the general rules stated that male patients were to be 'employed as much as possible, especially outdoors', noting specifically the role of farm work in 'occupying the minds of patients and inducing them to engage in physical exercise'.[46] This was reiterated in the rules for the government of Graylingwell Asylum.[47] Moreover, the medical superintendents and staff writing the case notes were often strong advocates of outdoor physical labour. Their rationale was deeply rooted in the notion of the curative nature of work, although they were also aware of its economic benefits. Mr T. Eccleston, surgeon-superintendent of the Lancaster County Lunatic Asylum at Rainhill, stated that 'one of the leading features in the treatment pursued in this asylum is the occupation of the inmates; and that such is the only humane and common-sense method of dealing with insanity in most of its varied forms, is now too well established a fact to need much comment'.[48]

His assertion was closely aligned with the principles of moral treatment and the shift from mechanical restraint.

This was further emphasised by his use of patient histories. Eccleston cited a patient who had been described as a 'most dangerous lunatic' and admitted in September 1851. On admission, he was 'securely bound by an ordinary cart rope, the removal of which gave no little trouble from the complexity of its attachments, a strait-waistcoat and a pair of transport leg chains completing the arrangement of the poor fellow's torture'.[49] This mode of restraint, which moral treatment sought to replace, was juxtaposed with his employment on the farm. It was noted that 'in the afternoon of the day of his arrival he was working on the farm with his fellow-patients, and has not been absent from employment a single day since that period'.[50] Moran and Topp argue that 'narratives of psychiatric progress were constructed rhetorically in the annual reports'.[51] Eccleston certainly used this narrative as justification for patients working on the farm, by demonstrating not only a positive association between this work and the patient's health and conduct, but also the stark contrast with his previous restraint. Eccleston's assertion that work was his 'chief remedial agent' was not without caveats. Eccleston, similarly to Conolly, highlighted that the employment of patients must be carefully managed. He emphasised the importance of giving 'the appearance of a favour granted, rather than a task imposed'. Moreover, he also explained the importance of selecting work most likely to improve the mental and physical condition of patients. Further, Eccleston stated: 'there are certainly no employments more generally adapted to meet the ends required than horticultural and agricultural pursuits'.[52]

As regards the alignment of suitable work to individual patients, medical superintendents initially oversaw the whole process. This included directly managing the farm, although this was gradually substituted by a farm bailiff and farm subcommittee who would oversee the day-to-day decisions on the farm. In 1862, Dr Wing, medical superintendent at Northampton Asylum, explained the rationale for the farm remaining under his direction, stating that it was deemed to be 'an arrangement which enables him with great advantage to regulate the work of the patients employed there according to their dispositions and the requirements of their mental states'.[53] Dr Wing used this opportunity to argue that the farm had other benefits. He alluded to the remuneration from the farm, but asserted that far more importantly they were 'supplied with good, choice, fresh, and early vegetables at a very moderate cost [...] a profit more in character with an asylum farm than endeavouring to make a little more money in the public market'.[54] This preoccupation with the value of farm work, both in terms of the labour undertaken by individual patients and the nutrition of the collective asylum population, shaped the way in which farm work was discussed in patient records.

Dr Palmer, medical superintendent at Lincoln County Asylum, similarly extolled the virtues of farm labour for patients in his annual report of 1854. He was pleased to report that no paid farm labourers were engaged and that patients under the direction of the farm bailiff had undertaken all the preparatory work. This included 'about 2000 tons of vegetable soil wheeled and spread, and spade husbandry applied to 10 acres of ground, besides which, about 10 acres of potatoes have been planted and dug, and nine acres of barley and oats harvested and prepared for market'.[55] He concluded that the patients were 'the true wizards of the soil'. The suitability of patients to undertake agricultural work was often determined by mental state and previous occupation. Lincolnshire was a largely agricultural district, with market towns and centres of agricultural manufacturing. In the same report, Dr Palmer acknowledged that 'in a county whose population is essentially agricultural, the admissions have included a large number of farm-labourers, their wives and families'.[56] Dr Palmer, fifteen years later, asserted that 'farm labour has continued to be the chief, as it is the most healthful and curative, employment of the male patients' and that 'the agricultural classes ... always seek their customary occupation with the earliest dawn of convalescence, healthier and happier for their exertions'.[57] In doing so, he positioned farm work not only as something patients contributed to and benefitted from, but in terms of work requested on account of their previous occupations. Both Dr Wing and Dr Palmer highlight the inherent dichotomy of institutional accounts of patient work, by emphasising the centrality of patient work and yet never actively foregrounding the patient 'voice'.

The institutional rhetoric was clear: farm work was curative, never imposed, and often requested. It is therefore perhaps not surprising to find case notes replicating these ideas, and often positioning the patient as passive in this process. Many casebook entries are admittedly enigmatic, commenting that a patient 'works well on the farm'. Joseph R., a stone and quarry labourer admitted to Carlton Hayes Asylum in 1896, worked on the farm between 1906 and 1908, having undertaken duties on the wards and assisting with 'feeble' patients for the preceding years.[58] Frederick M., a limekiln labourer also admitted to Carlton Hayes Asylum, was noted to be working as a 'Trojan'.[59] It is not clear in either case whether the notion of 'working well' or 'as a Trojan' was made in reference to therapeutic matters or the internal economy of the institution. They were, however, as Andrews argues, constructed within the wider context of institutional goals.[60] The language used in both instances is akin to that of moral treatment, valuing consistency and strength. The case notes for Francis G., a farmer, articulated the principles both of moral treatment and self-sufficiency. As he recovered, he worked on the farm where he 'made himself very useful, and while exerting himself for the benefit of the institution, he was improving his own health, and regaining his constitutional powers, at the same time hastening the period of his own recovery by the healthy occupation of outdoor employment, and he eventually left the asylum quite recovered'.[61] The patient voice appears to be silenced in such cases, with the emphasis on constructing a narrative that fulfils institutional objectives. Nevertheless, as outlined in the introduction to this chapter, there is potential not only to reconstruct the patient experience from case notes but also to see the ways in which patients 'narrated' their own experiences of work through their actions and reactions to work and to the farm environment.

The patient 'voice' appears strongest in two main categories: those patients requesting or refusing work and those for whom the work evoked a strong reaction in them. A strong occupational identity was sometimes evident among patients who were previously occupied on the land as farmers or farm labourers. Indeed, in some instances, a patient's occupational affinity was crucial in either making a request to work on the farm or shaping their experience of this work on the farm. References to patients requesting work could of course be an extension of institutions wanting to give the illusion of choice. Yet case notes also acknowledged negative experiences of farm work, which allow the patient experience rather than institutional priorities to come to the fore. Moreover, the nature of casebook entries, the product of construction and reconstruction or negotiation that involved the patient and often included references to what patients said or did, can demonstrate the role of the patient in the institutional understanding of work.

Joseph C., an agricultural labourer aged forty-two, was admitted to Carlton Hayes Asylum in January 1845. Casebook entries note that following an improvement in his condition, he requested he be allowed 'out of door employment from the circumstance of him being an agricultural labourer'.[62] Such occupation was considered beneficial and 'for nearly three months he worked indefatigably and well, and rapidly recovered his health and strength. He returned home quite recovered and I occasionally afterwards employed him as a labourer when he could not secure more regular work'.[63] While the beneficial effect of farm work on the patient's health may have been constructed to justify the rationale for the employment of patients, the 'voice' of the patient is intimated here, beginning with his 'request' to work outdoors. Not all patients requested work, and through his request Joseph C. highlighted the role that occupation prior to admission could play in that process. Farm work may have been curative and remunerative in the eyes of the institution, but from the patient's perspective it was familiar and perhaps reassuring. It might have been the only element of life outside the institution that was actively incorporated in his experience after admission. It could be indicative that he was aware of alternative work allocated to patients and thus asserted a preference using his previous occupation to provide a rationale. The entries therefore suggest that even within the constraints of institutional life, Joseph C. retained his occupational identity. Through his request for work while a patient and his subsequent employment on the farm, Joseph C. physically repositioned himself in relation to the institution. Agricultural employment was the constant throughout, while his status as a patient in an asylum was ephemeral. In other words, through his actions and reactions and the role of occupational identity, Joseph C. 'narrated' his own experience of farm work. Ultimately, the case notes for Joseph C. were an amalgamation of institutional priorities and patient experiences; the process of construction and reconstruction outlined in the introduction to this chapter. They were in line with institutional rhetoric, but the components from which they were constructed, such as the request to work on the farm, are evidence of how patients shaped their own experience of institutional life.

Not all patients who sought work on the farm had previously been employed in agricultural occupations (just as not all agricultural labourers or farmers requested work on the farm). Edmund C., a shoemaker aged fifty, was admitted to Carlton Hayes on 6 October 1866 with chronic mania. As early as 24 October 1866 the casebook entry noted that 'he asks to go out to work!'[64] The exclamation mark suggests surprise, perhaps due to his previous mental state and behaviour traits as he was found to be 'very wild and violent in his conduct' on admission. If requests to work on the land were simply included in case notes to provide a rationale for the employment of patients, the exclamation mark would become redundant. Shortly after this, Edmund C. went to work on the farm, but his case notes state that he was still 'rather intractable and threatening at times'. It is not clear whether this behaviour was exhibited while working on the farm, but later entries continue to record that he was working regularly on the farm until the end of the 1860s, and on 12 February 1869 it was noted that he was 'on the whole a well conducted patient. He goes to work on the farm regularly and is in good health'.[65] His continued farm work suggests that either his behaviour was manageable at first and then improved or that the aggression did not exhibit itself while on the farm. On the surface, these case notes reinforce the institutional rhetoric regarding the benefits of outdoor labour for patients, highlighting notable changes in behaviour and health. Nevertheless, the patient still played an active role in this process, characterised by the way in which the case notes studied an individual's reaction to their environment. No explicit reason was given as to why Edmund C. wanted to work on the farm, but over time he perhaps developed a sense of privilege arising from such work. Patients undertaking outdoor work often received 'bonuses' such as beer, and Edmund C. later assumed additional responsibility being 'employed carrying round beer to the various parts of the outdoor department', including the farm.[66] By focusing on his request to work outside, and charting his fluctuating behaviour during this time, the case notes allow us to see how Edmund C. 'narrated' his experience of the asylum through his actions and reactions.

This ability to 'narrate' experience through the actions and reactions of patients is particularly apparent in case notes that record a negative or indifferent outcome to working on the farm. Such entries defy institutional rhetoric about the benefits of farm work. Here, patients inform institutional understanding of the impact of work or exert their agency through resistance. Albert S., a framesmith, was admitted to Carlton Hayes on 19 December 1896.[67] In February and March 1897 there are references to him working on the farm. The first, on 18 February (just two months after admission), notes: 'Does not seem to alter at all, works on the farm, is looking forward to going home to pick gooseberries'. This entry moves beyond a purely medical narrative to include the patient 'voice', in this case a personal memory of life outside the institution triggered by farm work and a desire to return home. Moreover, his case notes do not equate to a progressive trajectory of farm work leading to improved health, as suggested by many institutional accounts. Instead, on 1 April his case notes state that 'he thinks he has a farm in his inside, can hear the hens cackling and the sheep bleating and the crows calling'.[68] The patient 'voice' is unequivocally recorded here, although the explicit connection between farm work and the voices heard was not reflected upon by the medical superintendent. This could be indicative of how case notes recorded the words of patients to illustrate 'madness', but it nevertheless suggests the profound psychological impact that working on the farm had on Albert S. and provides evidence of how patient reactions to their environment were included in case notes in order to understand and treat the patient. The inclusion of this patient 'voice' disrupted the institutional rhetoric regarding the benefits of work, which provides insight into patient–psychiatric relationships which Hazel Morrison asserts were 'mutually dependent and interrelated subjects of historical enquiries'.[69] The way Albert S. reacted and responded to the farm was no doubt influenced by his mental state, which on admission was recorded as mania and later described as a 'weak silly condition of mind'.[70] The inclusion of his reactions, both verbal and behavioural, in the case notes was, however, a product of the patient–medical superintendent dynamic, in which the patient 'voice' enabled greater understanding of work as 'treatment' and particularly its relative impact on different patients. Albert S. undertook no further work after this incident and his health deteriorated, until he died of meningitis on 23 August 1897.

Reluctance or resistance to work is another notable way in which the patient experience or 'voice' comes to the fore. As Natalie Mullen highlights, refusal to work was a means by which patients could exert some form of agency, and in some instances case notes provide insights that suggest it was 'a mechanism of resisting asylum authority'.[71] Often this was passive resistance rather than an explicit refusal to work. It was also perhaps indicative of patient awareness that work, although not subject to compulsion or coercion, was still imposed with little input from the patient. Reluctance or resistance through behavioural traits enabled them to show displeasure, and also suggest an understanding and negotiation of the institutional landscape and uses of work therein. For example, Walter Henry L., a railway signalman, admitted to Carlton Hayes in 1897, was noted to have worked on the farm with indifferent results during 1899.[72] His preference was to return to railway work, and his indifference to farm work was a way in which to assert this preference and to express dissatisfaction. This was in line with his behaviour on admission due to mania, when he would not listen to anything regarding why he had been admitted, and then ten days later, when it was recorded that 'he answers in an irritable defiant manner', conduct which would continue over subsequent months. A year later, on 1 July 1898, it was noted that he 'rarely does any work or occupation', and then on 9 January 1899 we find reference that he 'wants to be sent back to his work on the railway'. Walter Henry L. evidently contested his continued incarceration in the asylum and made it clear that he wanted to return to life outside the asylum. Perhaps this was interpreted as a desire to simply work outside that could be satisfied by farm work. This was clearly not the case for Walter Henry L., and on 14 April 1899 it was noted that he 'occasionally goes to work on farm, but needs watching and he is inclined to run away'. Here we see the patient's understanding of institutional space and opportunities for work shaping their behaviour and actions. The underlying desire to leave the institution and return to his regular employment manifested itself through his attempts to escape. Within two years of his admission, Walter Henry L. still retained an affinity with his life outside the institution and a strong dissatisfaction at remaining within the asylum. Interestingly, he continued to work on the farm and by January 1908 was considered to 'work well'. Just over a decade after admission, he had adjusted his behaviour in relation to an evolving understanding and negotiation of work and space, moving from a desire to return to his railway job and the use of farm work as a route to escape to a realisation that the farm enabled him to spend prolonged periods of time outside the main asylum building. This is in contrast to Joseph S., a farm labourer, who worked in 'a mechanical way on the farm' according to his case notes.[73] Here there is no evidence of resistance or reluctance, or indeed an alternative agenda such as escape, but rather his mental state determined his behavioural traits which were exhibited from the moment of admission.

In addition to requests for, or indifference to, farm work, occupational identity could trigger strong emotional responses in patients. Samuel C., a farmer, was admitted to Carlton Hayes in October 1896 with melancholia. The casebook entries suggest that he was both anxious and delusionary. His first entry notes that 'he is very anxious to get home as he says he has 80 acres of mangles rotting'. The patient voice, in this case what Samuel C. was reported to have said, was included as evidence of his delusionary state. Over the next year, his case notes oscillate between his continued work on the land and further delusions. For example, on 23 October 1896 he was reported 'to be full of business, says he has some land and wanted to buy some cattle to put on the land, the cattle were £100, but had not got 100 pence and thinks that must have worried him. Is now going out to work on the land'.[74] As Morrison emphasises, medical superintendents attempted to understand patients and their illness through involving them in the process and entering into dialogue, and in doing so, could reveal the inner lives of patients.[75] The case notes, as Kelly asserts, therefore reflect both the patient's behaviour and the institutional interpretation of this behaviour.[76] References made to farming by Samuel C. were presented as delusions yet reflected his occupational identity and to some extent determined the decision to use his labour on the farm. Indeed, sometimes his case notes focused exclusively on the productive work he undertook on the asylum farm. For example, on 4 April 1897 his case notes simply record that he 'remains about the same, and is in good health, works well on the farm'.[77] In contrast, on 1 July 1897 a longer entry refers only to the delusions, stating that Samuel C. 'Occasionally wants to be let out down the town to go and bargain in the cattle market, he has a deep scheme for becoming wealthy by buying beasts on credit and selling them again, he gets very mired in explaining the details'.[78] Such entries present a challenge to disentangle assumptions about patient delusions with Samuel C.'s own identity as a farmer, and thus as an agent in his experiences. Andrews explores how a growing interest in patients' delusions was reflected in case notes, and how these can provide a record of 'changes in patients' delusional systems'.[79] However, this was not mirrored by an interest in interpreting the apparent delusions; rather, they were referred to in a matter of fact way as evidence of 'madness'.[80] As such, the case notes make no connection between either this patient's previous occupation or his work on the asylum farm in terms of fuelling or alleviating these delusions. Delusions, however, often reflected some element of reality and were shaped by their context, especially when relating to something of great importance to a patient or where social challenges had previously been experienced.[81] Samuel C.'s 'delusions' were solely about farming and could conceivably have been grounded in his experiences prior to admission, and his experience of working on the institution's farm could have transported him back to life as a farmer and thus the challenges and opportunities he would have faced were 'voiced' through the 'delusions'. Although similar behavioural traits were recorded in later case notes, for example, 'he talks a lot of nonsense', specific references to farming were less apparent the longer he was confined within the institution, suggesting that the intensity to which his occupational identity shaped his experiences diminished over time.

The relationship between farm work and patient experience was therefore frequently observed in case notes, but it was not always fully understood or appreciated in terms of the patient perspective. Nevertheless, patients were clearly able to assert themselves and actively contribute to how their experiences of working on the farm were narrated through their actions and reactions. To understand further these experiences and the role patients played in shaping them, it is crucial to examine the space in which that work took place.

## Navigating institutional spaces

For patients who worked on the farm, it was a space in which their identity and experience of institutional life could be negotiated and shaped. The farm provided an opportunity for patients to 'navigate' institutional spaces and reposition themselves in relation to the institution. It represented a transitional space between the institution and the wider community, which is pivotal to understanding patient experiences. How and why patients experienced the farm spatially is particularly evident through two components: the separate living arrangements for patients working on the farm and the potential to escape from the institution via the farm.

The farm, for some people, was not only their place of work but also their home, with a few asylums erecting or converting buildings to accommodate them. The motivations were varied, and not always transparent, but were interlinked with institutional economies as it could save both time and money, burgeoning institutional populations, and case-by-case judgements about individual patients. At Graylingwell, West Sussex, in July 1896, Dr Kidd proposed the conversion of the farm house for use by patients who worked on the farm.[82] The house was a substantial two-storey property, with six bays, an additional wing and attic accommodation, and plans for its conversion were approved on 30 October 1896.[83] As such, the domestic aesthetics were instantly distinguished from the institutional appearance of the main asylum building. This was akin to the colony system, developed towards the end of the nineteenth and the beginning of the twentieth century, whereby villas were scattered across a site to diminish its institutional appearance.[84] This domesticity was further reinforced by the fact that psychiatric patients housed in separate farm accommodation lived with the farm bailiff and his wife, or a married attendant. Only a small proportion of patients who worked on asylum farms were permitted to live in separate accommodation, usually determined by mental state and behavioural traits. It was asserted, when the conversion at Graylingwell was first proposed, that this would enable sixteen 'quiet and harmless patients' to be accommodated.[85] The agreement for the conversion of the farm house also noted that these patients would be 'specially selected from among the cleanly quiet and well conducted class'.[86]

In contrast, increasing economic factors and pressure for acute beds in the asylum motivated the decision to create a separate 'farm residence' at Menston Asylum, West Riding of Yorkshire.[87] It was posited that the institution would obtain thirty-six beds at cheaper cost than those in the main institution and relieve beds in the main institution for thirty-six fresh cases. The spatial relationship between the farm and the main institution, where all farm patients were at that stage housed, was also highlighted as important. With approximately half-a-mile between the two locations, patients had to 'get up at 5 o'clock to be ready for their work at 6 o'clock – milking cows and attending to the farm and then they have to come back into the institution for their breakfasts and meals'. The County Surveyor, J. Vickers Edwards, argued that by having a new farm residence, the patients would be closer to their work, be able to get up later, and be better supervised in many ways. Correspondence highlighted that the only dispute over this accommodation was the cost and how elaborate the building should be.[88] This suggests that the main concerns were indeed economic in nature.

From an institutional perspective, 'farm residences' could save money and rationalise the movement of patients. For patients, living and working on the farm physically removed them from the main institutional buildings to a more natural setting and helped to create an occupational community in which space, routine and language distinguished them from other patients. This process of navigating institutional spaces and consolidating a sense of community could be disrupted by institutional regimes which sought to draw these patients back into the main institution. At Parkside Asylum, Cheshire, the conversion of the farm house in 1907 was to provide accommodation for '8 working patients', under the charge of a married attendant. Correspondence between the asylum and the Commissioners in Lunacy noted that this would entail a new dormitory for five patients and the use of two bedrooms for three more. It also noted that the kitchen would become the patients' day room and the back kitchen be used to prepare and consume meals, with the exception of dinner which would still be taken in the main asylum.[89] In spite of living and working in a separate environment, patients at Parkside Asylum were being brought back into the main institutional buildings for their evening meal. This was perhaps a symbolic action, as it could accentuate the dichotomy between incarceration and freedom, which the farms often straddled, and thus exacerbate feelings of oppression. It could also complicate the dynamics between staff and patients from within and between the wider institutional complex.

The complex relationships patients forged with institutional spaces, and how they navigated them, can be understood through the way in which the farm often constituted a space that facilitated the means of escape. As Natalie Mullen argues, outdoor work provided male patients with opportunities to escape, which in turn 'highlight the tension between control and cure'.[90] Notably, there is no indication that most patients were escaping from the farm due to problems arising from being in that environment, although it should be acknowledged that occasionally patients were subjected to physical injury and attack while working. In most instances, the farm was a transitional space they could use to escape from institutional confinement. Evidence of escapes from the farm can therefore provide an insight into how some patients perceived and navigated institutional spaces. This is particularly apparent when evidence of the patient experience is sought within the case notes. For example, Enos W., a farm labourer, was recorded as 'working well on the farm' at Carlton Hayes Asylum on the 1 April 1897, but also made two attempts to escape from the farm on 18 February and 1 May.[91] His case notes do not explicitly seek to explain the reasons for these attempted escapes. Nevertheless, the chronology of the aforementioned entries provides insight into the ways in which patients 'navigated' institutional spaces and thus 'narrated' their experiences. His attempts to escape were juxtaposed with his work on the farm. Whether 'working well' constituted health benefits or productivity, this nonetheless provided the impetus to continue allowing Enos W. to work on the farm in spite of his attempts to escape. This highlights the value attributed to outdoor work by the institution, but also suggests he was aware of how his behaviour influenced decisions taken about his treatment. By 'working well' on the farm, Enos W. could create opportunities to escape from the institution. Similarly, case notes make reference to George H., a brickyard labourer, also at Carlton Hayes, being 'put to work on the farm' on 4 August 1897, where he worked 'fairly well'. The following week, George H. was recorded as saying he was 'going to have a lot of money' and as such did not see why he should do any work while he was there. Apparent willingness to work on the farm could suggest compliance, but in this instance the case notes do not adequately engage with the patient experience or their understanding of space. George H. was in fact indifferent to the farm, which in his eyes constituted an opportunity to escape from the institution. He felt obliged to work and by September 1897 it was noted that he was 'Intent on escaping'. On 16 September the case notes state: 'This afternoon about 3.45, succeeded in slipping off the farm and made his way on to the London Road'.[92] The case notes reveal a great deal about how the patient navigated institutional spaces. His escape was not a spontaneous or impulsive action, but rather was planned and premeditated. The following July, George H. was still intent on escaping and his case notes recorded that he 'does no work now'.[93] While patients who refused to work were not punished or coerced to do so, in not allowing them to work on the farm, the institution removed the means to use this space to escape and thus disrupted how patients perceived and navigated institutional spaces.

The sense of agitation and desire to escape prompted by containment in psychiatric institutions is further evidenced in the minute book of the Visiting Committee to the East Riding Asylum in Beverley. J.W.W., a male patient, 'became excited because he was not discharged, and ran away from a farm working party', only to be brought back five hours later.[94] The same minutes also noted that T.R. 'escaped from a farm working party on the 27 October, and was brought back two hours later. He had been sent somewhere with a wheelbarrow, and his escape was not noticed for a quarter of an hour'.[95] An earlier escape was also mentioned in the minute book of the Visiting Committee when 'No. 3, a patient who had worked on the farm for many years, wandered away on 13 December. He was found by the East Riding Police, and brought back on 16 December. No one can be said to be in fault for his escape'.[96] Perhaps not surprisingly, the focus of these minutes is social control and managing the patient population. They nonetheless provide further evidence of how and why patients used this space beyond the intended purpose of farming, and how 'accepting' or 'requesting' farm work was a route to do so.

## Conclusions

Farms were an integral part of psychiatric institutions during the nineteenth and early twentieth centuries, and are a crucial space in which to uncover the patient experience of work. It was on the farm that the economy of the institution and the moral treatment of patients converged. Unsurprisingly, records of patients working on these farms were often constructed from an institutional perspective. As such, the patient 'voice' appears to have been silenced in order to provide a rationale for patient labour on these farms. Yet, as demonstrated in this chapter, it is possible to extrapolate the patient experience and in some instances the patient 'voice'. In spite of case notes being constructed within the wider context of institutional rhetoric, they were a product of both the institution and the patient. Underpinning the manifestations of 'madness' recorded in case notes are tantalising glimpses of people's lives before, during and sometimes after their time in the institution. The patient experience, and in some instances their 'voice', is asserted through their actions and reactions. Most notably this was expressed through requests or resistance to work, strong emotional responses and occupational identities. These experiences were nuanced, non-linear and often inconclusive, and as such do not coincide neatly with the institutional rhetoric. Patients also navigated institutional space and physically repositioned themselves in relation to the institution while working on the farm. Here was a distinctive community, integral to the institution but at the same time separate. It represented a transitional space, which redefined the patient experience. At some asylums, 'farm patients' lived together on the farm in specially converted premises, and while the motivation for this was often economic, it nonetheless shaped the experiences, and even the identities, of patients who lived and worked on the farm. Other patients used this space to escape incarceration. Through their actions and reactions to farm work, patients 'narrated' their own experiences and 'navigated' institutional space.

Nevertheless, in the absence of personal testimonies, official records will always present challenges regarding the experience and 'voice' of patients. This remains a challenge and struggle in the twenty-first century. Indeed, a lack of a 'voice' and sense of disempowerment has been a recurring theme in mental healthcare over the last decade. In 2012, the NHS Patient Experience Framework highlighted the importance of 'respect for patient-centred values, preferences and expressed needs', and yet 77 per cent of respondents to the 2019 community mental-health service survey said they had not been asked by NHS mental-health services to give their views on the quality of their care.[97] The 2019 survey noted further decline in areas identified as needing further improvement in 2018, which included giving patients sufficient time to discuss their needs and treatment and having opportunities to agree the care being received and being involved in the process. This sense of disempowerment and disengagement resurfaced in a survey published by the Parliamentary and Health Service Ombudsman in February 2020, asserting that patients were reluctant to 'speak up' or complain due to fear or a feeling it would be pointless, with poor communication being cited as a repeated problem.[98] Questions about how the patient voice is recorded and used have also been features of the contemporary research agenda. A study undertaken by the University of Sheffield School of Health and Related Research found that only a small number of NHS mental-health trusts in England were collecting patient feedback with a view to improving services. The recommendations put forward emphasised that service improvements should never be led by complaints alone but notably also listening to what works well for patients.[99] As such, it is evident that while official institutional records may provide opportunities for historians to identify 'agency' and 'voice' among those patients working on asylum and hospital farms, they also resonate with contemporary concerns about how and why the patient 'voice' is recorded and the extent to which patients feel empowered and engaged.

## Notes

* The author would like to thank Sheffield Hallam University for an Early Career Research grant that funded the archival trips for this research.
1 J. Andrews, 'Case Notes, Case Histories, and the Patient's Experience of Insanity at Gartnavel Royal Asylum, Glasgow, in the Nineteenth Century', *Social History of Medicine* 11:2 (1998), 255–81, 255.
2 Andrews, 'Case Notes', 258–9.
3 Ibid., 262, 265–6.
4 Ibid., 265–6.
5 B.D. Kelly, 'Searching for the Patient's Voice in the Irish asylum', *Medical Humanities* 42:2 (2016), 87–8.
6 Andrews, 'Case Notes', 280–1; Kelly, 'Searching for the Patient's Voice', 88.
7 Kelly, 'Searching for the Patient's Voice', 88.

8 H. Morrison, 'Constructing Patient Stories: "Dynamic" Case Notes and Clinical Encounters at Glasgow's Gartnavel Mental Hospital, 1921–32', *Medical History* 60:1 (2016), 67–86, 68.
9 S. Chaney, 'No "Sane" Person Would Have Any Idea': Patients' Involvement in Late Nineteenth-Century British Asylum Psychiatry', *Medical History* 60:1 (2016), 37–9.
10 Ibid., 39.
11 L.M. Thomas, 'Historicising Agency', *Gender and History* 28:2 (2016), 324–39, 335.
12 Ibid., 324.
13 J. Wallis, *Investigating the Body in the Victorian Asylum: Doctors, Patients and Practices* (Basingstoke: Palgrave, 2017), 34.
14 L. Topp, J.E. Moran and J. Andrews (eds), *Madness, Architecture and the Built Environment: Psychiatric Spaces in Historical Context* (Abingdon: Routledge, 2007).
15 Moran and Topp, 'Introduction', in Topp, Moran and Andrews (eds), *Madness, Architecture and the Built Environment*, 1.
16 B. Edginton, 'A Space for Moral Management: The York Retreat's Influence on Asylum Design', in Topp, Moran and Andrews (eds), *Madness, Architecture and the Built Environment*, 91.
17 C. Philo, 'Scaling the Asylum: Three Geographies of the Inverness District Lunatic Asylum (Craig Dunain)', in Topp, Moran and Andrews (eds), *Madness, Architecture and the Built Environment*, 113–14.
18 A. Scull, *The Most Solitary of Afflictions: Madness and Society in Britain, 1700–1900* (London: Yale University Press, 1993), 183–4.
19 Scull, *The Most Solitary of Afflictions*, 183–4; W. Ernst 'Introduction: Therapy and Empowerment, Coercion and Punishment. Historical and Contemporary Perspectives on Work, Psychiatry and Society', in W. Ernst (ed.), *Work, Psychiatry and Society, c. 1750–2015* (Manchester: Manchester University Press, 2016), 1–30, 7.
20 W.A.F. Browne, *The Moral Treatment of the Insane: A Lecture* (London, 1864), 7, 12.
21 G. Reaume, 'Patients at Work: Insane Asylum Inmates' Labour in Ontario, 1841–1900', in J. Moran and D. Wright (eds), *Mental Health in Canadian Society: Historical Perspectives* (Montreal: McGill-Queen's University Press, 2006), 69–96; Ernst, 'Introduction', 7; B. Arneil, *Domestic Colonies: The Turn Inward to Colony* (Oxford: Oxford University Press, 2017).
22 A. Borsay, *Disability and Social Policy in Britain since 1750: A History of Exclusion* (Basingstoke: Palgrave Macmillan, 2005).
23 Ibid., 66–71.
24 Ibid., 7.

25 P. Bartlett, *The Poor Law of Lunacy: The Administration of Pauper Lunatics in Mid-Nineteenth Century England* (London: Leicester University Press, 1999); S. Cherry, *Mental Health Care in Modern England: The Norfolk Lunatic Asylum* (Woodbridge, Suffolk: Boydell Press, 2003); R. Ellis, 'A Field of Practice or a Mere House of Detention? The Asylum and its Integration, with Special Reference to the County Asylums of Yorkshire, c.1844–1888' (unpublished PhD thesis, University of Huddersfield, 2001).
26 J.F. Saunders, 'Institutionalized Offenders: A Study of the Victorian Institution and its Inmates, with Special Reference to Late-Nineteenth Century Warwickshire' (unpublished PhD thesis, University of Warwick, 1983), 139–41.
27 Saunders, 'Institutionalized Offenders', 139–41.
28 M. Foucault, *Madness and Civilization: A History of Insanity in the Age of Reason*, with introduction by D. Cooper (London: Routledge, 2005), 55.
29 A. Digby, 'Moral Treatment at the Retreat, 1796–1846', in W.F. Bynum, R. Porter and M. Shepherd (eds), *The Anatomy of Madness: Volume II* (London, Routledge 1988), 52–72; Ernst, 'Introduction', 7.
30 Ernst, 'Introduction', 1, 6–8; Bartlett, *The Poor Law of Lunacy*; S. Rutherford, 'The Landscapes of Public Lunatic Asylums in England, 1808–1914' (unpublished PhD thesis, De Montfort University Leicester, 2003), 224–6.
31 Borsay, *Disability and Social Policy in Britain*, 13.
32 The emphasis on male patients working on asylum farms was at odds with the number of women with agricultural occupations in this period, from farm servants and agricultural labourers to farmers. For more about female farmworkers in Victorian and Edwardian England, see N. Verdon, *Rural Women Workers in Nineteenth-Century England: Gender, Work and Wages* (Woodbridge, Suffolk: Boydell Press, 2002) and N. Verdon, *Working the Land: A History of the Farmworker in England from 1850 to the Present Day* (Basingstoke: Palgrave Macmillan, 2017).
33 Edginton, 'A Space for Moral Management', 85.
34 Ibid., 89.
35 J. Conolly, *On the Construction and Government of Lunatic Asylums and Hospitals for the Insane* (London: John Churchill, 1847), 77.
36 Ibid., 77–80.
37 Ibid., 79.
38 C. Philo, *A Geographical History of Institutional Provision for the Insane from Medieval Times to the 1860s in England and Wales: The Space Reserved for Insanity* (Lewiston: Edwin Mellen Press, 2004); H. Parr, *Mental Health and Social Space: Towards Inclusionary Geographies*

(Oxford: Wiley, 2008); J. Walton, 'The Treatment of Pauper Lunatics in Victorian England: The Case of Lancaster Asylum, 1816–1870', in A. Scull (ed.), *Madhouses, Mad-Doctors and Madmen: The Social History of Psychiatry in the Victorian Era* (Philadelphia: University of Pennsylvania Press, 1981), 166–200; Bartlett, *The Poor Law of Lunacy*; Cherry, *Mental Health Care in Modern England*; Saunders, 'Institutionalised Offenders'; Rutherford, 'The Landscapes of Public Lunatic Asylums'; Ellis, 'A Field of Practice or a Mere House of Detention?'; Ernst, *Work, Psychiatry and Society*.
39 J. Laws, 'Crackpots and Basket-Cases: A History of Therapeutic Work and Occupation', *History of the Human Sciences* 24:2 (2011), 65–81.
40 Ernst, 'Introduction', 1, 3–4.
41 R. Porter (ed.), *Patients and Practitioners: Lay Perceptions of Medicine in Pre-Industrial Society* (Cambridge: Cambridge University Press, 1985), 1–3; R. Porter, 'The Patient's View: Doing Medical History from Below', *Theory and Society* 14:2 (1985), 175–98.
42 A. Bacopoulos-Viau and A. Fauvel, 'The Patient's Turn: Roy Porter and Psychiatry's Tales, Thirty Years On', *Medical History* 60:1 (2016), 1–18.
43 S.A. Pinto, *Lunatic Asylums in Colonial Bombay: Shackled Bodies, Unchained Minds* (Cham: Springer Nature Switzerland, 2018), 144.
44 The author also has a book, *Farming, Psychiatry and Rural Society: Asylum and Hospital Farms, England 1845–1955*, under contract with Routledge due for publication in 2022, which includes further analysis of patients undertaking farm work.
45 Borsay, *Disability and Social Policy in Britain*, 89.
46 Hull History Centre, C TCA/1/3, General Rules of Hull Borough Asylum 1884, 16.
47 West Sussex Record Office, HCGR 3/1/1, General Rules for the Government of the Asylum West Sussex 1898, 12.
48 First Annual Report of Mr T. Eccleston, surgeon-superintendent of the Lancaster County Lunatic Asylum at Rainhill, cited in the *Preston Chronicle* (24 April 1852), 4.
49 Ibid.
50 Ibid.
51 Moran and Topp, 'Introduction', 5.
52 First Annual Report of Mr T. Eccleston.
53 Minutes of the Annual Court of the Governors of Northampton Asylum, cited in *Northampton Mercury* (1 March 1862), 5.
54 Minutes of the Annual Court of the Governors.
55 Report for the Medical Superintendent, cited in the *Lincolnshire Chronicle* (28 April 1854), 3.
56 Ibid.

57 Annual Report of Committee of Visitors to Lincoln County Lunatic Asylum Including Extracts by the Medical Superintendent 1869, cited in *Stamford Mercury* (10 June 1870), 6.
58 Leicestershire Record Office, DE3533/202, Casebook 1896–97 (Carlton Hayes), entry 5788, 3 January 1908.
59 Ibid., entry 5821, 18 April 1897.
60 Andrews, 'Case Notes', 265–6.
61 Leicestershire Record Office, DE 3533/185, Casebook 1845–48 (Carlton Hayes), entry 706.
62 Ibid., entry 579.
63 Ibid.
64 Leicestershire Record Office, DE3533/191, Casebook 1865–68 (Carlton Hayes), entry 2699, 24 October 1866.
65 Ibid., 11 January 1867, 12 February 1869.
66 Ibid.
67 Leicestershire Record Office, DE 3533/202, Casebook 1896–97 (Carlton Hayes), entry 5797.
68 Ibid.
69 Morrison, 'Constructing Patient Stories', 68.
70 Leicestershire Record Office, DE 3533/202, Casebook 1896–97 (Carlton Hayes), entry 5797.
71 N. Mullen, 'Negotiating the Asylum: Agency and Authority in Lancaster County Asylum, 1840–1915' (unpublished PhD Thesis, University of Lancaster, 2019), 85–6.
72 Leicestershire Record Office, DE 3533/202, Casebook 1896–97 (Carlton Hayes), entry 5816.
73 Ibid., entry 5827.
74 Ibid., entry 5783.
75 Morrison, 'Constructing Patient Stories', 71.
76 Kelly, 'Searching for the Patient's Voice', 88.
77 Leicestershire Record Office, DE 3533/202, Casebook 1896–97, entry 5783.
78 Ibid.
79 Andrews, 'Case Notes', 259, 277.
80 Ibid., 277.
81 Kelly, 'Searching for the Patient's Voice', 89–90.
82 West Sussex Record Office, HCGR/MA/2, Minutes of the Visiting Committee of the West Sussex County Council 1894–1898, 24 July 1896.
83 West Sussex Record Office, HCGR 15/1/1, Graylingwell Mental Hospital, Chichester Illustrated Brochure, 1911 photograph of the farm house; West Sussex Record Office, HCGR/MA/2, Minutes of the Visiting Committee of the West Sussex County Council, 1894–1898, 30 October 1896.

84 Borsay, *Disability and Social Policy in Britain*, 89; Arneil, *Domestic Colonies*.
85 West Sussex Record Office, HCGR/MA/2, Minutes of the Visiting Committee of the West Sussex County Council 1894–1898, 24 July 1896.
86 West Sussex Record Office, HCGR/11/4/9, Agreement to convert farm house 1897.
87 The National Archives (TNA), MH 83 329, Menston Asylum, letter from J. Vickers Edwards, the County Surveyor, to the Commissioners in Lunacy, 28 October 1897.
88 Ibid.; *York Herald* (12 January 1899), 3.
89 TNA, MH 83 33, Correspondence re. Parkside Asylum, Macclesfield.
90 Mullen, 'Negotiating the Asylum', 90–1.
91 Leicestershire Record Office, DE 3533/202, Casebook 1896–97 (Carlton Hayes), entry 5807.
92 Ibid., entry 5870.
93 Ibid.
94 East Riding of Yorkshire Archives, NH6/10/8, Minute Book of the Visiting Committee 1913–19, 12 November 1913.
95 Ibid.
96 East Riding of Yorkshire Archives, NH6/10/1, Minute Book of the Visiting Committee, 2 January 1893.
97 Care Quality Commission, Community Mental Health Survey 2019, www.cqc.org.uk/publications/surveys/community-mental-health-survey-2019 (accessed 12 August 2020).
98 Parliamentary and Health Service Ombudsman, '1 in 5 Mental Health Patients Don't Feel Safe in NHS care', www.ombudsman.org.uk/news-and-blog/news/1–5-mental-health-patients-dont-feel-safe-nhs-care-ombudsman-finds (accessed 12 August 2020).
99 University of Sheffield, 'NHS Needs to Act on Patient Feedback', www.sheffield.ac.uk/news/nr/nhs-act-patient-feedback-sheffield-health-researchers-1.868251 (accessed 12 August 2020).

# 5

# The patient's view as history from below: evidence from the Victorian poor, 1834–71*

*Paul Carter and Steve King*

It is almost thirty-five years since the publication of Roy Porter's 'The Patient's View'.[1] Since then, the article has often been styled as 'seminal'. It has a firm place in the historiography of 'patient' related historical study being 'a modern day classic [...] and virtually every chapter, article or monograph on medical practice published since 1985 seems to refer back to it'.[2] In essence, Porter was concerned that histories of medicine did not simply ossify into a series of corporate-style accounts of groundbreaking medical science, innovative surgeons and the steady march of professionalism against amateur 'folkloric remedies'. For Porter any medical encounter takes at least two (and sometime more than two) people: the sick person or sufferer and the doctor or healthcare professional. His unease focused on the way in which the sufferer's role, voice or view of healing and healthcare had been routinely underplayed.[3]

This call for a more nuanced and balanced understanding of doctors, patients and their relationships has been partly met, with innovative new studies of the nature of professionalisation, the extraordinary longevity of herbal remedies, and the complex world of the medical marketplace which both doctors and consumers were obliged to navigate.[4] Porter's wider call to reclaim 'the voice of the voiceless', or perhaps more properly to discover and foreground that voice (repeated by Peter Bartlett in terms of lunatic voices), has achieved less traction.[5] Alexandra Bacopoulous-Viau and Aude Fauvel note that for the history of psychiatry, patient narratives are a vital tool in understanding the experiences and construction of lunacy, even if in practice we more often hear and analyse the voices of relatives than we do lunatics themselves.[6] Some of the contributors to this volume remedy that situation, notably through the use of the voices of ex-patients. In the wider history of medicine literature, however, Mary Fissell was able to suggest in 1993 that the patient's narrative had actually *lost* ground to histories of doctors and the institutions that they increasingly populated.[7] Subsequent work has not recovered this position, particularly in the context of working-class people as opposed to the middle-class consumers whose voices and experiences dominate current understandings of the nature and constellation of healthcare. The sense that the ordinary patients' presence is obscured and available largely through accounts produced by clinicians or administrators remains strong.[8] It is also misleading, as historians who are now focusing on the dependent poor have begun to show. Thus, for the Old Poor Law (the national system of parochially based welfare established in 1601 and running to 1834), Steve King has used pauper letters – the authentic texts of marginal people and sometimes their advocates – to recover and analyse the voices of the sick and disabled poor.[9] Those who have worked on the New Poor Law in the post-1834 period have also begun to find similar material.[10] In this broad context, it has become increasingly clear that the voices of ordinary patients emerge most firmly in the historical record when things went wrong with healthcare and they were obliged to contest their care (or lack of it), provide evidence in the event of medical scandals, or complain about medical professionals. Jessica Meyer and Alexia Moncrieff, Sarah Holland and Burkhart Brückner have already made similar points in earlier chapters of this collection.

We return to these themes below, but for now it is important to note that similar imperatives have driven the possibilities for capturing patient voices in the very recent historical past. Sustained attempts to elicit, analyse and preserve patient views ensure that future researchers will have much easier access to relevant data for the late twentieth and early twenty-first centuries.[11] Yet even in this context the patient voice emerges most powerfully, frequently and viscerally when ordinary people have to contest healthcare. Examples would include instances of the near impossibility of securing timely appointments with general practitioners. This has recently led to patients in Northamptonshire queuing outside surgeries simply to book in appointments for a later date. In Leicestershire people found themselves being turned away from walk-in centres because they did not have appointments, in contradiction to the centres' intended purpose.[12] Some outpatients with hospital appointments are finding it necessary to travel long distances for care as smaller local hospitals have been closed.[13] Reporting of inadequate funding for assisting the chronically ill to live comfortably at home is frequent. Determined that lives should be lived to the fullest extent, one mother, frustrated at the inability to secure a walking frame for her son who suffered with cerebral palsy, declared that he 'wants to stand up. He wants to see what's going on. He is meant to be upright, not crawling all his life.'[14] Some voices of contestation are even heard beyond the grave. In one of many similar cases, an inquest heard in June 2019 that a forty-eight-year-old man committed suicide after his benefits were cut and he was declared fit to work.[15] Moves to silence claims of abuse and neglect invariably backfire, as for instance with the Staffordshire hospital scandal, leading to a torrent of patient and family voices.[16] The difficulties in understanding the detail of healthcare mean that thousands of people annually turn to the Patients Association for advocacy or advice, with many of those original voices subsequently preserved.[17] Brückner traces a similar rationale behind the emergence of pressure groups supporting supposedly lunatic patients in the early twentieth century, a clear signal of the timelessness of this sort of observation.[18]

These frameworks – contestation, scandal and complaint – are then important for any study of the patient voice in whatever period we wish to hear it. The fact that we can trace these long-term continuities, however, also reflects the fact that many of the piercing questions about healthcare that political and medical elites, planners or policy experts and even patients see as essentially 'current' have deep historical roots too. These include, *inter alia*: how much trust should we place in doctors and the interest groups that they embody and represent? How much can and should be spent on healthcare by the state? How should a healthcare system be organised? In particular what is the appropriate balance of centralisation versus localism? Are the sick consumers, or are they patients? Are the relatives of the sick merely relatives, or are they/do they have to be advocates? How can the expectations of patients in the face of ever-expanding medical possibilities (and thus costs) be controlled and limited? Who should make all of these decisions? Above all, what role should class play in healthcare systems? Crudely, if the wealthy and middle class pay disproportionately into the healthcare system should there be limits on the amount that they can get out of it? Turned on its head, the question might become: should we care about persistent health inequalities? Can society afford to act, or can it afford not to?

For modern stakeholders these are essentially presentist questions, a consequence of a health service funded from general taxation and free at the point of contact. More than this, the questions appear to emerge from the operation, stresses and failures of the most recent variant of the National Health Service (NHS) and associated services such as GP practices. This is simply wrong. These questions stem not from the particular organisation and funding of a healthcare system, but from universal tensions in the provision of healthcare, tensions that are not easily or obviously bounded by organisational chronologies. The poor have always had the greatest susceptibility to sickness, the worst mortality rates and slowest recovery times, so who should pay the bills?[19] Conflict between the authority of doctors and that of the state emerged well before the NHS, and the disjuncture that we currently see between the highest medical need being in poor areas while resources are over-concentrated in middle-class areas clearly emerged in the nineteenth century rather than being a purely modern phenomenon.[20] Above all, how far supply-side stakeholders (doctors, hospital staff, civil servants, administrators, taxpayers and politicians) should have to take note of the voices of the poor (as opposed to vocal clients such as the middle classes) is a foundational question in any healthcare system. For the latter question to be answered in the affirmative, those same stakeholders have to create the mechanisms to both hear and act upon the poor voice. To understand how they did and do so, our chapter shifts attention back to the nineteenth century when systematic institutionalised provision for the sick poor started to become a reality under the New Poor Law.

This is not an unproblematic exercise. The number and overall size of published and archival sources multiply exponentially as we reach the modern period and the arrival of a maturing information state.[21] Crudely, the archival 'haystack' becomes ever larger and more complex and the poor patient voice 'needle' thus even harder to locate. It is perhaps for this reason that, while Porter claimed that the 'history of the sick should [not] prove any more intractable than the history of the labouring classes, of women, criminals, the illiterate, of Outcast London, or any other sort of history "from below"', he gave few examples of the socially and economically poor sufferer. Indeed, he asserted that 'underdogs such as paupers and criminals in previous centuries were often illiterate, or silenced, or were vocal only in ways leaving few traces in the archives'.[22] Yet, and as we have already begun to suggest, it is possible to use the overlapping lenses of complaint, contestation and scandal to explore very directly the words of the poorest of the sick poor if we look for them. While in their examination of medical care at the Birmingham workhouse between 1733 and 1900, Jonathan Reinarz and Alistair Ritch found that, 'during most years, very little additional evidence about the patients at the workhouse, other than their number, is included in the guardians' minutes', we have found more than six thousand advocate letters, pauper witness statements, and pauper or poor peoples' letters in the central archives of the New Poor Law.[23] While not all of these were from or about sick people, many were and they provide a richly detailed factual, rhetorical and strategic source base through which we can explore both how ordinary people understood and negotiated healthcare in the nineteenth century and some of the resonances with modern patient concerns and experiences. In particular, we explore four broad questions through the lenses of contestation, complaint and dispute. First, how might poor people know what 'rights' they had to medical care? Second, who decided if someone was too sick to work? Third, how did poor people feel about being expected to travel to secure medical assistance? Finally, how did poor people contest decisions made in the context of chronic sickness? These questions, we argue – embodying as they do issues of the patient as a consumer, the relative power of doctors/elites and poor patients, the reasonableness of the conditions attached to medical welfare for the most needy, and the agency of poor patients – were and are central to the way that the poor experience healthcare systems irrespective of the way those systems are organised and financed or their chronological specificity. Before we turn to this wider agenda, however, some sense of the administrative process of the New Poor Law and the sources thus generated is necessary.

## An archive and process

We take as our chronological starting point the welfare reforms enshrined in the 1834 Poor Law Amendment Act. The Act was founded on the establishment of a central poor law authority based in London, and the creation of hundreds of local poor law unions (collections of parishes) across England and Wales.[24] These unions were in effect new local government authorities managed by parish representatives (styled 'guardians') who were elected on a ratepayer franchise. The unions were staffed by paid officers such as the workhouse master and matron, clerks, porters, relieving officers, rate collectors and others as welfare was 'professionalised'. With reference to the sick and their care under the new welfare arrangements from 1834, the law was surprisingly quiet. The founding legislation of the Old Poor Law in 1601 had said nothing about medical relief. Similarly the poor law report and legislation of 1834 said little about the types and levels of medical provision that should be delivered, in significant part because the disciplinary and coercive powers of guardians under the New Poor Law were never meant to be aimed at the sick and other groups of the broadly and historically conceived 'deserving poor'.[25] The 1834 Act simply stated that medical assistance might be given 'where any Case of sudden and dangerous Illness may require it'.[26] Obviously, such an opaque statement left many potentially contentious issues unresolved and afforded much ground for contestation over local decisions and scandals arising from neglect or inadequate spending.

In terms of the administrative history of poor law unions, it is important that we understand that poor law unions, as new supra-local entities under centralised supervision, were themselves immediately divided for the provision of medical services, with medical officers appointed to each of these newly formed so-called 'districts'. These – not unlike modern GP practice demarcation areas – were usually organised on the basis of district population size. Some poor law medical officers who, in the guise of parish doctors, prior to 1834 had worked across one or two parishes, now found themselves spread thinly across a much larger area. Smaller unions might have only a couple of medical officers, but larger ones could have many more. Generally, although not always, a separate district was based on the union workhouse itself. Medical provision thus grew organically from the bottom up rather than being imposed by the central authorities and the law. It is clear, however, that a New Poor Law focused ideologically and philosophically on crushing the claims and entitlement assumptions of the able-bodied poor was rapidly overtaken by the needs and claims of the traditional client groups of the English and Welsh welfare system, among whom the sick were the largest and most expensive.[27] The balancing (and often lagging) expansion of medical provision under the New Poor Law was accidental, piecemeal, slow-moving and unevenly spread across the indoor and outdoor poor. The substantial geographical imbalances in the scale of medical need versus the locus of spending that we construct as essentially 'modern' begins here. Notwithstanding these caveats, the post-1834 English and Welsh poor had the right to apply for the local medical services supplied under the New Poor Law, just as had been the case pre-1834.[28]

Following the establishment of the London-based central poor law authority and the hundreds of local poor law unions across England and Wales, these two bureaucracies did what bureaucracies of this size do: they created millions of pieces of paper and sent them backwards and forwards to each other.[29] The parallels to the modern NHS are firm and striking. They also created a complex registry system predicated on paper numbers (individual unique identifying numbers) by which the bureaucratic staff were able to search for, find and retrieve, individual pieces of correspondence.[30] This correspondence is now to be found at The National Archives (TNA) under record series MH 12. It is the largest series held under MH (Ministry of Health), running to almost 17,000 individual large bound volumes and it is this source which forms the archival focus of our chapter.[31] Although the series is mainly made up of correspondence between the central and local authorities covering finance, pauper discipline, staff appointments, official returns and clarifications to law and process, other 'non-authority' correspondence, such as that from local landowners and occupiers, tradesmen, ratepayers, paupers and other local poor, is included and filed alongside the authority paperwork. This was done on a union-by-union basis in year and paper-number order. The result of bringing together this authority and non-authority paperwork into a single 'union correspondence' series within the central authority provided the government of the time with a detailed account (and thus one that could be monitored, much as was the case with the NHS) of the state of locally managed but centrally directed welfare.

Examining some of this non-authority paperwork in consort with other specific types of authority records provides us with a step-change in revealing the sick pauper's view. In general we can identify three major types of records produced or co-produced by ordinary poor people.[32] Simply put, these are advocate letters, witness statements, and pauper or poor peoples' letters.[33] These three types of records appear in the archive covering a diverse range of subject matters such as complaints about categories and levels of relief, refusals of applications for relief, physical or verbal ill-treatment of paupers, unequal treatment of workhouse inmates, unfair punishments, illegal appropriation of goods by union officers, unfit under-weighted dietaries, and more general attempts to contest the decisions taken by officers and guardians in localities. But the poor sick in mind or body (or both) appear as the backbone of this element of the correspondence. This group, then, was not voiceless. For the purposes of this chapter we have combed the thousands of letters collected as part of our AHRC project (aimed at producing a New Poor Law history from below), in order to identify case studies that can throw particular light on questions of agency, power, complaint, scandal and patient rights. While all case study approaches face questions of representativeness, the particular stories that we use here stand out not in terms of the rhetoric, strategy or experience of writers, but rather the intricacy of the detail which individual writers provide. The advantage of such an approach of course is that we can emblematise the remarkable similarities in terms of rhetoric and strategy between historical actors and modern patients.

## Contesting rights

We turn first to the question of how a group whose welfare needs were not really covered by the law of 1834 established, maintained and enforced their rights. While any poor person meeting certain residence criteria had a right to apply for relief from their union, the New Poor Law was a discretionary welfare and healthcare system and such applications could be and were turned down. This notwithstanding, it is clear from our material that the sick poor and their advocates often wrote about the poor's 'rights' or referred to the law or regulations to back up a variety of welfare claims. Thomas Henshaw, from Ilkeston in the Basford Union, wrote to the Poor Law Commission (PLC) on 5 February 1842 to set out a case for relief. He described himself as 'a poor Man by trade A Frame worknitter', with a wife and three children. His recent underemployment had worsened to unemployment and the family had become 'completely destitute of food since February the $1^{st}$ to the present time'. Henshaw related how he had applied for relief but was refused. He then approached a local magistrate who provided a 'positive order' to give to the local officers, but again to no avail. Henshaw submitted his case to the central authorities asking for 'redress' as he had followed the regulations they had set out for securing relief and he felt his case was wrongly dismissed. He also understood the relevant legislation, referring in his letter to the $54^{th}$ clause in the Poor Law Amendment Act 1834, which allowed for relief in 'Cases of sudden and urgent Necessity' such as sickness.[34] Demonstrating further comprehension of the workings of the New Poor Law, Henshaw also referred in his letter to a circular he had seen from Edwin Chadwick, the 'clark to the poor law commissioners', stating that neglect of this section could see union and parish officers held to account in law.[35]

Such claims of law and right can be seen in many of the statements and letters of the poor and their advocates. Thus the Reverend Hugh Metthie, in his letter from the Wrexham Union in Denbighshire to the PLC in February 1835, disputed their answer to an earlier letter he had sent. The PLC had claimed they were unable to interfere in the matter of individual cases of relief. Metthie said that he understood the point they made but that he had referred 'to the $15^{th}$ section of the Act, & find by it that the Commissioners *have* the power of making rules for the administration of relief to the poor; and, though they cannot interfere in any *individual* case, yet a *general* rule issued to them would apply to *individual* cases'. Furthermore, claimed Metthie, by section 27 of the Act in any union formed under it, two magistrates could order relief to an aged person disabled from working without that person being required to reside in the workhouse.[36] Clinical legal discourse such as this was more common than might perhaps have been expected of this period, but most writers (pauper and advocate) melded together both moral and legal claims on the welfare authorities. Advocate letters are particularly important in this sense for our understanding of the position and agency of the sick poor. While such letters are theoretically separate texts from those sent by the poor themselves, in practice there are good reasons to think that the sick had direct input into the stories, rhetoric and strategy embodied in advocate texts, in a form of co-production. Thus, in early 1837 William Passey wrote from the Kidderminster Union to the PLC on behalf of Benjamin Hughes. Passey couched his complaint as a case of maladministration of the New Poor Law, claiming himself to be 'an advocate of those clauses which order immediate relief to the necessitous, aged and infirm'. He then complained that Hughes, described as 'a poor, deserving old man, 72 years of age, who has been unable to gain or procure a livelihood for the last two years', had lost his job 'through his general debility and deficiency of sight; which was represented by his late employers to the Reliving-officer here'. When the relieving officer attended Hughes in his lodgings, the old man was 'very ill in bed' and Passey claimed that at that time he had only part of a halfpenny's worth of oatmeal to eat. In turn, Hughes was told by the relieving officer that he could have nothing and advised him to make the twenty-two-mile journey to his home parish of Ludlow in Shropshire. Passey, in stressing the importance of those 'clauses which order immediate relief to the necessitous' (echoing Henshaw's contention above) claimed that the central poor law authorities should have acted:

> to prevent the new system of relief falling in general disgrace and abhorrence. The poor old man presents the picture of the most dire destitution, his face, legs and other parts of his body has begun to swell and hourly he becomes more alarming ill through total destitution![37]

It is simply inconceivable that Passey could garner and deploy this level of detail had he been a passive bystander. At the very least Hughes must have related the detail, but more than this it seems likely that Hughes was there as Passey wrote and actively participated in the production of the letter.

Also claiming knowledge of what the law allowed was James Hoare, an ex-serviceman living in Colyton in the Axminster Union in Devon, who wrote to the PLC in July 1844. Hoare hoped that the Commission would 'excuse my Boldness' but that, as he had 'arrived at the advanced age of 64 years, and totally dissabled with rupture and loss of one Eye, while serving in the Defence of my country [sic]', he must correspond with them. He disputed the legality of his current allowance of only two loaves a week 'with regard to my old age pay'. The local officials, he claimed, did not allow him his due 'by the act of the Poor law'. He asked the central authorities to intercede 'by, ordering, what is allowed by the Poor Law act, to Be paid to me weekly'.[38] We find a similar letter from Daniel Rush, who lived at Bethnal Green. He wrote to the Poor Law Board (PLB), 'Implorin of you to take my Case into your most seirous Considration [sic]'. Rush was a seventy-one-year-old silk weaver but now considered himself as 'Past Labour'. He and his sixty-eight-year-old wife earned about 3s. per week and having applied for relief locally were only offered the workhouse. When they arrived there, the staff insisted that the couple, who had been married for forty-nine years, were separated. He claimed that 'soner then We Would be seperated We Will Perish for Want [sic]'. Rush quoted (albeit inaccurately) from the 1847 Consolidated General Order: 'in the Act for the Administration of the Laws in England 23 July 1847 Chap 109 Verse 23 any two Persons being Husband and Wife shall not be ness be Compeld to be separate [sic]' and asked the Board to ensure they would not be separated.[39] Here Rush was referring to that part of the Order that allowed that there was no compulsion on any union 'to separate any married couple, being both paupers of the first and fourth classes respectively'.[40] This linguistic register of law, oppression, moral right and reasonable expectation plays out across our sample, but it also has a remarkable resonance with how modern patients dispute, directly or mediated through the media, the decisions of healthcare authorities on issues across a spectrum from drug rationing to the legal and moral failings of care homes. Increasingly in the late twentieth and early twenty-first centuries intertwining (and sometimes contradictory) imperatives, such as seeing patients as consumers, containing costs, closing local hospitals, devolution of GP services and an inexorable increase in health and safety legislation and associated compensation cultures, has resulted in a dwindling of informal contestation and more legalistic and formulaic challenges to the authority of doctors and politicians and the depth and quality of healthcare. In this context, rhetoric, strategy and method for such contestation seems to have had a pattern which transcends

## The patient's view as history from below

geography and chronology.[41] Whether this sort of template is specific to the voices and the experiences of the poor (as opposed, for instance, to being generalised also to the middling classes, however we define them) is more difficult, but a consideration of historical material clearly points to the adaptability of the poor in terms of their acquisition of new narrative and rhetorical threads when faced with healthcare challenges. We see very similar experiences in the morphing of modern hospital scandals from individual concerns into concerted campaigns with a legal and compensatory basis.

### Contesting exclusion

Equally contentious, in a modern sense, have been post-2010 reforms to a broadly conceived basket of 'disability allowances'. These have resulted in many more people being classified as fit for some work, although systematic legal challenges on the part of patient and advocate groups have seen the rolling back of many individual decisions. The essential question behind these processes (who can decide if someone is too sick to work?) was played out equally firmly by the poor under the New Poor Law. Managing the sick poor may have been opaquely included in the 1834 Act, but the profile of workhouse inmates and outdoor poor suggest that the very young, the elderly and the sick predominated pauper populations.[42] This notwithstanding, union and central authority staff continuously spent time setting out what type of work might be undertaken by different categories of pauper in receipt of relief. This juxtaposition of the enfeebled or sick pauper and the allocation of work tasks led to complaints that paupers were allocated labour tasks unfairly or illegally. In particular, the sick poor and their advocates argued that they were given work that they were unable to perform or that would further endanger their health. Complaints were commonly raised directly by paupers themselves. In May 1843, one J. Lazenby, an indoor pauper at the Bethnal Green Workhouse in Middlesex, wrote to the PLC complaining that 'about five weeks ago the Master Compelled the Age[d], Cripples, and Infirm Males to laber [sic] at the Pump instead of the able Bodied Men, under 60 years of age (which is I presume against the Poor Law Act)'. Lazenby claimed that he and other aged men were threatened that their food allowances and agreed periods of leave on Sundays would be stopped if they did not undertake this task work. Furthermore, he asserted that through fear many men who were too elderly (between seventy and eighty years old), feeble and sick to work undertook the tasks as the threats were being enforced because the medical officers who might have supported the sick poor in their resistance to labour were by law not allowed to interfere in the allocation of workhouse tasks. He provided details of his own medical conditions, which included spitting quantities of blood, shortness of breath, 'fungus flesh in both Ears and my Nostrils', and his ears continually discharging some form of foetid matter. Refusing the task work himself on medical grounds, Lazenby claimed he was 'deprived of my liberty' and had been 'most grossly and infamously insulted'.[43] A similar concern over work being imposed on those unable to labour can be seen in the letter from James Holmes, who wrote from Calverton in the Basford Union in Nottinghamshire in August 1846. Stating that he had recently been reduced to applying for poor relief on account of his and his wife's ages (being sixty-nine and sixty-five, respectively), he was told that he would need to work on the roads to receive relief, but claimed his advanced years and impaired constitution (caused by military service in the West Indies and Egypt) made this impossible. Holme's service rendered his constitution:

> so impaired that I am quite unable to bear any Exertion Under these Circumstances, it is hoped my deplorable situation will meet with your sympathy It is hoped you will attend to my Case I cannot do without relief and they with-hold it what am I to do? [...] I would just add that they would not admit me into the House nor relieve me.[44]

Sometimes the very medical men employed to treat the sick were the subject of complaints about the injurious effects of work on those who were already at their lowest ebb. Thus, William Morgan wrote to the PLB a few days after leaving the Cardiff Union workhouse in May 1852 and was 'under the Disagreable. Necessety of Lodgings a Complaint Against the Surgeon of the union, As regards his Inhumain treet-ment for poor patients afflicted by the hand of God [sic]'. He painted a very dark picture of the porter who made it his 'perticular business [sic]' to complain about paupers to the doctor and guardians. This led to the sick poor being given 'work at the pumps and also to break stones when Entirely unable', while others were 'put to break stones for several Days some with wounds in their legs'. Morgan concluded by offering to assist the PLB should they 'feel Disposed to make Any further inquiry in the matter'.⁴⁵

The link between unemployment and hopelessness explicitly developed in these letters also has real resonance with modern health discourses. In a recent study, redundancy and periods out of work were said to account for around one-fifth of suicides across a sample of sixty-three countries in the first dozen years of the twenty-first century.⁴⁶ Commenting on the research in 2015, Roger Webb and Navneet Kapur cautioned that suicide cases attributed to the financial crisis of 2007–8 were only 'the tip of the iceberg' of a greater suite of social and psychological problems associated with exogenous shocks to employment and status.⁴⁷ That the mid-nineteenth-century poor were also aware of such pressures is further demonstrated in the case of John Knight, a labourer of Thorncombe in the Axminster Union in Devon, who gave sworn evidence as part of an investigation in June 1837 into the suicide of his father, James Knight. John had returned home from work and, going upstairs, found his father dead. He described the scene: James had a rope round his neck placed over his chin and up behind his ears forming a noose. Another piece of rope could be seen on a beam above him (the rope had at some time apparently snapped). James had been out of work about a fortnight and prior to this he used to earn 3s. or 3s. 6d. a week at weeding corn, supplemented by 1s. 6d. and two loaves per week from the local poor law authorities. He had just been informed that his bread allowance was going to be halved in future and had been heard to comment that he would 'be starved now he could get no work'. James had sought work from several farmers but could secure none. He also unsuccessfully asked the Axminster guardians for additional relief. John blamed Haskell, the relieving officer, for his father's death: 'I believe that the cause of my Fathers [sic] putting an end to himself was the being unable to get work & the Refusal to give him any further relief and shortening what he had from the Union'. Moreover, John was very clear that his father's mental state deteriorated concluding that 'the fear of starving prayed on my Fathers [sic] mind'.⁴⁸ The rhetorical infrastructure of these claims matches almost perfectly that used by relatives of those who have taken their own lives in response to the withdrawal or downgrading of benefits through reforms to Disability Living Allowance or Universal Credit.

## Distance and timeliness

One of the most controversial aspects of Universal Credit has been the fact that delays to sick people applying for and receiving benefits are written into the very fabric of the system. Equally, even a cursory glance at most modern newspapers reveals innumerable complaints of sick people having to wait for doctors' appointments or patients having to undertake long journeys for medical care.[49] Many of our nineteenth-century writers also faced and contested similar problems. Thus, although medical districts were originally meant to have medical officers located within their boundaries, this was not always possible. Applications for any given district may not have attracted interest from a local doctor.[50] In such cases medical officers could reside many miles from the district they served, making timely access difficult or perhaps even impossible. The reverend James Rudge of Hawkchurch in the Axminster Union complained to the central authorities in March 1842 after he had visited Samuel Quentin, who was confined to his bed by typhus. Quentin complained directly to Rudge of the inconveniences the sick poor suffered on account of the distance that the newly appointed medical officer lived from them. Rudge pointed out that the new man lived at Chard and that from his house to Chard was about nine or ten miles. Indeed, there was no part of Hawkchurch from which it was less than six or seven miles. Thus:

> the result of any application for medical assistance, must be as follows. A messenger, in going and returning, will have to walk about eighteen miles – the medical Gentleman to see his patients will have to ride the same distance and another journey of the same extent must be undergone to fetch the medicine; and I need scarcely add, that, from the length of time these journeys will take, the disease of the patient may be accelerated, and death, in some cases, may ensue. The medical officers, to whom such important interests are entrusted, should certainly not live three or four miles or farther from the residences of the poor.[51]

The frequency of very strong advocacy on the subject of timely treatment (or rather its absence) is a striking feature of our letter corpus, which has its analogue in modern letters to newspapers and media reporting. Thus in early 1864 Frederick T. Velly wrote from Chelmsford in Essex to the PLB concerning an unnamed man who walked from Borham to Chelmsford, a distance of about four-and-a-half miles, to call on the union surgeon and who was 'completely covered with the small pox'.[52] The surgeon secured an order for the man to be admitted into the workhouse. However, after making his way there, he was refused entry and travelled back to the town. A second order for admission was secured, but once again the man was denied. The surgeon then personally sought out and spoke with the chairman of the local guardians, but he refused to intervene in the case. Eventually, a half-open shed was found for the man where he was able to sleep. Velly was convinced that the time spent on the journey added to the man's misery. On top of the initial trip from Borham, further 'hours [...] a greater part of which time the poor man was in the open air either standing about in the market place [...] or travelling to and from the Union house a distance of one mile or thereabout each way' were added to his burden.[53]

For some of the sick poor, as with modern patients, delays to treatment resulted in tragedy, enquiries and lessons to be learned. Thus, in late 1849, Martha Barker, a pregnant thirty-one-year-old from Ilkeston in Derbyshire, was taken ill. After she complained to her husband, Thomas, 'of feeling very bad' and expressly wanted medical assistance, he sought out Marshall, the local parish overseer, and obtained an order for the medical officer to see Martha. However, Edgar Henry Longstaff, one of the local medical officers, refused to attend and instructed Thomas to bring Marshall to his (Longstaff's) house. Longstaff claimed that the order was invalid and instructed Thomas to go to Bulwell to secure a new order from Topliss, the Ilkeston district relieving officer, as the case was not an 'urgent one'. Thomas disagreed and argued that the case was urgent and that his wife was likely to die. Furthermore, Thomas refused to undertake the journey, saying he did not know the way and that he could not leave his wife alone in her current state as it would be a round trip of some fourteen miles. Taking offence at 'my Sauce', Longstaff refused to provide medicine for Martha, although he later relented.[54] In the event Martha died and Longstaff, who claimed to have misunderstood his duties as medical officer, was officially cautioned to attend all lawful orders as soon as they have been served on him.[55] The aged were also susceptible to this sort of treatment, as Joseph Manderston, an unemployed collier aged seventy-eight in Northumberland, found out in December 1855. Residing at that time in the Berwick-upon-Tweed workhouse, he gave an account of his experiences of a couple of months earlier, when he had unsuccessfully visited the Detchant Moor Colliery to seek employment. While there, Manderston picked up what he thought was a bottle of coffee. He removed the cork close to the cabin fire and the contents, being gunpowder, exploded. He was struck on the forehead by the blast, his clothes were on fire in several places and both of his hands, his face and neck were severely burnt. Manderston dressed his hands with Florence oil, which some of the pitmen gave him.[56] He left the colliery a couple of days later and made for Belford, being advised by the colliery workmen that the workhouse there would be bound to take him in. On arrival, and with all his clothes soaked by rain, he visited Mr Scott, the relieving officer, but found him not at home. Scott's wife *'said that I could be taken in only for the night, but that I could not be allowed to stop'*, telling Manderston to inform the doorkeeper at the workhouse that she had sent him for a night's lodging.[57] At the workhouse, Manderston was placed in a room which had 'only sloping boards for sleeping on – There was no Bedding and no Bed Clothes except two old coverlets'. Later the workhouse doorkeeper returned with Mr Scott, who said:

> 'Who sent you here and what right have you to come here' He jumped round me like a man either drunk or mad and said 'You have no right here and you must go out. I tried to speak, but he would not listen – "He said you have imposed upon my wife and if I had been at home you should not have got in here for I would not have let you". He told me several times to go about my business – I said will you have no mercy upon a poor old man in the situation I was in and with my hands in such a state'. He said again that I was to go about my business – I asked him for mercy's sake to allow me to stay a few days and get medical assistance.[58]

When Manderston asked Scott if he was to die 'in a Christian land without medical aid', Scott replied that he did not care either way. The party then left and around thirty minutes later a doctor came and examined Manderston's left hand. He ordered a poultice, which was done but without the hand being washed. Although Manderston thought the doctor's manner to be civil, he refused to examine the right hand or his face and neck. Put to bed with a supper of porridge and treacle, Manderston described feeling feverish and having to walk across the room throughout the night to keep warm. A breakfast of porridge and treacle (again) was followed by an order from an unidentified female to leave the workhouse. It was, claimed Manderston, 'a very coarse stormy and wet day – I left with tears in my eyes', and he was eventually admitted to the Berwick workhouse having walked the thirty-five miles there.[59] Even by the standards of the nineteenth century, these events signalled neglect of duty and failures of process. It is important that, much as with modern equivalent stories, such failures generated complaint and scandal, and with them insistent and powerful patient voices.

## Dealing with chronic sickness

Chronic sickness, both in our period and for modern healthcare consumers, presents the most acute problems for patients and their families. It was and is also the territory on which complaint, contestation and scandal (and with them patient voices) emerges most strongly, as Brückner has also shown in relation to familial treatment of supposed lunatics.[60] For many nineteenth-century writers facing a landscape of medical science in which definitive cures were rare, chronic sickness was intricately tied up with the question of having or not having the resources simply to manage their own or a relative's condition. Children who were born disabled or became incapacitated in some way during infancy posed a particular problem. In August 1863, Joseph Smith, from the Bethnal Green Union, wrote to the PLB, concerning his son Joseph John Smith. Joseph John was then aged twenty-five and regarded as physically and intellectually weak. He was 'afflicted with general debility, his back having grown out through an accident in his infancy, unable to do any Kind of work'. Joseph (the father) had made four separate applications on his son's behalf to the Bethnal Green guardians and on each occasion they refused to admit Joseph John to the workhouse. The young man's father was apparently caring for his son on the scant income of a journeyman silk weaver's wage, which at the time was around 8s. a week. Furthermore, the father was caring as a lone parent:

> [My] wife [was] a drunken dissolute woman [who] has separated from me having involved me in debt so much that I know not how to extricate myself. I waited on the Magestrate [sic] of Worship Street Police Court who advised me to write and explain my case to the Poor law Commissioner.[61]

Much as with modern families who have exhausted their reserves of money and emotional support and thus seek institutional care for their disabled children, Joseph Smith played on the moral conscience of those with the power to order welfare in a discretionary system.

Some of our writers sought to retain children in the home, although they required additional financial resources as the child became older or during periodic downturns in family finances. In June 1856, John Bacon wrote from Arnold in the Basford Union to the PLB. He stated that he had a daughter aged fourteen 'that is totally dark'.[62] Up until the time of the letter, he had managed to care for her, but he 'cannot do it any longer without some assistance somewhere'. Bacon had approached the local authorities but they would not allow any relief 'Unless we all go into the Union house and we should not like to break up our home and go into the house, we only want a little relief for the Girl'.[63] A similar letter, again from a father concerning a daughter, was written by Joseph Fletcher in January 1859. Living in Walmgate in the York Union, he apologised for writing :

> but my reason for so doing is, because I have a Child upwards of five Years of Age, whose Limbs are Paralised [sic] she was Born in that State, and has no use whatever of herself she cannot talk nor anything, and is likely to be a burden as long as she lives, and as I am but a working Man, I have not much to stir on, therefore I beg to ask your Advice about applying to the Board of Guardians, for a little support for her. I wish to know if they can take her from me, I have not yet applied to them nor do I intend until I have your Advice on the subject, as I am willing to do what I can for her, I have now been out of employ for some weeks past and have had no Assistance from any one, and would be very glad to do without entirely if I could, but I find I am unable to do so any longer, therefore I ask your Advice whether I must Apply for myself or the Child.[64]

Again here the emphasis was on his having looked after the child for as long as possible without help, but now needed some assistance.

Fletcher, like Bacon, was unwilling to break up the family home to secure assistance, even though the strain of looking after a paralysed child must have imposed significant economic and emotional stress. Fearful that the guardians could forcibly remove his child, Fletcher refrained from asking for relief locally until he had received advice from the PLB confirming whether the guardians would have such authority. Much as with modern families who challenge the refusal to provide attendance allowances or their withdrawal, chronic sickness and disability provided a rich canvas of protest and complaint through which patient agency in shaping the healthcare they received emerges.

## Conclusions

Our corpus of complaints, contesting letters and statements given in the wake of medical disputes speaks very directly to Porter's 1985 call to give voice to the voiceless ordinary patient. Such material, either produced or co-produced by ordinary poor people, allows a sharper picture to emerge of their experiences, their concerns and their views on being sufferers seeking medical care. What emerges from this material is the insistent voice of the sick pauper and their advocates, informed by law, a sense of legal and moral right and above all a sense that the central authorities had a duty to listen and act given the suffering described. The thousands of witness statements in the central archive – produced under the direction of union or central-authority investigations but with much the same authenticity as letters – provide explicit evidence that the sick poor were willing to contest their treatment right the way through the system to which they were notionally subject. Nowhere is this better demonstrated than in the case of Thomas Hartley, who wrote to the PLB in April 1848 to set out a series of complaints around general conditions in the workhouse. One of the most serious of these was that the elderly and infirm were set to hard task work, with one 'Old Man which is 80 years of age or upwards forc'd to the stones sometime carried up on a mans back some[times] Weeld down in a wheelbarrow [sic]'. Hartley was clear he had no faith in the guardians' desire or ability to deal with such criticisms and believed that: 'I have enough to inform you gentlemen that [this] place wants much investigation, I wish [an] inquiry before I procede farther [sic]'.[65]

The fact that, at least episodically, sick paupers did get their requested inquiries signals an important level of patient agency of the sort that Porter suspected but could not prove when he wrote on the need to resurrect the ordinary patient voice.[66] There is also, however, and as we have argued above, important resonance in the rhetoric, attitude and expectations of our sick paupers with modern patient voices. Both groups use complaint, scandal and the forum of the inquiry to contest (for themselves, families or others without power) refusals to grant medical aid or to challenge late, inadequate, hard-to-access and grudgingly given healthcare. In doing so, they challenged and challenge the administratively powerful, very often to great effect. Individually and collectively, then, the voice of the patient demonstrates considerable continuity, both in terms of what is said and how. All of this, of course, reflects something that is often missed by medical and welfare historians, which is that the nineteenth-century sick poor shared with their modern counterpart a clear sense and associated rhetoric of rights.

This sort of chronological connectivity is important. The nineteenth-century poor had and could articulate many of the same concerns about health and medical welfare as their modern counterparts. More than this they rhetoricised those concerns and framed their disputes (for instance via references to law and accepted practice) in very similar ways. There are many readings of this experience and its meaning, but one is that there is a timelessness to the basic conundrum for poor people: how to confront the power of those who run systems of welfare and medicine and who thus have the scope to impose experiences on others. In the context of healthcare there was and is plenty to go wrong in that imposition, and thus for scandal and intense contestation to develop. Ultimately, however, standing above the detail of individual cases we can see both that the presentism of so much recent commentary on 'modern' healthcare conundrums is unwarranted, and that ultimately the poor inevitably seek ways to limit the power of the executive. In this sense, we end our chapter with the anonymous voice of a complaint for 'the old inmates of Bethnal Green at Spitalfields Workhouse [who] are very harshly treated, the poor old men being set to break stones, which is quite beyond their strength, & the old Women being very scantily clothed & fed'. The author warned that if such practices were not ended then those in authority 'will hereafter be called to account', much as modern patient groups seek to hold governments to account.[67] Once patients found a voice and could sustain it, they felt no compunction in holding those responsible for safeguarding health to the highest standards.

## Notes

* Material used in this chapter was drawn from the work of our AHRC-funded project 'In Their Own Write' (grant no. AH/R002770/1). We are grateful for the support of the AHRC.
1 Roy Porter, 'The Patient's View: Doing Medical History from Below', *Theory and Society* 14:2 (1985), 175–98.
2 Alexandra Bacopoulous-Viau and Aude Fauvel, 'The Patient's Turn: Roy Porter and Psychiatry's Tales, Thirty Years On', *Medical History* 60:1 (2016), 1–18; Flurin Condrau, 'The Patient's View Meets the Clinical Gaze', *Social History of Medicine* 20:3 (2007), 525–40.
3 Porter, 'The Patient's View', 175.
4 Michael Brown, *Performing Medicine: Medical Culture and Identity in Provincial England c.1760–1850* (Manchester: Manchester University Press, 2011); Elaine Leong and Alisha Rankin (eds), *Secrets and Knowledge in Medicine and Science 1500–1800* (London: Ashgate, 2011); Anne Digby, *Making a Medical Living: Doctors and Patients in the English Market for Medicine, 1720–1911* (Cambridge: Cambridge University Press, 1994).
5 Peter Bartlett, *The Poor Law of Lunacy: The Administration of Pauper Lunatics in Mid-Nineteenth Century England* (Leicester: Leicester University Press, 1999), 132–41. The process of reclamation has also been chronologically uneven, with more (and more nuanced) work undertaken for the early modern period than for the nineteenth century. See Hannah Newton, *The Sick Child in Early Modern England, 1580–1720* (Oxford: Oxford University Press, 2012).
6 Bacopoulous-Viau and Fauvel, 'The Patient's Turn', 1; Louise Wannell, 'Patients' Relatives and Psychiatric Doctors: Letter Writing in the York Retreat, 1875–1910', *Social History of Medicine*, 20:2 (2007), 297–313; Catherine Smith, 'Living with Insanity: Narratives of Poverty, Pauperism and Sickness in Asylum Records, 1840–1876', in Steven King, Elizabeth Hurren and Andreas Gestrich (eds), *Poverty and Sickness in Modern Europe: Narratives of the Sick Poor, 1780–1938* (London: Bloomsbury, 2012), 117–41.

7 Mary Fissell, 'The Disappearance of the Patient's Narrative and the Invention of Hospital Medicine', in Andrew Wear and Roger French (eds), *British Medicine in an Age of Reform* (London: Routledge, 2015), 92–109.
8 Jonathan Gillis, 'The History of the Patient History since 1850', *Bulletin of the History of Medicine*, 80:3 (2006), 490–512.
9 Steven King, *Sickness, Medical Welfare and the English Poor 1750–1834* (Manchester: Manchester University Press, 2018); Steven King, *Writing the Lives of the English Poor, 1750s to 1830s* (Montreal and Kingston: McGill-Queen's University Press, 2019).
10 Samantha Shave, '"Immediate Death or a Life of Torture are the Consequences of the System": The Bridgwater Union Scandal and Policy Change', in Jonathan Reinarz and Leonard Schwarz (eds), *Medicine and the Workhouse* (Rochester: Rochester University Press, 2013), 164–91, 174–5; Elizabeth Hurren, *Protesting about Pauperism: Poverty, Politics and Poor Relief in Late-Victorian England, 1870–1900* (Woodbridge, Suffolk: The Boydell Press, 2015).
11 Maren Klawiter, 'Breast Cancer in Two Regimes: The Impact of Social Movements on Illness Experience', *Sociology of Health and Illness* 26:6 (2016), 845–74; Fadhila Mazanderani, 'The Patient's View: Perspectives from Neurology and the "New" Genetics', *Science as Culture* 23 (2014), 135–44, which also credits Porter's 'The Patient's View' as a prime mover in changing the focus from the medical establishment towards the patient.
12 'Queuing at NHS GP Surgery in Wellingborough "a Bit 19th Century"', BBC News, 8 May 2019, www.bbc.co.uk/news/uk-england-northamptonshire-48200555 (accessed 13 January 2020); 'People Are Being Turned Away From Walk-In Centres Because They Don't Have an Appointment', *Leicester Mercury*, 12 May 2019, www.leicestermercury.co.uk/news/health/people-being-turned-away-walk-2855717 (accessed 16 February 2020).
13 'Swathes of Countryside Becoming "Healthcare Deserts" with £100 Trips for Hospital Care', *The Telegraph*, 22 May 2019, www.telegraph.co.uk/news/2019/05/22/swathes-countryside-becoming-healthcare-deserts-100-trips-hospital (accessed 16 December 2019).
14 'Campaign to Buy Frame for Boy, Seven, to Stand at Home', BBC News, 12 May 2019, www.bbc.co.uk/news/uk-wales-48205285 (accessed 11 August 2019).
15 'Chronically Ill Father Died by Suicide after DWP Declared Him Fit to Work and Cut His Benefits', iNews, 6 June 2019, https://inews.co.uk/news/dwp-benefits-man-declared-fit-to-work-death-suicide (accessed 11 July 2019). In their chapter in this collection, Jessica Meyer and Alexia

Moncrieff deal with the thorny question of whether the existence of such narratives means that they can be ethically used.
16 David Holmes, 'Mid Staffordshire Scandal Highlights NHS Cultural Crisis', *Lancet* 381 (16 February 2013), 521–2.
17 www.patients-association.org.uk (accessed 22 April 2020).
18 See Burkhart Brückner's chapter in this collection.
19 King, *Sickness, Medical Welfare*, passim.
20 Digby, *Making a Medical Living*, passim; Brown, *Performing Medicine*, 68–76.
21 Edward Higgs, *The Information State in England: The Central Collection of Information on Citizens since 1500* (Basingstoke: Palgrave, 2004), 64–98.
22 Porter, 'The Patient's View', 178.
23 Jonathan Reinarz and Alistair Ritch, 'Exploring Medical Care in the Nineteenth-Century Provincial Workhouse: A View from Birmingham', in Jonathan Reinarz and Leonard Schwarz (eds), *Medicine and the Workhouse* (Rochester: Rochester University Press, 2013), 140–63, 151, 153. The material for this chapter is drawn from our current AHRC project, 'In Their Own Write: Contesting the New Poor law 1834–1900' (AH/R002770/1). For more information see https://intheirownwriteblog.com/about (accessed 20 January 2021). Our corpus has been taken from a sample of some eighty poor law unions.
24 The numbers of poor law unions fluctuate from the mid/late 1830s onwards. In 1838, there were 594 poor law unions across England and Wales and this had increased by the early 1860s to 646 unions. See *Annual Report of the Poor Law Commissioners* Vol. IV (1838); *Annual Report of the Poor Law Board* Vol. XIII (1860–61).
25 Anne Crowther, 'Health Care and Poor Relief in Provincial England', in Ole Peter Grell, Andrew Cunningham and Robert Jütte (eds), *Health Care and Poor Relief in 18th and 19th Century Northern Europe* (London: Ashgate, 2002), 203–19, 212.
26 Ruth G. Hodgkinson, 'Poor Law Medical Officers of England 1834–1871', *Journal of the History of Medicine and Allied Sciences* 11:3 (1956), 299–338, 300.
27 For a summary see Steven King, 'Thinking and Rethinking the New Poor Law', *Local Population Studies* 99:1 (2017), 5–19.
28 Kim Price, *Medical Negligence in Victorian Britain: The Crisis of Care under the English Poor Law, c.1834–1900* (London: Bloomsbury, 2015), 10.
29 Paul Carter and Natalie Whistance, 'The Poor Law Commission: A New Digital Resource for Nineteenth-Century Domestic Historians', *History Workshop Journal* 71:1 (2011), 29–48; Paul Carter and Natalie

Whistance, *Living the Poor Life: A Guide to the Poor Law Union Correspondence, c.1834 to 1871*, held at The National Archives (British Association for Local History, 2011); Paul Carter and Steve King, 'Keeping Track: Modern Methods, Administration and the Victorian Poor Law', *Archives* 40:128 (2014), 31–52.

30 The central register to these papers, and the correspondence itself from c.1900 onwards, no longer survives, being destroyed during the Second World War. See Carter and King, 'Keeping Track'.

31 TNA's online catalogue lists 16,745 volumes. When using this material below we have retained all spellings and punctuation as in the original documents.

32 By co-produced we mean records produced with the active participation of poor people, who we now understand were adept at seeking and finding others who held socially superior positions to them, who would listen to their accounts or complaints of welfare and would then take up their cause.

33 Witness statements are interchangeably referred to as statements, witness statements, evidences and depositions. The distinction between letters from paupers and letters from poor people is also problematic. While being in receipt of relief defined one as a pauper, an application for relief did not. Letters complaining of a lack of relief while destitute, followed by a subsequent one acknowledging inadequate relief had been given, and perhaps a third complaining that even this has been withdrawn, therefore embodies a fluid position where the poor might slip from poverty to pauperism and then back quite quickly. For ease of argument we have deemed all such texts as pauper letters.

34 Section 54, 'An Act for the Amendment and Better Administration of the Laws Relating to the Poor in England and Wales, 1834'.

35 TNA, MH 12/9232/46, paper number 1356/B/1842, Thomas Henshaw, Ilkeston, Basford Poor Law Union, to the PLC (7 February 1842).

36 TNA, MH 12/16104, paper number 4244/C/1835, Reverend Hugh Metthie, Wrexham Poor Law Union, to the PLC (9 February 1835), emphasis added.

37 TNA, MH 12/14016/68, paper number 780/C/1837, William Passey, Kidderminster Poor Law Union, to the PLC (30 January 1837).

38 TNA, MH 12/2097/207, paper number 10898/A/1844, James Hoare, Axminster Poor Law Union, to the PLC (20 July 1844).

39 TNA, MH 12/6846, paper number 35021/1851, Daniel Rush, Bethnal Green Poor Law Union, to the PLB (22 August 1851).

40 PLC, 'The Consolidated General Order', 1847, article 93 section 3. These classes were men and women deemed infirm through age or any other cause.

41  As outlined, for example, in Ros Levenson, *The Challenge of Dignity in Care: Upholding the Rights of the Individual* (London: Help the Aged, 2007) and K. Walshe, *Inquiries: Learning from Failure in the NHS* (London: Nuffield Trust, 2003).
42  Andrew Hinde and Fiona Turnbull, 'The Population of Two Hampshire workhouses, 1851–1861', *Local Population Studies*, 61 (1998), 38–53; David Jackson, 'The Medway Union Workhouse, 1876–1881: A Study Based on the admission and Discharge Registers and the Census Enumerators Books', *Local Population Studies* 75 (2005), 11–32.
43  TNA, MH 12/6844, paper number 5914/1843, J. Lazenby, Bethnal Green Poor Law Union, to the PLC (21 May 1843).
44  TNA, MH 12/9236/266, paper number, 11970/B/1846, James Holmes, Calverton, Basford Poor Law Union, to the PLC (29 August 1846). The rhetorical and tonal overlap with the letters of recovering VD patients noted by Lloyd (Meadhbh) Houston later in this volume are unmistakeable, pointing to a wider understanding of the linguistic register of appeal, service and hopelessness. See Lloyd (Meadhbh) Houston's chapter in this collection.
45  TNA, MH 12/16249/212, paper number, 18153/1852, William Morgan, Cardiff Poor Law Union, to the PLB (19 May 1852). The local union responded that Morgan 'was insubordinate in his conduct and on one occasion was found haranging the paupers into the view of creating a mutiny'. TNA, MH 12/16249/236, f 324, 22954/1852, Thomas Watkins, Clerk to the Guardians of the Cardiff Poor Law Union, to PLB (15 June 1852).
46  Carlos Nordt, Ingeborg Warnke, Erich Seifritz and Wolfram Kawohl, 'Modelling Suicide and Unemployment: A Longitudinal Analysis Covering 63 Countries, 2000–11', *Lancet Psychiatry* 2:3 (2015), 239–45.
47  Sarah Boseley, 'Unemployment Causes 45,000 Suicides a Year Worldwide, Finds Study', *The Guardian* (11 February 2015).
48  TNA, MH 12/2095/158, Witness statement of John Knight, in Harry Burrard Farnall, Assistant Poor Law Commissioner, to the PLC (19 June 1837).
49  See, for example, Denis Campbell, 'One in Five Patients Waits Two Weeks to See a GP, Finds Report', *The Guardian* (7 December 2018).
50  Alan Kidd, *State, Society and the Poor in Nineteenth-Century England* (Basingstoke: Palgrave, 1999), 41.
51  TNA, MH 12/2096/269, paper number 2937/A/1842, Reverend James Rudge, Axminster Poor Law Union, to the PLC (22 March 1842).
52  TNA, MH 12/3405, paper number 3930/1864, Frederick T. Velly, Chelmsford Poor Law Union, to the PLB (29 January 1864), original emphasis.

53 Ibid.
54 TNA, MH 12/9239/202–203, paper number 36390/1849, witness statement of Thomas Barker, Ilkeston, in Richard Birch Spencer, Clerk to Basford Poor Law Union, to the PLB (13 December 1849).
55 TNA, MH 12/9239/249, paper number 15938/1850, draft letter from the PLB, to Edgar Henry Longstaff, Medical Officer for Ilkeston in the Basford Poor Law Union.
56 This was an oil-based tincture incorporating salt, alcohol and (in some versions) herbal essences including rosemary.
57 TNA, MH 12/8983, 46155/1855, witness statement in W. and E. Willoby, Union Clerks, Berwick Poor Law Union, to the PLB (4 December 1855), original emphasis.
58 Ibid., original quotation marks.
59 TNA, MH12/8983, 46155/1855, witness statement in W. and E. Willoby, Union Clerks, Berwick Poor Law Union, to the PLB (4 December 1855).
60 See Burkhart Brückner's chapter in this collection.
61 TNA, MH 12/6850, paper number 29994/1863, Joseph Smith, Bethnal Green Poor Law Union, to the PLB (3 August 1863).
62 The phrase 'dark' in this context signals blindness from birth. See Carol Beardmore, Steven King and Geoff Monks, *Disability Matters* (Rutland: Call of Crows, 2018), 18–21.
63 TNA, MH 12/9245/96, paper number 25337/1856, John Bacon, Arnold, Basford Poor Law, to the PLB (19 June 1856).
64 TNA, MH 12/14405, paper number 2512/1859, Joseph Fletcher, York Poor Law Union, to the PLB (18 January 1859).
65 TNA, MH 12/16248/140, paper number 11120/1848, Thomas Hartley, Kidderminster Poor Law Union, to the PLB (17 April 1848).
66 Porter, 'The Patient's View'.
67 TNA, MH 12/6847, paper number 45369/1857, anonymous, Bethnal Green Poor Law Union, to the PLB (10 December 1857).

# III

User-driven medicine

# 6

# Respiratory technologies and the co-production of breathing in the twentieth century*

*Coreen McGuire, Jaipreet Virdi and Jenny Hutton*

In 1933, Nobel prize-winning physicist William H. Bragg (1862–1942) was worried about his neighbour, Capt. Samuel Crosby Halahan (1869–1939), who lived in West Sussex and suffered from what Bragg described as a 'terrible wasting of the muscles'.[1] Not much is known about Halahan's life other than his military service and that his friendship with Bragg resulted in the design of a new homemade 'breathing machine'. In 1926, Halahan began gradually to lose weight as well as all 'power of moving his limbs' until he was unable to drive a car or write. Halahan also lost the ability to breathe unaided, therefore eventually requiring the care of two nurses:

> For a long time two nurses were employed giving artificial respiration continually: the wife felt very much the disability of being unable to speak to him except in the presence of a nurse because her strength had considerably diminished due to the strain of her husband's illness, and she was unable therefore to give artificial respiration herself.[2]

It is unclear what kind of artificial respiration Halahan was given, though the nurses probably employed a manual lung-inflation device such as the McKesson resuscitator, rather than attempting to maintain purely manual inflation. Halahan needed such continuous artificial respiration from the onset of paralysis in 1931 until his death in 1936 at the age of sixty-six.[3] His respiratory paralysis was diagnosed as resulting from progressive muscular atrophy.

Given the strain that continuous artificial respiration placed on Halahan's relationship with his wife, Bragg 'had the idea that [he] could ease matters by a simple system of india [sic] rubber bladders, football bladders in fact' to substitute the human effort. To devise this automated system, he bandaged one of the bladders under a binder on Halahan's chest and the other to a pair of hinged boards on the ground, then connected the two with a long tube. This bellows device applied rhythmic pressure directly to the chest, forcing the diaphragm to contract and air to enter and leave the lungs. Rather than continuously pressuring the chest with her hands, a nurse or Halahan's wife, Maud (1872–1967), could apply pressure, by simply pressing down on the hand lever that connected to the pulsating rubber bellows.[4] Bragg's invention used positive pressure which meant that it enforced expiration of air by forcing the ribs in, much like the manual ventilation methods more commonly associated with drowning. The device's mechanism, however, only lasted three days before the rubber burst, eventually being replaced by a hot water bottle used as an airbag. Again, the materials proved to be insufficient. The revised design lasted just another three weeks after being replaced and patched. Then the hinges attached to the original boards became loose.[5] A substitute was created by a 'firm of organ builders', but this proved too hard for the nurse to manoeuvre, especially since no means of electric supply was available.

Despite the mechanical improvement, the labour remained arduous for the nurses and Maud, so Bragg commissioned instrument maker Robert W. Paul (1869–1943) to construct a small hydraulic machine that relied on the main water supply.[6] This new design worked effectively – except on occasions when the water pipes froze or the water supply was shut off for repairs without notice – and was estimated to have caused 15 million involuntary respirations in Halahan's lifetime.[7] It was discreet, as the hollow bandage that replaced the football bladder could be hidden by the bedcovers so 'that there was no evidence of anything unusual except the quiet click-clack of the pulsator in another part of the room'.[8] Furthermore, it made Halahan's relationships easier, as Maud could 'give artificial respiration while she sits and reads to her husband' and only one nurse was required to assist.[9] He wore the device up to seventeen hours each day, as he could not 'bear the constriction of the bandage' all day; the remaining hours were filled with manual respiration.[10] Bragg's portable system offered Halahan more mobility and privacy. It also gave him more control over his breathing. The system was adjusted to fit to Halahan's body, leaving him 'free to do as much as he could have done if it had not been applied'.[11] It was even allegedly modified so that it could be used while driving.[12]

As Coreen McGuire and Havi Carel have elucidated, the elements of co-production in its origins of design involved engagement with the patient's needs beyond the strictly medical.[13] The story of Bragg and Halahan's friendship and collaboration encapsulates many of the themes we explore in this chapter, in which we analyse how bodily knowledge and insight influenced the design of technological support for respiratory disability. Our chapter is primarily focused on twentieth-century developments to respiratory technologies in Britain and will analyse the extent to which consideration of users and user involvement featured in technologies designed to facilitate breathing. We use this user-focused framework to examine respirators like Bragg and Paul's device, which became commercialised as the 'Pulsator' during the interwar period, as well as oxygen-based therapy used in the hospital and the home.[14] With the exception of Halahan's story, recovering these machine users' voices is challenging as they are often filtered in the historical record through the voices of designers, physicians and family members. We refer to patients in this chapter primarily as users for manifold reasons, applying a 'social construction of technology' approach to highlight the contributions of patients to design. In this way, our examination of breathing and assistive technologies links directly to the new ways of locating patient voices outlined in this collection. Following historically appropriate terminology outlined by the Medical Research Council (MRC), we refer to 'breathing machines' for apparatuses used to stimulate breathing artificially over prolonged periods of time. The term 'respirator', however, is also commonly applied to machines that supply oxygen (or oxygen and carbon dioxide).[15] The terminological conflation of the two is rooted in the longer history of artificial respiration. Respirators originally referred to mask type coverings that were popularised in the Victorian era as a health tool used to warm the air prior 'to its entering the mouth, or nose, in respiration' especially in cold weather and for users 'in delicate health'.[16] Rudimentary homemade respirators were also used (to little effect) by firefighters and coalminers attempting to keep their lungs free from dust and debris. However, by the 1930s, the term respirator was more commonly used in relation to the 'mechanical respirators' that were used to stimulate artificial breathing in patients with respiratory paralysis, which generally occurred as a result of polio. These 'breathing machines' are like modern-day ventilators in the sense that they 'breathe' for those who cannot; but differ in that ventilators of today use masks or (more often) breathing tubes inserted into the windpipe or through a tracheostomy. We also discuss the ambulatory oxygen devices which provide supplemental oxygen to people with low oxygen levels.

All such devices are characterised by an intimate proximity to their users' bodies and both mediate the reception of oxygen into the body and thus have a symbolic relationship to our understandings of breath as associated with voice, life and death.[17] These technologies followed disparate pathways of development: while mechanical respirator designs were characterised by user involvement, ambulatory oxygen was initially designed within emergency medicine for use on patients as passive recipients in a hospital setting. This approach can lead to lack of consideration of the lived experience of patients using such devices.

For instance, in the early stages of the COVID-19 pandemic there were worldwide shortages of the ventilators necessary to treat patients suffering from the worst effects of the virus, and British government officials were criticised for commissioning non-specialist engineering firms without consulting medical experts.[18] Reliance on a hastily assembled industry consortium means that the resulting basic design does not include key features, most notably those intended to ensure the comfort of patients such as 'spontaneous breathing modes' which allow the patient to breathe in synchronicity with the device, making it easier for them to be weaned off the machine.[19] Prioritising cost efficiency over patient need is especially dangerous because breathing, while universal, is characterised by extreme subjectivity and variability. One size will never fit all when it comes to breath prosthetics. We can see this by reviewing the discussions of ambulatory oxygen for home use after its introduction in 1968, through which we can assess the extent to which concerns about costs and the possible dangers of oxygen toxicity outweighed consideration of patient's non-medical needs. Consideration of the weight of the object, its portability, appearance and noise level, was secondary to its cost efficiency. As disability scholars have demonstrated, the frequent disjunct between the medical design of prosthesis and the needs of intended users has often stemmed from the medical model of disability.[20] The medical model paradigm defines disability as a loss of function or impairment, which medical intervention ideally would be able to cure. This is in opposition to the social model of disability, which attributes the discrimination and problems faced by disabled people as wholly resulting from the society in which they live. Prosthetic technologies have thus been criticised as being a 'technological fix' for problems which are in fact more social than medical.[21]

Not all prosthetic designs fit easily within the medical/social model binary. Hearing assistive devices, for instance, rely on the embodied knowledge of the user and have often been designed in co-production with people with hearing loss.[22] The process of co-production then, may be particularly important in devices used in conditions like breathlessness, which is usually personal, invisible and intimate. However, the crucial role of the patient/user is frequently devalued within the medical model paradigm.

In what follows, we start our chapter by outlining the twentieth-century developments to mechanical respirators which set up use of the Bragg-Paul Pulsator in opposition to iron lung style devices. The dichotomy presented between these two machines reflected the tension between the heterogeneity of individual breathing and the need for a standardised breathing machine. This need for technological consistency was especially important to the MRC. Indeed, their interwar report on 'breathing machines' reveals that their drive for standardisation worked in opposition to patients' diverse experiences of these machines. As well, there are many parallels between the current ventilator procurement programme and the interwar debate over respiratory technologies. Who ought to be responsible for providing and perfecting such technologies? Should respiratory technologies be designed by engineers or by medical men? Or by those using the technologies themselves? How were users' voices heard in the context of this debate? These questions crystallised around the MRC's crucial interwar debate about which breathing machines were best: those using negative pressure or those using positive pressure. In this chapter we analyse the extent to which users were involved in this debate. We also explore how the eventual emergence of the iron lung as the standard 'breathing machine' shaped patients' experiences in hospitals in the post-war period. And, finally, we reflect on how diverse patient needs were incorporated into the administration of portable oxygen concentrators in the context of the National Health Service (NHS).

## Mechanical respirators, 1930–39

In the 1930s, the application of respiratory technologies increasingly focused on respiratory paralysis caused by the polio epidemics that seasonally ravaged Britain. The MRC estimated in 1939 there were at least 600 cases of respiratory paralysis a year that required technological intervention to assist in breathing.[23] The term 'iron lung' respirator – a negative pressure ventilator to assist in breathing when muscle control is lost or limited – was often used in general terms as an eponym in the interwar period for any kind of respirator, but the machine was actually one of many technologies adapted at the time to enable artificial breathing. The first 'iron lungs' were designed in the United States at Harvard University by Philip Drinker (1894–1972) and Louis Agassiz Shaw Jr. (1886–1940). These machines used negative pressure to create a vacuum and force a patient's diaphragm to expand and contract to exert alternating pressure through a push-pull motion.[24] By regulating the rate and depth of respiration, the device allowed for prolonged artificial respiration, either until the patient recovered muscle strength or until an alternative method of treatment became available.

The Drinker respirator, as it became known, was first used in Britain in 1930.[25] However, it was expensive: costs ranged from £200 to £2,000 depending on export fees. Bulky and heavy, it was difficult to transport. Moreover, some hospitals lacked the necessary funds and space for obtaining the machine. Indeed, even though Drinker and Edgar L. Roy offered instructions for building an emergency makeshift respirator with common hardware materials, the apparatus was not as widely used in Britain as in the United States.[26] It was eventually superseded by Australian inventor Edward T. Both's (1908–87) plywood-based iron lung, which was presented as a more affordable alternative.[27] Like the Drinker respirator, the Both iron lung required the patient to be entirely encased in a cabinet with only their head protruding out with only the capacity to eat, drink and sleep.[28] The depth and rate of breathing was controlled by an attendant, not by the patient.[29] One user described the challenge of moderating eating and breathing patterns to the machine by explaining that:

> You can eat in the iron lung because your head is outside but the rest of your body is inside, although since you are flat on your back you really need to be careful when you swallow; you have to swallow in rhythm with the machine because it's pulling your diaphragm in and then pushing it out again. You just wait until it's breathing out and then you swallow. Coughing was a bit more difficult because you don't cough in rhythm with the iron lung. It was something you had to work around.[30]

By comparison, through using positive pressure to force expiration of air, the Bragg-Paul Pulsator represented a cheap and *portable* alternative to the iron lung respirators, designed so that it could be carried by a single porter for use in a private home or ward.[31] Bragg's initial iteration worked through manual rhythmical manipulation of the pump, with Paul ensuring that the bellows could also be actuated by hand if needed. Yet, even though their design provided greater agency to the patient by freeing them from completely mechanised enclosure, the breathing was still controlled by an attendant. This reliance and the need to protect the Pulsator against any unforeseen complications (e.g. electrical or water failures) meant that Halahan was never left alone. He was also to use his tongue and teeth without breath to sound an alarm 'resembling that of a bird' to alert the attendant.[32] This technique holds parallels with the 'frog breathing' described by Daniel Wilson, which involved patients with paralysed chests utilising the muscles of the neck instead to breathe in a gulping fashion 'like a frog'.[33]

The benefits of a portable, semi-mechanical respirator being widely available were not lost on Bragg and Paul. Indeed, as early as 1933, Bragg contacted several hospitals to inquire as to whether there was any medical interest in the Pulsator. One reply, from K.N. Knapp of Swindon and North Wilts Victoria Hospital, agreed that it would be beneficial to have the device in the hospital and that such 'a semi-mechanical respirator would often be most useful, and would save labour and Staff'.[34] Knapp also advised Bragg to contact physiologists to improve the mechanisation of the device. In January 1934, Bragg invited physiologist A.V. Hill (1886–1977) to inspect the machine and asked whether he had any suggestions for its improvement.[35] Hill suggested Paul contact Dr Edward Poulton at the London School of Hygiene and Tropical Medicine, to help work out how to standardise the measurements of ventilation efficiency needed for different patients.[36] This was a necessary step for allowing large-scale usage of the respirator and for its incorporation into a hospital setting.

Intrigued by the device, Poulton agreed that the Pulsator should be widely distributed to hospitals, but before this could be done, the device needed to be put through a series of rigorous physiological tests to determine its efficacy and safety. Subsequently, Poulton hoped to make clinical tests with the device at Guy's Hospital, perceiving its potential value for treating asphyxia in newborns.[37] To this end, Poulton recommended that Paul should consult physiologist Dr Phyllis Kerridge (1901–40), who would play a pivotal role in making the respirator viable for widespread hospital use and adaptable to different bodies.

After testing the physiological parameters of the device, Kerridge suggested simplifying the 'waistcoat' by adding an airbag lined with canvas and vulcanised together, thereby allowing the lining to circumvent the awkward bellying of the bag.[38] She suggested this form and mode of application as well as working out the best position of the airbags and the measurements of ventilation efficiency needed to introduce it to the medical profession.[39] The pressure of the belt could be adjusted, with several sizes available to suit different patients, including infants; the belt was to be worn over an undergarment which would not crease and cause discomfort to the patient's skin.[40] It also allowed for adjustment to suit individual respiratory rate.[41]

To ensure the Pulsator was available to hospitals, and to popularise it as an alternative to iron lungs, Paul assumed the financial responsibility to order six devices for hospitals using his personal limited funds. Both Bragg and Paul explained that they were not 'financially interested' in their machine and thus chose not to patent it or request royalties.[42] The machine was then manufactured by the firm Siebe Gorman and Co. (who had made the Haldane gas masks) and they proposed a cost of £30 which would be worth approximately £1,500 today.[43] They also substituted steel for brass in certain parts to 'strengthen the design of the apparatus'.[44] By this stage the Pulsator was electrically driven and Bragg emphasised that this meant it was 'practically noiseless' – an attractive improvement over the Drinker respirator, which was notoriously loud.[45] Its externally audible noisiness was amplified further for users, who could also feel the pump vibrations. Thirteen Pulsators were installed in British hospitals by 1937 (a further six were sent overseas) and another sixteen were on order.[46] Even more were placed on backorder, perhaps because in 1938 there were several polio outbreaks and an increased number of diphtheria cases requiring ventilators.[47]

The Pulsator's highest profile promotion was given by the BBC on a Friday night on 8 July 1938. The BBC sent out an emergency SOS for a Bragg-Paul Pulsator needed at an Ipswich Hospital to save the life of a child.[48] One was immediately sent by car from a London Hospital, but the patient died while it was in transit.[49] On 14 July 1938, this case was discussed in the House of Commons and the Minister of Health was asked whether he could provide more Pulsators to hospitals throughout Britain to extend coverage from the eighteen already in use.[50] Similarly, on 24 July 1938, a fifty-eight-year-old man died in the Royal Infirmary in Liverpool after a plane was sent to rush a Bragg-Paul respirator from Ipswich to Liverpool.[51] Presumably, the respirator had been in Ipswich since it was sent from London previously, and it was immediately sent back by train for another patient. Such well-publicised crises generated a media furore but there was some initial confusion in the press between the Drinker respirator and the Pulsator. Paul hastened to write to Dr Sommerville Hastings following the broadcast to explain the advantages of the Pulsator: 'I, personally, find it hard to imagine the continuous use of the other type for three years on a patient'.[52] However, Hasting replied that the Drinker respirator was thought by physiologists to be better because it used negative pressure (creating a vacuum) which more closely imitated natural breathing.[53]

## Patient experiences in the machine

The debate over positive versus negative pressure led to the MRC appointing a committee to investigate the best mechanical apparatus for 'preventing asphyxia due to respiratory paralysis'.[54] This subject demanded immediate attention, as a serious polio epidemic had hit England and Wales in 1938.[55] Kerridge initially suggested to the Ministry of Health that there should be a large-scale survey on infantile paralysis and the potential of artificial respiration.[56] The Ministry, however, rejected the survey but inquired on the position of the Pulsator in comparison to other artificial respirators, thus forming a 'Respirators (Poliomyelitis) Committee' comprised of eight medical professionals, including Kerridge, and a secretary.[57] Patients and users were not considered as possible members of this committee, which was convened to 'examine the various forms of machine available and to consider the problem from the physiological point of view'.[58] The study aimed to analyse and compare the relative merits of all available mechanical apparatus for preventing asphyxia following the request from the Ministry of Health. Initially, the committee aimed to evaluate which pressure was best for artificial respiration and thereby conclude whether the Bragg-Paul Pulsator or the iron lung device should be recommended as standard. However, the variability of respiratory conditions under consideration and the complexities of individual cases meant that the report expanded to consider a wide variety of 'breathing machines'.

The committee divided power-driven machines into three categories: first, machines that enclosed the full body of the patient; second, machines that enclosed the body and head; and finally, machines that did not involve total enclosure of the body. These categories suggest how bodily autonomy and movement of the patient were factored into the usefulness and effectiveness of the machines. The Barospirator was invented in 1906 and was the only device that enclosed both the body and the head. It worked like the earlier oxygen rooms, through strict atmospheric controls applied to a large chamber which the patient and up to two others could remain in. The control of carbon dioxide that this necessitated was considered by the committee to be too onerous and so this invention was not given detailed consideration.

Thus, the main debate was between full-body enclosure or not. Full-body enclosure devices included the Drinker respirator, the Drinker-Collins respirator, the Emerson respirator, the Henderson respirator, the Siebe-Gorman 'drinker' respirator and the Both respirator. Devices that worked without full-body enclosure included the Biomotor of Dr Eisenmenger, the Bragg-Paul Pulsator, the Burstall Jacket respirator, the London County Council Cuirass respirator, the Turner Jacket respirator, the Laffer Lewis Apparatus and Eve's Motor Rocking Bed. The latter device worked on a different principle from the others: rather than using negative or positive pressure, it used gravity and the weight of the patient to force the diaphragm to move in and out. Such rocking beds were used regularly in the United States on partially paralysed polio patients but this one was presumably included under power driven machines because it used an electronic motor to rock the bed.[59]

In the section of the MRC report on 'preparing the patient for the machine' we find details about what kind of clothes the patient should wear in a box style device. Only pyjama trousers and an undervest were allowed until the patient was secured inside the machine and then the pyjama jacket was put on back to front to avoid skin irritation due to the neck rubbing against the rubber neck-hole.[60] A thin layer of cotton wool was also applied (and held in place with a bandage) to avoid such skin irritation. It was crucial that 'bedsocks' were then worn to avoid chilled feet from the air that rushed in from the suction hole at the end of the machine and blankets were strategically placed to prevent patient complaints of 'cold spots' and to avoid bed sores. Careful consideration of clothing and handling of the patient was important because of patient complaints of extreme tenderness and 'hyperaesthesia' (excessive skin sensitivity) which could make any handling very painful and distressing.[61] Adjusting the temperature of the patient within the machine was clearly an issue of some concern, and heated lamps within the cabinet were utilised alongside hot water bottles and bellows (for cooling). Learning to eat and drink also required adjustment, as users had to learn how to adjust their swallowing to fit with the rhythms of the machine.[62] The complicated relationship between breathing and eating was memorably described by home ventilation user David Brooks in 1990:

> In addition to breathing, body movements, walking and talking, the most energy sapping activity is surprisingly eating. Having lost so much weight following lung cancer, the removal of my right lung and radiotherapy, it rather added insult to injury to find that the mechanics of eating, swallowing and digesting so intimately involved the respiratory system. Exhausted swallowing muscles and pain filled chest muscles convulse along with my uselessly flapping diaphragm. They are my accompaniments to meal times, a constant battle ground between the requirements of nutrition and the insistent distress of respiratory despair.[63]

The MRC report also highlighted significant concerns about how best to synchronise an individual's breathing with the rhythm of the machine. If conscious, patients could 'frequently' indicate what pressure felt most comfortable and best matched their personal breathing rate.[64] However, it seems that this did not always lead to a perfect fit, as:

> the Patient's breathing will usually be, for a short time, irregular and 'out of step' with the regular breathing of the machine, but cases with respiratory insufficiency readily adapt themselves to the rate of the machine. If the patient's breathing persistently fails to synchronise, it means that he has an adequate power of natural breathing and does not require treatment in the machine.[65]

This reveals the difficulty inherent in standardising measures for a process as individual and variable as breathing. Moreover, the suggestion that users adapt themselves to the rate of the machine indicates that they were expected to modify themselves to fit the technology rather than the other way around. If patients were continually unable to adapt themselves in this way or were apprehensive of doing so, the breathing rate was adjusted slowly and without their knowledge.[66] Alternatively, they were simply given a sedative, which was 'not required for long, as most patients soon learn to co-operate with the machine'.[67] Clearly, there was awareness of how distressing these breathing machines could be for users. However, the MRC report insisted that for seriously ill patients 'the relief afforded is so great and so sudden that any psychological stress is quickly banished'.[68] Perhaps surprisingly given Bragg's reference to noise as a problem, the rhythmical noise of the motor was suggested here to be soothing and conducive to deep sleeping. This assessment is in marked contrast to Brooks' (admittedly much later) description of sleeping in an assisted ventilation unit: 'the noise at night of all these pumps, huffing and puffing, inevitably at different tempos, was rather like a poorly syncopated orchestra with a demented wind section'.[69] The impact of the noise of the various breathing machines discussed in this chapter is a resounding theme, and the impact that noise had on patients' ability to integrate these machines into their lives has been consistently underestimated by designers. The possibilities for sleeping, holding conversations and disguising prosthetic devices are all diminished as sound is increased.[70]

Indeed, the MRC's optimistic analysis is not wholly supported by the details provided in the appendix to their report, which provides quantitative and qualitative details in relation to individual case reports involving use of the Drinker respirator and the Bragg-Paul Pulsator.[71] There are repeated instances of user rejection in these tables. For instance, one patient survived treatment with the Both type respirator but 'objected strongly to being put in it'.[72] One patient using the Bragg-Paul Pulsator 'tended to breathe against it' and died after a day of its use. Similarly, another user of the Bragg-Paul Pulsator had difficulty adjusting to its breathing rate: 'Difficulty in synchronisation of artificial and natural respiration caused discomfort and led to cessation of treatment.'[73] Many patients simply refused to use the machines. Although some patients survived, in other cases this refusal was noted as contributing in their death. In certain cases, the patient is simply noted to have found the machine either a source of 'relief' or as 'uncomfortable', though one specific case noted 'discomfort in machine so severe that patient's removal from it was ordered'.[74] Another patient was described as 'so terror-stricken by machine that he had to be removed'.[75] Overall, user experiences of these 'breathing machines' varied considerably. Crucially, the user's inability or unwillingness to use the machines was a repeated motif and clearly affected the viability of this kind of treatment.

One key appeal of the Pulsator was that once worn, the patient was not hindered or inconvenienced by its movements. With an attachment, moreover, it could also be used by two patients at the same time, forcing them to literally conspire together in the original sense of the Latin, *con* (with) and *spirare* (breathe).[76] However, there was concern that positive pressure respiration could depress circulation and reduce cardiac output and blood pressure, a concern which was heightened for bulbar polio patients suffering from circulatory damage.[77] It was crucial then, the MRC decided, for patients using an artificial respirator to be under the expert management of doctors, nurses and other attendants who were 'acquainted with certain points and difficulties which arise during the use of mechanical aids to respiration', especially when repair was required.[78] Care was also necessary to ensure that infections, bed sores, vomiting and constipation were managed so as not to cause serious complications, especially in patients with respiratory paralysis.

PLATE I                                              *To face page 12*

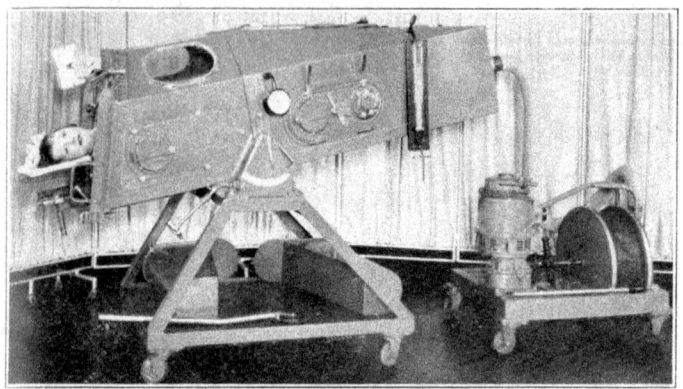

Fig. A.—Drinker Respirator, English Model, as made by Siebe Gorman & Co., Ltd.

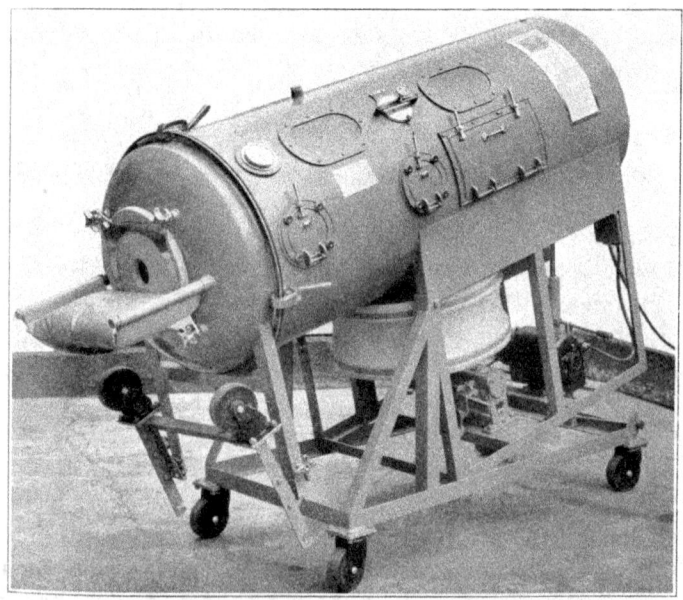

Fig. B.—Drinker-Collins Respirator, Tilting-Rotating Model.

**6.1** The Drinker Respirator and Drinker-Collins Respirator (1939)

The MRC report on '"Breathing Machines" and their Use in Treatment', came out in 1939, just as William Morris, the later Lord Nuffield (1877–1963) announced his intent to distribute free of charge 800 Both respirators throughout Britain. Morris manufactured the iron lungs in his car factories and eventually donated more than 5,000 of these devices.[79] The donation of iron lungs to hospitals throughout Britain allowed for free and easy institutional usage, especially as the MRC recommended that it was more beneficial to bring patients to the hospital rather than to bring equipment to the home. By the end of March 1939, there were approximately 1,000 respirators in the British Isles: 965 Both respirators, 43 Bragg-Paul Pulsators and 30 Drinker respirators.[80]

## From home to hospital

Bringing patients to the hospital and placing them in these machines became standard practice after the Second World War. However, this solution (while medically and economically advisable) could lead to added distress for families who lost the ability to communicate with their loved ones. Not only were patients quarantined (physically isolated), but it was also difficult for them to communicate with the medical team due to their encasement and reduced visibility in the iron lung. This encasement literally impeded patient voice, as they could only talk on the out-breath of the machine. We can determine the practical consequences of such isolation from cases like that of Dorothy (aged sixteen), who woke in the night of 28 September 1950 with severe back pain.[81] Over the next two days her pain worsened, until she was vomiting from agony and forced to go to the now-obsolete Ham Green Hospital in Bristol. The attending doctor noted that she had widespread paralysis and diagnosed APM (acute poliomyelitis). Her subsequent isolation caused severe anxiety to her mother, who wrote to the hospital to explain:

> when Dorothy was taken away I had 2 shocks first was to be told by her own Dr, that Dorothy was 10 weeks pregnant, second was to hear she had Polio, this has drove me nearly crazey [sic] with worry, as Dorothy was in such awful pain I decided not to say anything to her about being pregnant until she was better, but instead she got worse and was taken away.[82]

Plate III

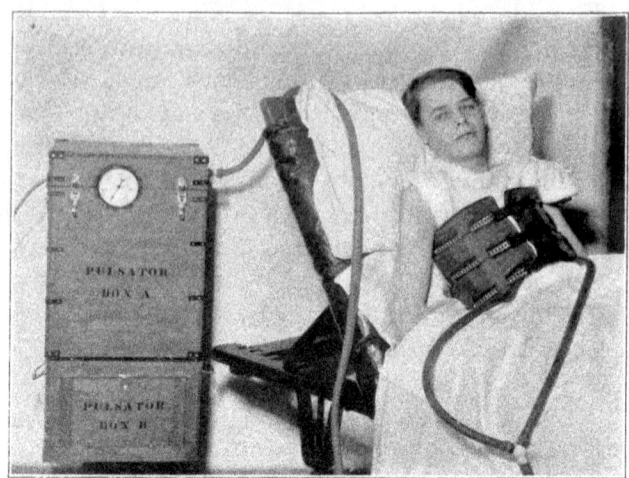

Fig. A.—Bragg-Paul Pulsator.

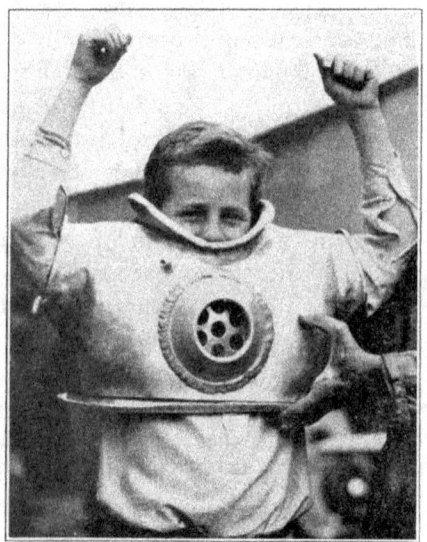

Fig. B.—Burstall Jacket Respirator (being fitted).

**6.2** The Bragg-Paul Pulsator and Burstall Jacket Respirator (1939)

The physician treating Dorothy replied somewhat caustically that 'I can hardly doubt but that Dorothy knows quite well that she is pregnant', but reassured her mother that the paralysis was improving and that Dorothy had not lost the baby. However, by the end of November he decided that it was necessary to terminate the pregnancy to save the patient. It was clear that the patient would not survive artificial respiration while pregnant. In the context of our current struggle against COVID-19 – another virus that compromises respiratory function – Dorothy's suffering is a sobering reminder of the need for accessible emergency abortion and contraception services, even in the midst of a global pandemic. After her abortion, Dorothy's condition rapidly improved, she was able to undergo physiotherapy and after ninety-four days in hospital, she was discharged. Although her experience was undoubtedly traumatic for her and her family (she was described twice in the notes as hysterical), Dorothy's case at least ended with recovery.

By contrast, polio patient Rose (aged twenty-nine) was admitted to the same hospital on 16 October 1950 and was immediately placed in a mechanical respirator.[83] Her abdominal reflexes were described as 'absent' and she had 'little movement' in her diaphragm. Her distress was such that she was only partially examined before being placed straight into the respirator. While in the respirator, she was given physiotherapy 'in so far as can be managed with patient in respirator'.[84] By December, she could be taken out of the respirator for controlled periods, only initially managing two–three minutes but up to four–five minutes by the end of the month. On 31 December 1950 there was an electricity failure in the hospital which meant Rose 'almost died' before it was possible to get the 'manual operation working'. This may be the reason that six days later she was transferred from the Drinker respirator to the Both respirator – a change which made her both more cheerful and comfortable. However, over the following month she contracted pneumonia and, despite rallying towards the end of January, she had a 'sudden attack of dyspnoea' (breathlessness) at midnight on 1 February 1951, became unconscious, was briefly revived to be described as 'terrified' and subsequently died.

The practice of gradually building up the time the patient spent breathing unaided outside the respirator was a standard treatment for polio patients with respiratory paralysis, especially as it allowed them to participate in physiotherapy.[85] Patients using the respirator were encouraged to stay out for longer periods and once they could remain out for forty-five minutes, they started taking their meals outside the machine. Although adult patients were relatively isolated and relied on epistolary correspondence to communicate with the outside world, parents were able to visit younger children living in the iron lungs, often for extended periods. One such child patient spent 218 days in the hospital in the Drinker respirator. When he died, the attending physician at the hospital described it as a 'welcome event', noting that he 'would never have lived independent of respirator' but that he was 'quite cheerful up to end. Parents helped a great deal by visiting daily without fail'.[86] The child's GP agreed with this assessment and wrote to the hospital physician to thank him for his care and noted, 'I agree with you that it was the best thing that could have happened to the poor child, under the unhappy circumstances'.[87] These notes illuminate the changing conception of the respirator, from a prosthetic enabling the user to continue life at home, to emergency hospital equipment in which life was considered untenable. Even though these patients were described as cheerful, the iron lung was not being used in the hospital as a prosthetic in the way that Halahan had used his Pulsator at home. However, there is evidence that some contemporary users were using iron lungs to live full and productive lives in this period, as in the case of Mr Fred Suite, who lived in an iron lung for three years before getting married in 1939 and going on honeymoon in a specially weight adapted trailer.[88] There are also accounts of users of iron lungs and their family members designing home-made personalised machines during this period in Britain. For instance, in 1949 Mr A.F. Evans, a motor engineer in Coventry designed a specific style of iron lung for his daughter which would allow her to live at home. He explained that he had built the device in his garage with some assistance from his employees and his daughter's friend, and emphasised that, 'This new lung I have made covers only the abdomen and chest. It keeps Ann breathing and allows the physiotherapist to give massage and to exercise the limbs to bring fresh life into them'.[89] Another twenty-six-year-old man in Essex who had virtually no movement except of his head and neck lived at home and was reported to 'frog-breathe for up to three hours but otherwise needs a Tunnicliffe respirator and pump'.[90] In a letter to the editor of the *Lancet*, his doctor detailed the different organisation involved in his care: 'The County Health Department provide a special nurse; the local council have altered the house; the GPO installed a telephone within 24 hours; the next-door neighbour services the pump; and the Association for the Physically Handicapped have helped in many ways.'[91]

However, while some users emphasised the greater portability and independence that chest-only devices offered, others preferred the all-encompassing relief offered by the standard iron lung's negative pressure. For example, Marshall Barr contracted polio in 1949 and began using an iron lung in 1971. He described the experience of encasement as a 'relief' and highlighted the relaxing qualities of its sounds and vibrations, 'Like: ... breathing, bump; breathing, bump ... It was not quite like a smooth breath'.[92] Paul Alexander, who started using an iron lung in 1952, used it in his university dorm in the United States to pursue a successful career as a lawyer; he still remains in the machine.[93] In 2017, Martha Lillard, one of three people still using iron lungs in the United States described how the lung provided relief by taking away the effort of breathing for her: 'Imagine if you were real tired of breathing, how good that would feel – if you were struggling to take a breath'.[94] For Martha and others still reliant on these older technologies, one of the main challenges is finding technicians willing to repair the iron lungs, as the private companies which originally designed them no longer take responsibility for maintaining them.[95]

As this chapter has emphasised, the heterogeneity of respiratory disability experiences proved challenging for the development of standardised treatments. Assorted 'breathing machines' facilitated patient breath while simultaneously impeding patient voice. This historical analysis highlights the importance of prioritising patient voices today, especially when making judgements about quality of life. Caution in this respect is highlighted by the existence of 'the disability paradox'. That is, the fact that many disabled people rate their quality of life as good or excellent although external observers imagine them to have an 'undesirable daily existence'.[96] This was illuminated by a seminal 1999 investigation in which the disabled people surveyed reported problems related to discrimination, day-to-day activities and society, but nevertheless reported excellent or good quality of life.[97] At the same time, when asked to imagine the wellbeing of disabled people, non-disabled people tend to imagine it to be far worse than it is. This error is exacerbated if the non-disabled person is a healthcare professional and corrected if they have spent time with disabled people. Recent studies have shown that even in states of illness that healthy observers rate as being worse than death, the people with the actual conditions reported similar levels of wellbeing as the healthy counterparts.[98] Given these findings, this historical episode highlights the crucial importance of centring patient voices and especially disabled voices in all discussions about prosthetic technology. Amplifying disabled voices is especially crucial in situations where resources are scarce. Amid attempts to mitigate the worst effects of the COVID-19 pandemic, the prospect of scarce ventilator resources has meant that decisions to deny life-saving treatment to some disabled people are normalised as an inevitable result of 'triage'.[99] In such cases it is key, as journalist and disability activist Frances Ryan has argued, that we differentiate decisions about *treatment efficacy* from judgements about quality of life.[100] More awareness of the high quality of life experienced by disabled people might change the way we make these assessments. More awareness, too, of the long history of disabled innovation (without which we would lack most of the communication technology we currently rely on so heavily) might also help. Indeed, there is a lot we could learn from disabled people should we chose to listen. However, highlighting the triumphs and innovations of disabled people should not be necessary. Disabled life does not have to be useful to 'count'. As Ryan explains:

> In recent days, I have seen disabled people take to social media to list their achievements, as if trying to make the case that they are worth saving. A disabled person who has their ventilator removed during this crisis may have gone on to cure cancer. But then, they may have just been loved. A mum with heart disease who always burns her daughter's birthday cakes. An accountant born with muscular dystrophy who watches *Doctor Who* every Sunday. Disabled people, like all minorities, are only fully human when we are permitted to be as wonderfully average as anyone else.[101]

Providing adequate funding to enable disabled people to live full lives in their own homes has been a key part of facilitating autonomy and full participation in society. The development of portable oxygen has been a key part of that story, as we will see in the following section.

## Oxygen in the home, 1940–present day

While the mechanical respirators were a tremendous advance on manual methods previously available for assisting respiration or treating respiratory failure, the eventual confinement of these machines to the hospital posed a challenge for patients facing life-long respiratory paralysis. The shift from hospital to home also coincided with a greater need for patient autonomy, especially as most poliomyelitis and diphtheria survivors were young when first afflicted with the disease. Moreover, when routine polio vaccination was introduced in the 1950s, cases of polio were dramatically reduced and breathing machines for paralysis became less necessary. Thereafter, home respiratory medicine focused more on the use of oxygen to support people who could breathe, but whose lungs could not absorb enough oxygen.

Between 1940 and 1968 oxygen for clinical use was primarily stored in liquid form, kept in cylinders that could be refilled either from a central dispensary, at depots belonging to the British Oxygen Company, or from a larger cylinder stored in patients' homes.[102] The British Oxygen Company was at that time mainly concerned with providing oxygen and other gases for industry and commerce and its provision of portable oxygen devices was only 'a tiny part of its activities'.[103] There were repeated calls for new methods of administering clinical oxygen due to difficulties with supply and transportation. However, alternatives to oxygen cylinders (such as oxygen concentrators) were still in the early stages of development. In 1968, a landmark American study showed that oxygen was safe to use in the home in a controlled fashion and argued that portable oxygen concentrators would allow users with Chronic Obstructive Pulmonary Disease (COPD) to increase their activity levels.[104] However, there were concerns over the cost of developing these new technologies in Britain.[105]

Oxygen usage in Britain was also delayed because of concerns about potentially dangerous side-effects. An increasing number of cases of blindness caused by retrolental fibroplasia in premature infants led to great concern over the use of oxygen therapy. At the start of this period, there was a general consensus that there was almost no risk of oxygen poisoning from continual oxygen use.[106] However, in the 1950s studies emerged which confirmed a link between the development of retrolental fibroplasia in premature infants and overly high levels of oxygen concentration administered during therapy for respiratory issues.[107] A simple solution to this problem was found by reducing the environmental concentration of oxygen used to treat premature infants. This resulted in a huge reduction in the number of these cases and in addition there appeared to be no adverse effect on mortality rates due to respiratory illness.[108] However, these incidents created a lasting fear around clinical oxygen usage which persisted into later years and limited the development of certain therapies.

These fears were augmented by concerns over oxygen prescription. Such concerns were highlighted in a House of Commons debate on 10 December 1974, which outlined case studies of patients undergoing home oxygen therapy and discussed the best ways to administer and distribute oxygen systems. Peter Hardy, MP for Rother Valley, instigated this debate due to the plight of one of his constituents, Mr J. Aisbitt. Mr Aisbitt suffered from a severe case of pneumoconiosis owing to his time as a miner and because of this illness he had extremely poor quality of life. Hardy explained that Aisbitt was unable to leave his home for months at a time because he needed to stay close to the large oxygen cylinders at his home.[109] Eventually the local branch of the Royal British Legion purchased a portable oxygen appliance (a Portogen appliance from the British Oxygen Company) for Aisbitt so that he might have greater freedom and independence. However, Mr Hardy was greatly concerned that this equipment had to be acquired privately and was not widely available through the NHS. Although patients could be prescribed domiciliary oxygen therapy for the home, Hardy emphasised that there were very few portable oxygen appliances available (less than a dozen in the east of England in 1972–74) and that the devices that were available were used only in the hospitals for emergencies and midwifery cases, 'and not for people who spend most of their time in their own home'.[110] While Hardy acknowledged that such equipment could be bought privately, he argued that 'many of those disabled by chest disease have been among the poorest in the community for years, perhaps decades, and the £40 or so involved in purchasing the appliance and recharging equipment could not easily be found by them'.[111] In response, Alec Jones, the Under-Secretary of State for Health and Social Security, acknowledged problems about the lack of portable oxygen devices but emphasised 'that the prescription of breathing appliances is a medical matter'.[112] As a result, he argued that their administration was best confined to the hospital and warned about the risk of fire hazards from oxygen users refilling portable devices from their main cylinders. He also highlighted possible risks of user dependency and outlined the potential problems associated with supplying portable oxygen outside the hospital.[113]

Primarily these problems related to the administration, maintenance and supply of oxygen therapy. These tripartite concerns reflect those outlined in a 1969 *Lancet* article on domiciliary oxygen, which discussed both the cost of maintaining oxygen supply as well as the physical inconvenience of the equipment. Its authors maintained that these difficulties were not as insurmountable as commonly perceived.[114] However, they were also concerned about the variability of user responses and the fact that even those who responded positively to the treatment found the equipment uncomfortable.[115]

Problems related to user response and comfort were also superseded by concerns about equipment costs. Petty and Finigan's original study on continuous oxygen therapy in the United States for the treatment of patients with COPD concluded that, while highly effective as a treatment for COPD, the cost and maintenance of the equipment was a disproportionate financial burden for patients already suffering from a disability which inhibited their ability to work and earn.[116] Cost efficiency was thus prioritised over usability in the development of newer systems, such as oxygen concentrators.[117] The oxygen concentrator was first discussed in depth in 1973 by Stark and Bishop in an article that focused on the Rimer-Birlec oxygen concentrator, which was cheaper than the cylinders, but louder and less reliable. While its economic benefits were undeniable, its large size and excessive noise levels meant that few individuals could realistically use this system, as they found the loudness of the noise unbearable.[118] Though patient comfort was discussed here, it was addressed (as in most studies of this period) in one or two sentences which outlined the need for improvement without offering suggestions for how such improvements could be accomplished. The overriding concern of these studies was not user experience, but rather the challenge of marrying clinical sufficiency with economic sustainability. User experience was considered in terms of the impact of different systems on patient quality of life, which was measured using the proxy of hospital visits. For example, one 1975 study demonstrated the positive effect of home oxygen therapy on patients' quality of life by showing the reduction of hospital visits and thus demonstrated that patient benefits were aligned with economic concerns through decreases in hospitalisation.[119]

Cost reduction was a constant concern for those administering oxygen therapy, as they struggled to connect the expense with the variable and individual medical benefits. For instance, a 1978 study in the *British Medical Journal* praised users who relied on oxygen only intermittently as 'a relatively small drain on resources'.[120] This study described in detail the process of receiving home oxygen at this time, which involved the user handing in their prescription to the chemist, who would then obtain the cylinder from the British Oxygen Company. At this time the British Oxygen Company enjoyed a virtual monopoly over NHS oxygen usage – something that was criticised in a 1984 debate in the House of Lords during which Lord Young of Dartington pointed out that the company controlled 'nearly 100 per cent of the medical gases which are supplied to the National Health Service' at a cost of £35 million each year.[121]

Thus, in Britain the focus on patient use and experience was centred around the practicality of administering oxygen and maintaining the equipment in an economically efficient fashion, whereas studies in the United States more seriously considered patients' personal experiences of using the equipment, including the experience of stigma. For example, Petty, Nett and Lakshminarayan's 1973 study was one of the few which discussed patients' reluctance to use two nasal prongs because they were more conspicuous compared to a single prong which could be more easily disguised and afforded a less visible treatment.[122] British studies offered more focus on the practicality of using these systems. For instance, a 1973 study by Stark, Finnigan and Bishop into long-term domiciliary oxygen for patients with chronic bronchitis gave definite consideration to practicable long-term oxygen treatment in the home and the best methods of administration to allow for a fuller life, though the emphasis was still very much on the medical aspects of the treatment.[123] A more considerate approach to patient use was previously offered in a 1969 study which evaluated multiple oxygen therapy devices. This study concluded that the nasal cannula was the most effective method not because of its clinical benefits, but because it was preferred by patients. That it was the most comfortable method for users made it more effective.[124] Another *Lancet* article suggested that for use in public places the apparatus could be made less stigmatising through adaption of 'an inconspicuous palm breathing device instead of a mask'.[125] Such considerations are crucial. Today, breathlessness is often normalised in communities where smoking is prevalent, which are often low socio-economic areas.[126] This adds to the invisibility and stigmatisation of COPD, which arises from its association with both smoking and ageing, meaning that users who are prescribed ambulatory oxygen often reject or conceal its use to 'pass' as well.[127] Management of breathlessness without fear of stigma is critical to successful self-management and the ability to retain a strong sense of self: 'For those with chronic dyspnoea, there is ultimately a sense of the diminishment of identity; of not being able to be the person that they once were or wish to be'.[128]

There were further attempts to improve patient experience when using oxygen therapy in the 1980 Nocturnal Oxygen Therapy Trial (NOTT) of the US National Heart Lung and Blood Institute. This study investigated shorter therapies and took into consideration the need to monitor patients' overall quality of life.[129] It established that long-term oxygen could improve survival, especially if given continuously (as opposed to only nocturnally or intermittently). The year after this was published (1981) the MRC Working Party released findings from a three-year multi-centre-controlled trail meant to determine whether long-term domiciliary oxygen could improve mortality and quality of life for its users. This was an important and oft-cited study, which demonstrated no evidence of oxygen toxicity and showed reduced mortality in both men and women. Patients in this trail reported 'general improvement in the sense of wellbeing, improved appetite, and general alertness' although the researchers cautioned that these 'subjective impressions, although doubtless very important, could not be quantified' and were not correlated with the proxy measure for quality of life usually used – number of hospital stays.[130] It also highlighted the fact that oxygen usage seemed to have a greater impact on women, as the 'mortality of the control women was significantly more than that of the treated women from the start of the study', but the low numbers of women in the trail (twenty-one versus sixty-six men) meant that it was difficult to determine why this was.[131]

Administering home oxygen therapy to patients proved difficult during this period, as were evaluations of its efficacy. Though there was general agreement that it was beneficial, in many cases concerns over cost, possible risk to patient health and complications with the equipment made it hard for studies to form conclusive results. Concerns over ease of use centred around balancing what was best for patient quality of life with cost limitations. There were concerns about over-administration of oxygen and cost-cutting efforts focused on making sure that the right people were prescribed oxygen therapy and that they were then monitored to ensure proper and consistent use for the most effective results.[132] One study assessed prescription and usage in the home through questionnaires and home visits from respiratory nurses and found that in some cases patients had not actually been assessed by a respiratory physician, only diagnosed and prescribed treatment of oxygen cylinders 'as standard' to be used sporadically to decrease breathlessness. It claimed that 'although there are established indications for the provision of long-term oxygen therapy with concentrators the indications for treatment with intermittent oxygen using cylinders are less clear'.[133] Another study called for patients to be reassessed at three months and then again at a year after starting treatment.[134] Such inconsistencies in the practice of assessing and prescribing oxygen treatment to patients fuelled clinical concerns about over-administration.

Concerns about how patients were being assessed for oxygen therapy merged with concerns about the subsequent rate of compliance. Patient co-operation became an issue at this point only because very little attempt had previously been made to monitor their co-operation. A 1985 article in the *Lancet* on domiciliary oxygen criticised the guidelines for failing to emphasise strongly enough the importance of patient co-operation. For instance, difficulties arose because many users of oxygen were smokers, who needed to scrupulously avoid smoking while using oxygen to avoid accidental self-immolation. In one study, patients 'denied smoking' but some had not been told how to use their oxygen and two participants used their oxygen less than 'four feet away from an open or gas fire'.[135] Not only did patients need to be able to understand the controls to operate the system; they also needed to be 'dedicated to the continuous wearing of nasal prongs or an oxygen mask for fifteen hours a day which will inevitably alter their lifestyle'.[136] Domiciliary oxygen was still not compatible with what we would consider normal day-to-day activity, thus making it difficult for many patients to accommodate it into their lives. For example, although domiciliary oxygen was supposed to raise activity levels in its users, 'unlike studies in the laboratory' the lengths of tubing were too short to allow them to actually use the oxygen while exercising.[137] In practice, the tubing was only long enough to allow users to move from one room to another. One 1997 study pointed out that the concentrators short tubing restricted mobility to within six metres and that users found the devices excessively noisy.[138] Crucially, there was a trade-off between the amount of time the devices could be used and their weight. The 'lightweight' portable oxygen devices (1.5 kg) lasted for less than half an hour which precluded usage away from the home, whereas the longer lasting devices were too heavy (at 4.5 kg) for users with severe respiratory illness to use with any success.[139] Although the general attitude expressed by medics was that 'half an hour to one hour [...] is adequate for most activities', this limitation did preclude users from making full use of their devices.[140] Subsequent user resistance presented a problem for those prescribing it as the treatment was only effective when used properly.

Ease of use was an important factor in oxygen administration only so far as it was affordable. Moreover, the individual nature of this treatment made it difficult to create standardised guidelines for assessing and prescribing. Worries that oxygen was becoming a blanket treatment had little impact on the way in which it was prescribed other than to restrict it in ways that were often less than helpful to users. Though more user-friendly administration techniques were developed, they were subject to regional inequalities and often restricted to the private healthcare sector. Poor tolerance to the equipment available often led to patients failing to use their home therapy correctly. Yet the solutions offered were limited, focusing on designing better criteria for assessing and identifying appropriate candidates, as well as better education on use and purpose of oxygen therapy during the course of treatment to promote effective use.[141] These are hardly solutions developed with users' quality of life in mind.

## Conclusions

Device usability and patient co-operation remain key factors in the successful uptake of oxygen. Compliance with prescribed oxygen in Britain is very low (just 22 per cent) with one study citing up to 51 per cent of oxygen users still smoking, despite the very high risk of fire and burn injury.[142] In 2002, another study demonstrated widespread user rejection of ambulatory oxygen from COPD patients who lacked the confidence and instruction to use the devices and were inhibited by the stigma attached to their use. It concluded by emphasising the need to consider the lived experience of people using oxygen and argued that its widespread rejection illustrated 'the pitfalls associated with designing technologies without reference to the ultimate end users'.[143] As McGuire and Carel have outlined, such rejection often stemmed from the perceived stigma attached to ambulatory oxygen usage, which is noisy and difficult to disguise:

> The connotations of severe illness and the accompanying fear of contagion further exacerbate the user's sense that the equipment is stigmatizing. A further sense of shame may arise from the association between respiratory disease and smoking (possibly attributing to the user responsibility for her condition). The relative rareness of such equipment seen outside a hospital increases the interest of and thus questions and comments from strangers, so the user also suffers some loss of privacy and anonymity.[144]

The lack of co-production in initial design has led to ongoing problems around portability, comfort, consideration of stigma and the everyday life of the patient.[145] Home oxygen has thus been described as simultaneously life-giving and burdensome.[146] This dual way of relating to oxygen has led sociologist Megan Wainwright to refer to it as a 'limiting enabler' that represents independence and dependence concurrently.[147] One early adopter of portable oxygen articulated this sense of reluctant attachment to her portable oxygen system, which she named 'Harvey'. She explained:

> I cannot get along without Harvey, yet I find I cannot get along with him either [...] Harvey and I have what you would call a love/hate relationship. I call him my friend; but he is not really my friend when I trip over his cord, forget to turn him on [...] he misbehaves and gets tangled up in the market shopping cart.[148]

Anthropomorphising oxygen machines in this way is not uncommon. David Brooks, for instance, discussed his relationship with his oxygen machine, Fifi, as that of man and wife.[149] Another user discussed her oxygen cylinder as if 'she' was a naughty pet and named her Gwendolin. This practice may be related to the need to control the machine and to moderate one's attachment to it.[150]

Although companies such as Invacare have developed much more advanced lightweight mobile oxygen concentrators, these are neither in widespread circulation nor available on the NHS.[151] In 2006, following the Linde group's takeover of the British Oxygen Company (now BOC), four private companies took over control of the NHS oxygen service in an attempt to both save the NHS money and allow users easier access to oxygen. As part of the privatisation of the service, the country was divided into regions, which went out for tender. Today, Air Liquide meets most of Britain's medical oxygen requirements, but some regions are supplied by BOC or Baywater. In the first month of this transition to a wholly privatised service, one woman died because the delivery of her oxygen was delayed. Many other users reported problems (ranging from inconvenient to life threateningly problematic) because of delayed access to oxygen.[152] Each company has their own procedures and protocols and they do not communicate with each other. Like trying to use a train ticket bought from one train company on a train run by another train company on the same line, this results in great bureaucratic difficulties when users attempt to work or travel in another company's area. Users must request their oxygen cylinders directly from the oxygen company and this change has had the unintended consequence of destroying the vital social networks that had developed between the pharmacist and the oxygen users.[153] Users today point out that the current system is designed for the convenience of the oxygen companies rather than its users. It may also exacerbate social difficulties for more precarious users of oxygen as they are personally responsible for informing their landlords if they are using oxygen, but the risk of fire means that private landlords are more likely to refuse leases to oxygen users.[154] Not only is the timing of oxygen delivery non-negotiable, but the company's scheduling is also predicated on the ableist idea that the oxygen user is non-working and housebound, thus making it even harder for users to lead lives with normal educational or working patterns. Users have a distinct lack of control over their oxygen supply, even though its effective provision can be quite literally a matter of life and death. The resulting anxiety often results in users attempting to conserve their supplies by 'hoarding' their oxygen.[155] Thirteen years later, after that isolated incidence of privatisation, many other parts of the NHS are now under threat from just such 'patchwork privatisation'. Yet the case of oxygen provision and the abandonment of the iron lung users in the United States does not suggest that we should be either optimistic or complacent about this process.[156]

This privatisation and division of medical oxygen has led directly to oxygen shortages in hospitals treating COVID-19 patients, as multiple hospitals have declared critical shortages and some have been forced to limit the number of people treated on mechanical ventilators.[157] GPs have advised patients who normally use oxygen at home through the NHS to buy it privately because it is so scarce.[158] This is especially egregious given that we know that most users come from lower socio-economic backgrounds and may be particularly isolated and unable to ask for support. Moreover, an article in the *Health Service Journal* has argued that while the amount of medical oxygen available in Britain was sufficient, there were problems specifically around the co-ordination of deliveries and availability of engineering staff.[159] It seems clear that these problems of co-ordination across regions would be mitigated by a nationalised service with standardised practices and easy ability to communicate. Disabled users have been highlighting these problems out for years. It is past time for us to start listening.

## Notes

\* This chapter was written with the generous support of a Wellcome Trust Senior Investigator Award (grant no. 103340; www.lifeofbreath.org). We are grateful to the Trust for supporting the Life of Breath project and to the University of Bristol Faculty of Arts for funding Jenny Hutton's research as the Life of Breath Intern. Coreen McGuire would like to thank Manchester University Press for allowing her to use material from her monograph *Measuring Difference, Numbering Normal: Setting the Standards for Disability in the Interwar Period*.

1 Bragg described Halahan as his friend and his 'neighbour in the country', Bragg was working in London at this time but may have

had a second home/main base in West Sussex. Letter from W.H. Bragg to Leonard Hill (4 January 1934), William Henry Bragg RI Admin Correspondence 1933–39, RI MS WHB/27E/5, Royal Institution of Great Britain (thereafter WHB). Information on Samuel Crosby Halahan was retrieved from GENi, www.geni.com/people/Samuel-Halahan/6000000015282798567 (accessed 16 February 2021).
2   Letter from Bragg to Hill (4 January 1934), WHB.
3   P. Kerridge, 'Artificial Respiration for Three and a Half Years', *Lancet* 227:5870 (1936), 504. The discussion of the nurses' continuous artificial respiration is discussed in a newspaper clipping titled 'Iron Lungs' in the William H. Bragg Miscellaneous Correspondence, Bragg-Paul Pulsator (15 March–15 August), RI MS WHB/8B/9, Royal Institution of Great Britain (henceforth WHBMC). See also U. Blackwell, 'Mechanical Respiration', *Lancet* 254:6568 (1949), 99–102.
4   Maud Ethel Halahan (neé Galton), www.geni.com/people/Maud-Ethel-Galton/6000000015282765918 (accessed 16 February 2021).
5   Kerridge, 'Artificial Respiration', 504.
6   Paul was internationally renowned for his scientific instruments: including the galvanometer, early wireless telegraphy sets and devices for submarine warfare; he is also famous today as a pioneer of British film, devising cameras and projectors for motion pictures.
7   'Iron Lungs', WHBMC.
8   W.H. Bragg, 'Bragg-Paul Pulsator', *British Medical Journal* (30 July 1938), 254.
9   Letter from Bragg to Hill (4 January 1934), WHB.
10  Bragg, 'Bragg-Paul Pulsator', 254.
11  Copy of letter from William H. Bragg to Secretary of the British Red Cross Society, addressed to Col. Day (11 July 1938), WHB/8B/4–5, WHBMC. The Red Cross was also interested in Bragg's creation, especially since they helped to commercialise oxygen tents, as indicated by a 17 July 1938 letter from Sir Harold B. Facus, the Director-General of the British Red Cross Society to Bragg, WHB/8B/6, WHBMC.
12  'Iron Lungs', WHBMC.
13  C. McGuire and H. Carel. 'Stigma, Technology and Masking: Hearing Aids and Ambulatory Oxygen', in D. Wasserman and A. Cureton (eds), *Oxford Handbook of the Philosophy of Disability* (Oxford: Oxford University Press, 2019), 598–615.
14  The branding of the Bragg-Paul device as the 'Pulsator' was owed to physiologist Phyllis Kerridge who worked to improve the physiological dimensions of the machine.
15  For a historical discussion of this nomenclature, see, L.J. Witts, G.R. Girdlestone, R.G. Henderson, P.M. Tookey Kerridge, G.W. Pickering,

C.L.G. Pratt, E. Schuster, A. Topping and N.F. Smith, '"Breathing Machines" and Their Use in Treatment: Report of the Respirators (Poliomyelitis) Committee', *Medical Research Council Special Report Series, No. 237* (London: His Majesty's Stationery Office, 1939), 1–91, 6.
16  Anon., 'On the Comparative Inutility and Extravagant Cost of the Patent Metallic Respirators', *Lancet* 30:765 (1838), 167–8
17  K. Binnie, C. McGuire and H. Carel, 'Objects of Safety and Imprisonment' (under review with *Journal of Material Culture*).
18  P. Foster and M. Pooler, 'Muddled Thinking Punctures Plan for British Ventilator', *Financial Times* (17 April 2020), www.ft.com/content/5f393d77-8e5b-4a85-b647-416efbc575ec (accessed 16 February 2021).
19  Ibid.
20  For a review of the divergences between medical history and disability history in the United States, see B. Linker, 'On the Borderland of Medical and Disability History: A Study of the Fields', *Bulletin of the History of Medicine* 87:4 (2013), 499–535.
21  For an overview of the shortcomings of the social model in this respect, see T. Shakespeare, 'The Social Model of Disability', in Lennard J. Davis (ed.), *The Disability Studies Reader* (New York: Routledge, 2010), 195–203. For a discussion of the problems of the social model for historians, see J. Anderson, *War, Disability and Rehabilitation in Britain* (Manchester: Manchester University Press, 2011), 5–6.
22  Cf. the amplified telephones described in C. McGuire 'Inventing Amplified Telephony: The Co-Creation of Aural Technology and Disability', in C. Jones (ed.), *Rethinking Modern Prostheses in Anglo-American Commodity Cultures, 1820–1939* (Manchester: Manchester University Press 2017), 70–90; Oliver Heaviside's work in long distance telephony and radio signals explored in G. Gooday and K. Sayer, *Managing the Experience of Hearing Loss in Britain, 1830–1930* (Basingstoke: Palgrave, 2017), 8.
23  Witts et al., '"Breathing Machines"', 4.
24  D.M. Oshinsk, *Polio: An American Story* (Oxford: Oxford University Press, 2006), 61.
25  Ibid.
26  J.E. Klein, J. Echtenkamp, V. Alvin and N. Baird, 'Emergency! An Iron Lung in a Hurry', *Iron Lung Web Exhibit*, University Of Virginia, Health Collections at the Claude Moore Health Sciences Library (2005), http://historical.hsl.virginia.edu/ironlung/ironlung/pg6.cfm.html (accessed 16 February 2021).
27  The device was originally requested by the South Australian Government in 1938 to combat a devastating poliomyelitis epidemic.

28 P. Drinker, 'Prolonged Administration of Artificial Respiration', *Lancet* 217:5622 (1931), 1186–8.
29 The attendant was also essential for enabling toilet function, through bedpans and enemas, see Drinker, 'Prolonged Administration of Artificial Respiration', 1187.
30 M. Barr, 'The Iron Lung: A Polio Patient's Story', *Journal of the Royal Society of Medicine* 103:6 (2010), 256–9, 256.
31 'Iron Lungs', WHBMC.
32 Kerridge, 'Artificial Respiration', 504.
33 This technique is called glossopharyngeal breathing. See Daniel J. Wilson, *Living with Polio: The Epidemic and its Survivors*. (Chicago: University of Chicago Press, 2005), 91.
34 Letter from K.N. Knapp to William Bragg (18 September 1933), WHB/27E/4, WHB.
35 Hill mentioned that a similar German apparatus was in existence but had failed because the positive pressure could be injurious to patients, at times inflating the heart with mucus and blood.
36 Poulton also invited Bragg and Paul to present their device at the Therapeutic and Pharmaceutical Section of the Royal Society of Medicine.
37 Letter from Dr Poulton to William Bragg (15 February 1934), WHB/27E/7, WHB.
38 Furthermore, Kerridge suggested to Bragg and Paul that an article published in the *Lancet*, detailing the clinical features of the device – without going into too much technical detail – would appeal to general practitioners who would otherwise not learn of it. Letter from Phyllis Kerridge to William Bragg (19 March 1934), WHB/27E/10, WHB.
39 Letter from Paul to Editor of *British Medical Journal* (30 July 1938), WHB/8B/16, WHB.
40 C.J. McSweeny also argued for the benefits of different sizes, arguing that with the Pulsator, 'the rate of compression can be modified to suit the respiratory rate of the patient – 18, 20, or 22 strokes per minute, as the case may be'. C.J. McSweeny, 'The Bragg-Paul Pulsator in Treatment of Respiratory Paralysis: Report on Thirty-Four Cases', *British Medical Journal* (1938), 1206–7, 1206; Cf. Witts et al., '"Breathing Machines"', 45.
41 'Artificial "Lungs"', *Public Health* (1938–39), 69–70.
42 Letter from Bragg to Secretary of British Red Cross Society, WHBMC.
43 Letter from William Bragg to S.C. Dyke (7 June 1934), WHB/27E/20, WHB. In 2017, £30 was worth approximately £1,519.88 according to the national archives currency converter, www.nationalarchives.gov.uk/currency-converter/#currency-result (accessed 16 February 2021).

44 Letter from Siebe Gorman & Co. Ltd to Robert W. Paul (21 May 1936), WHB/27E/29, WHB.
45 The same company that designed the oxygen mask equipment. Bragg, 'Bragg-Paul Pulsator', 254. On the noisiness of the Drinker respirator see A.A. Gilbertson, 'Before Intensive Therapy?', *Journal of the Royal Society of Medicine* (1995), 459–63, 461.
46 Letter from Paul to Hutchinson (12 August 1938), WHB 8B/24–26, WHB. Pulsators were distributed to hospitals in Manchester, Birmingham, London, Norwich, Ipswich and Liverpool.
47 The bacteria causing diphtheria releases a toxin that causes a thick grey film (the pseudomembrane) to develop in the throat. As the disease advances and the film sticks to tissues, breathing is obstructed; severe complications include damage to the heart muscles and nerve damage, including paralysis and respiratory failure. Breathing obstruction was such a notable feature of the disease, that it was often called 'The Strangler' or 'Kiss of Death'. In Britain, cases of children admitted with respiratory failure were frequently identified as 'post-diphtheric respiratory paralysis'.
48 'Bragg-Paul Respirator', HC Deb (14 July 1938), 1517–18, https://api.parliament.uk/historic-hansard/commons/1938/jul/14/bragg-paul-respirator (accessed 16 February 2021).
49 Letter from Robert Paul to C.J. McSweeny (17 July 1938), WHB/8B/8, WHBMC.
50 'Bragg-Paul Respirator', HC Deb (14 July 1938).
51 'Plane's Vain Dash with Respirator', *The Scotsman* (25 July 1939), accessed via British Newspaper Archive.
52 Letter from Paul to Dr Somerville Hastings (2 January 1938), WHB/27E/66, WHB (re. BBC Broadcast). Paul was sent the transcript by Bragg.
53 Letter from Dr Somerville Hastings to Paul, WHB 27E/66, WHB.
54 Witts et al., '"Breathing Machines"', 3.
55 Review, 'Medical Research Council. Special Report Series no. 237', *Indian Medical Gazette* (1940).
56 Letter from Robert W. Paul to William Bragg (16 August 1938), WHB/8B/28, WHBMC.
57 Witts et al., '"Breathing Machines"'.
58 Ibid., 2.
59 Wilson, *Living with Polio*, 91.
60 Witts et al., '"Breathing Machines"', 46.
61 Ibid., 47.
62 Ibid., 51.
63 D. Brooks, 'Living with Ventilation: Confessions of an Addict', *Care of the Critically Ill* 8:5 (1990), 205–7, 206; D. Brooks, 'The Route

to Home Ventilation: A Patient's Perspective', *Care of the Critically Ill* 6:3 (1992), 96–7.
64 Witts et al., '"Breathing Machines"', 48.
65 Ibid.
66 Similar tactics were used to wean nervous patients off the machines in which case 'the pressure can, without their knowledge, be gradually reduced until finally the motor is running but no negative pressure is being produced'. See Witts et al., '"Breathing Machines"', 52.
67 Ibid., 49.
68 Ibid.
69 Although there is a fifty-one-year gap between these two reports it is clear from Brooks' description of the machines that there was more continuity of this type of technology than might have been expected. Brooks, 'Living with Ventilation', 207.
70 Victoria Bates' UKRI-funded project (2020–24) on the senses and the modern healthcare environment will provide a welcome intervention into the healthcare soundscape and its impact on user experiences.
71 That these were the only two machines that this kind of data was available for indicates that they were two most widely used machines in Britain at the time of the reports compilation.
72 Witts et al., '"Breathing Machines"', Appendix 'Table A – Continued', 76.
73 Ibid., 90.
74 Ibid., 88.
75 Ibid., 89.
76 'Iron Lungs Will Help Save Midland Kiddies', *Birmingham Gazette* (4 November 1938), accessed via British Newspaper Archives. Note that, although the headline refers to iron lungs, it was a Bragg-Paul Pulsator which was gifted. Iron lung was often used in the popular press to refer to a variety of style of respirators.
77 J.G. Wilson, 'A Continuing Battle Against the Virus of Polio', *The Municipal Journal* 59:3 (1951), 1577–81, 1577.
78 Witts et al., '"Breathing Machines"', 43.
79 S. Hurley 'The Man Behind the Motor – William Morris and the Iron Lung', *Science Museum Blog* (2013), https://blog.sciencemuseum.org.uk/the-man-behind-the-motor-william-morris-and-the-iron-lung (accessed 16 February 2021).
80 A.A. Gilbertson, 'Before Intensive Therapy?', *Journal of the Royal Society of Medicine* 88:8 (1995), 459–63, 462.
81 In an exception to the practice not to anonymise in this collection, this patient's name has been changed to preserve her anonymity because the date of this record means that she could potentially still be alive.

82　Ham Green Hospital Bristol, Records of Poliomyelitis Chicken Pox Herpes Zoster Rubella Mumps 1951, Patient Reg No. 1236/50 Letter to Resident Physician James Macrae inserted into patient records 10/1/1950–1/1/1951.
83　Ham Green Hospital Bristol, Records of Poliomyelitis Chicken Pox Herpes Zoster Rubella Mumps 1951, Patient Reg No. 1298/50 patient records 16/10/1950–2/2/1951.
84　Ibid.
85　Wilson, *Living with Polio*, 92.
85　Ham Green Hospital Bristol, Records of Poliomyelitis Chicken Pox Herpes Zoster Rubella Mumps 1951, Patient Reg No. 1360/50 patient records 30/10/1950–3/6/1951.
87　Ibid. Letter inserted from Gloucester Road surgery 7/6/1951.
88　Anon., 'Iron Lung Man Wed', *Telegraph and Independent*, Sheffield (11 August 1939), accessed via British Newspaper Archive.
89　'Home-Made Iron Lung Speeds Girl's Recovery', *The Coventry Evening Telegraph* (24 August 1949), accessed via British Newspaper Archive.
90　J.C. Graves, Letter to the Editor, 'Domiciliary Rehabilitation of the Respiratory Cripple', *Lancet* 274:7110 (1959), 1033.
91　Ibid.
92　M. Barr, 'The Iron Lung – A Polio Patient's Story', *Journal of the Royal Society of Medicine* (2010), 256–9, 256.
92　J. Brown, 'The Last of the Iron Lungs', *Gizmodo* (2017), https://web.archive.org/web/20190411011054/https://gizmodo.com/the-last-of-the-iron-lungs-1819079169 (accessed 16 February 2021).
94　Ibid.
95　Ibid.
96　G.L. Albrecht and P.J. Devlieger, 'The Disability Paradox: High Quality of Life Against All Odds', *Social Science and Medicine* 48 (1999), 977–88, 977.
97　Ibid., 982.
98　H. Carel, 'Ill, But Well: A Phenomenology of Well-Being in Chronic Illness', in J.E. Bickenback, F. Felder and B. Schmitz (eds), *Disability and the Good Human Life* (Cambridge: Cambridge University Press, 2014), 243–70, 253.
99　F. Ryan, 'It Is Not Only Coronavirus that Risks Infecting Society – Our Prejudices Do, Too', *The Guardian* (9 April 2020), www.theguardian.com/commentisfree/2020/apr/09/nice-guidelines-coronavirus-pandemic-disabled (accessed 18 April 2020).
100　Ibid.
101　Ibid.

102  J.E. Cotes and G.E. Gilson, 'Improved Portable Oxygen Apparatus with Detachable Cylinders for Domiciliary Use', *Lancet* 271:6947 (1956), 823.
102  Lung Disease (Breathing Appliances), H.C. (10 December 1974), vol. 883, cols 481–482 (col. 475).
104  T.L. Petty and M.M. Finigan, 'Clinical Evaluation of Prolonged Ambulatory Oxygen Therapy in Chronic Airway Obstruction', *American Journal of Medicine* 45:2 (1968), 242–52.
105  N. Capener, 'Domiciliary Rehabilitation of the Respiratory Cripple', *Lancet* 274:7104 (1959), 677–8.
106  Annotations, 'Pros and Cons of Liquid Oxygen', *Lancet* 235:6088 (1940), 842.
107  N. Roberton, J. Gupta, G. Dahlenburg, J. Tizard, 'Oxygen Therapy in the Newborn', *Lancet* 291:7556 (1968), 1323–9.
108  R.M. Forrester, E. Jefferson and W.J. Naunton, 'Oxygen and Retrolental Fibroplasia: A Seven-Year Survey', *Lancet* 264:6832 (1954), 258–60.
109  Lung Disease (Breathing Appliances), H.C. (10 December 1974), vol. 883, cols 481–482.
110  Ibid.
111  Ibid.
112  Lung Disease (Breathing Appliances), H.C. (10 December 1974), vol. 883, col. 477.
113  Ibid., col. 482.
114  Leading article, 'Domiciliary Oxygen', *Lancet* 293:7594 (1969), 560.
115  W. O'Donohue, J. Baker, G. Bell, O. Muren and J. Patterson, 'The Management of Acute Respiratory Failure in a Respiratory Intensive Care Unit', *Chest* (1970), 603–10.
116  T.L. Petty and M.M. Finigan, 'Clinical Evaluation of Prolonged Ambulatory Oxygen Therapy in Chronic Airway Obstruction', *American Journal of Medicine* 45:2 (1968), 248–9.
117  M.J. Fox and G.L. Snider, 'Respiratory Therapy: Current Practice in Ambulatory Patients with Chronic Airflow Obstruction', *JAMA* 241:9 (1979), 937–8.
118  R.D. Stark and J.M. Bishop, 'New Method for Oxygen Therapy in the Home Using an Oxygen Concentrator', *British Medical Journal* (1973), 105–6.
119  B.N. Stewart, C.I. Hood and A.J. Block, 'Long-term Results of Continuous Oxygen Therapy at Sea Level', *Chest* 68:4 (1975), 486–92, 486.
120  M.M. Jones, J.E. Harvey and A.E. Tattersfield, 'How Patients Use Domiciliary Oxygen', *British Medical Journal* (1978), 1397–1400.
121  'British Oxygen Company: Prices', HL Deb (8 February 1984), vol. 447 cols 1141–1144 (col. 1142).

122  T. Petty, L. Nett and S. Lakshminarayan, 'A Single Nasal Prong for Continuous Oxygen Therapy', *Chest* 64:1 (1973), 146–7.
123  R.D. Stark, P. Finnigan and J.M. Bishop, 'Long-term Domiciliary Oxygen in Chronic Bronchitis with Pulmonary Hypertension', *British Medical Journal* (1973), 467–70.
124  M.S. Shulman, G. Schmidt and M.S. Sadove, 'Evaluation of Oxygen Therapy Devices by Arterial Oxygen Tensions', *Diseases of the Chest* 56:4 (1969), 356–9, 357.
125  Leading article, 'Domiciliary Oxygen', 560.
126  R. Oxley and J. Macnaughton, 'Inspiring Change: Humanities and Social Science Insights into the Experience and Management of Breathlessness', *Current Opinion in Supportive and Palliative Care* 10:3 (2016), 256–61, 258.
127  McGuire and Carel, 'Stigma, Technology and Masking'.
128  Oxley and Macnaughton, 'Inspiring Change', 259.
129  The NOTT study group, 'Is 12-Hour Oxygen as Effective as 24-Hour Oxygen in Advanced Chronic Obstructive Pulmonary Disease with Hypoxemia? (The Nocturnal Oxygen Therapy Trial – NOTT)', *Chest* (1980), 419–20.
130  Medical Research Council Working Party, 'Long Term Domiciliary Oxygen Therapy in Chronic Hypoxic Cor Pulmonale Complicating Chronic Bronchitis and Emphysema', *Lancet* 317:8222 (1981), 681–6.
131  Ibid., 682. There is not sufficient scope to explore this issue in depth here, but for more consideration of historical developments in terms of gendered differences in care see C. Mcguire, *Measuring Difference, Numbering Normal: Setting the Standards for Disability in the Interwar Period* (Manchester: Manchester University Press, 2020).
132  Anon., 'Long-term Domiciliary Oxygen Therapy', *Lancet* 2:8451 (1985), 365–7; J. Escarrabil, R. Estopa, M. Huguet and F. Manresa, 'Domiciliary Oxygen Therapy', *Lancet* 326:8458 (1985), 779.
133  A.A. Okubadejo, E.A. Paul and J.A. Wedzicha, 'Domiciliary Oxygen Cylinders: Indications, Prescription and Usage', *Respiratory Medicine* (1994), 777–80.
134  G.H. Guyatt, M.L. Nonoyama, C. Lacchetti, R. Goeree, D. Heels-Ansdell and R. Goldstein, 'A Randomised Trial of Strategies for Assessing Eligibility for Long-Term Domiciliary Oxygen Therapy', *American Journal of Respiratory and Critical Care Medicine* 72:5 (2005), 573–80.
135  Jones, Harvey and Tattersfield, 'How Patients Use Domiciliary Oxygen', 1398.
136  Anon., 'Long-Term Domiciliary Oxygen Therapy', 367.
137  Jones, Harvey and Tattersfield, 'How Patients Use Domiciliary Oxygen', 1399.

138 R.J. Shiner, U. Zaretsky, M. Mirali, S. Benzaray and D. Elad, 'Evaluation of Domiciliary Long-Term Oxygen Therapy with Oxygen Concentrators', *Israel Journal of Medical Sciences* 33:1 (1997), 23–9.
139 Jones, Harvey and Tattersfield, 'How Patients Use Domiciliary Oxygen', 1399.
140 Leading article, 'Domiciliary Oxygen', 560.
141 S. Booth, H. Anderson, M. Swannick, R. Wade, S. Kite and M. Johnson, 'The Use of Oxygen in the Palliation of Breathlessness: A Report of the Expert Working Groups of the Scientific Committee of the Association of Palliative Medicine', *Respiratory Medicine* 98:1 (2004), 66–77, 73.
142 A.J. Lindford, H. Tehrani, E.M. Sassoon and T.J. O'Neill, 'Home Oxygen Therapy and Cigarette Smoking: A Dangerous Practice', *Annals of Burns and Fire Disasters* 19:2 (2006), 99–100, 99. For interesting analysis of UK regional inequalities in oxygen and cigarette related burns, see B.G. Cooper, 'Home Oxygen and Domestic Fires', *Breathe* 11 (2015), 4–12.
143 E. Arnold, A. Bruton, M. Donovan-Hall, A. Fenwick, B. Dibb and E. Walker, 'Ambulatory Oxygen: Why Do COPD Patients Not Use Their Portable Systems as Prescribed? A Qualitative Study', *BMC Pulmonary Medicine* 11:9 (2011).
144 McGuire and Carel, 'Stigma, Technology and Masking', 605.
145 Ibid.; Arnold et al., 'Ambulatory Oxygen'.
146 A. Collier, K. Braeden and J. Phillips, 'Caregivers' Perspectives on the Use of Long-Terms Oxygen Therapy for the Treatment of Refractory Breathlessness: A Qualitative Study', *Journal of Pain and Symptom Management* 53:1 (2017), 33–9.
147 M. Wainwright, 'Exploring Ambivalent Oxygen-Machine-World Relations Through the Lens of Post Phenomenology', *Journal of Material Culture* 23:4 (2018), 426–47, 433.
148 T.L. Petty, *Adventures of an Oxy-Phile* (AARC, 2004), 60.
149 Brooks, 'Living with Ventilation', 205–7.
150 Binnie, McGuire and Carel, 'Objects of Safety and Imprisonment'.
151 Invacare Platinum Mobile Oxygen Concentrator, www.invacare.ie/respiratory/portable-oxygen-concentrators/invacare-platinum-mobile-portable-oxygen-contentrator (accessed 16 February 2021).
152 'Patients Hit by Oxygen Shortage', BBC News (17 February 2006), https://web.archive.org/web/20190128152905/http://news.bbc.co.uk/2/hi/health/4722700.stm (accessed 16 February 2021).
153 Ibid.
154 See BOC Home Oxygen Service UK, www.bochomeoxygen.co.uk/en/patients/introductiontobochealthcare/introduction_to_boc_healthcare.html (accessed 16 February 2021); Rosen Law Office, 'Smoking and

Medical Oxygen: What's a Landlord to Do?', www.rosenlawoffice.com/smoking-and-medical-oxygen-whats-a-landlord-to-do (accessed 16 February 2021).
155 McGuire and Carel, 'Stigma, Technology and Masking'.
156 A. Nunns. 'The Patchwork Privatisation of our Health Service: A Users' Guide', *Keep our NHS Public Report* (2007), http://image.guardian.co.uk/sys-files/Education/documents/2007/01/19/Liste Patchworkprivatisation.pdf (accessed 16 February 2021).
157 D. Campbell, 'Coronavirus: London Hospital Almost Runs Out of Oxygen for Covid-19 Patients', *The Guardian* (2 April 2020), www.theguardian.com/society/2020/apr/02/london-hospital-almost-runs-out-oxygen-coronavirus-patients (accessed 17 April 2020); S. Marsh and R. Booth, 'Hertfordshire Hospital Forced to Consider Who Should Be Refused Oxygen', *The Guardian* (5 April 2020), www.theguardian.com/world/2020/apr/05/hertfordshire-hospital-forced-to-consider-who-should-be-refused-oxygen (accessed 17 April 2020).
158 G. Pogrund and T. Ripley, 'GPs Tell Patients to Buy Their Own Oxygen as NHS Supplies Run Low', *The Times* (12 April 2020), www.thetimes.co.uk/article/gps-tell-patients-to-buy-their-own-oxygen-as-nhs-supplies-run-low-dmznjgs0h (accessed 17 April 2020).
159 B. Clover, D, West, J. Illman, 'Oxygen Supply Problems 'the New PPE', Warn Hospital Bosses', *Health Service Journal* (6 April 2020), www.hsj.co.uk/oxygen-supply-problems-the-new-ppe-warn-hospital-bosses/7027333.article (accessed 17 April 2020).

# 7

## The patient's new clothes: British soldiers as complementary practitioners in the First World War

*Georgia McWhinney*

The patient voice in First World War medicine is a well-known concept. The emphasis on military patients over practitioners in many recent works has allowed historians to explore and unpack traditional biomedical understandings and hierarchies. Notable leading scholars like Mark Harrison have used the voices of patients to understand and critique past biomedicine.[1] Other historians, such as Ana Carden-Coyne and Fiona Reid, have explored the position of the patient within the political landscape of Great War medicine, documenting their agency and occasionally their resistance.[2] Yet, while these studies provide important insight into Great War medicine in many ways, the consumer perspective still often tells us about professional practice and the authoritative practitioner. The patient is a mirror for biomedicine.

Channelling the words of Roy Porter, often it is more desirable to speak of 'sufferers' or 'the sick', rather than patients, as not all who are ill engage with professional medical practitioners.[3] The First World War soldier was not an exception. Flurin Condrau has argued more broadly that historians have not paid enough attention to patient agency, stating that the 'issues of how to write the patient's history, how to deal with subjectivity, experience and perhaps even choice is still very much uncharted territory for historians of medicine'.[4] Thus this chapter strides decisively into patients' lived experience to explore medical possibilities and to broaden our understanding of healthcare and the patient voice in the First World War.

The Western Front of the First World War provides a compelling canvas for the exploration of this theme. Large numbers of soldier-patients kept records of their daily thoughts, emotions and activities. The wealth of personal diaries, letters and oral histories of British Great War soldiers provide an extensive corpus that relates not only the patient's view, but their subjectivity, agency and choices. As argued by Jessica Meyer, the importance of these sources lies in their nature as 'personal, self-reflexive texts' that convey the subjective experiences, understandings and practices of the soldier.[5] These personal records challenge the notion of a patient–practitioner binary and suggest that patients were more than merely mirrors for biomedicine. Rather, patients functioned as complementary practitioners. Individually and communally, soldiers established their own vernacular medical system.

Fiona Reid notes that soldiers' understandings and practices are the most marginalised aspect of First World War medicine. It is interesting, then, that she provides no further explanation for this historical lacuna.[6] It may be that medical historians' methodological approaches have, thus far, coloured how they conceive of the patient.[7] New insight into the medical lives of patients is only possible when the historian distances them from biomedicine, and thus shifts the dynamic of power beyond Porter's initial call in 'The Patient's View' and into new avenues of study in the history of medicine.

As a case study, 'exposure diseases' – spurred by the environmental effects of lice, mud and gas – provide insight into preventive medical knowledge and practice. Both medical professionals and soldiers understood 'exposure diseases' to be one of the worst aspects of trench life.[8] Body lice (*Pediculus humanus corporis*) caused diseases such as trench fever, typhus and relapsing fever. Mud and water in the trenches gave rise to trench foot and secondary gangrene. Exposure to gases caused bodily harm and discomfort through asphyxiation and, in the case of mustard gas, chemical burns. While doctors and patients both understood and engaged with the environment and the exposure diseases it spurred, the manner in which they crafted their health systems contrasted greatly. For medical professionals, soldiers' ailments were physiological disorders to be cured. For soldiers, healthcare knowledges and practices were important coping functions for the traumatic experiences of day-to-day life in the trenches.[9]

Soldiers' vernacular medicine was a local social system.[10] The meaning of vernacular, as 'using plain, every-day, ordinary language', conveys how soldiers developed their own form of medicine as a local system.[11] The term 'vernacular medicine' is not a catch-all descriptor for practices outside biomedicine, but denotes medicine initiated by the individual, spread by word of mouth, through unpublished texts and other shared practices. This recognises the subjectivities and choices of its practitioners and reshapes understandings of healthcare systems in the Great War and beyond. Vernacular medicine was coloured by soldiers' social roles, interpersonal relationships, external environment and access to preventative measures and resources for self-care. These components form the basis of a unique – and demotic – healthcare system.[12]

This emerging history forces us to reconceptualise soldiers as more than reflections of biomedicine.[13] It opens avenues to escape traditional hierarchies and to broaden historical understandings of both the patient and of what constitutes a healthcare system. In particular, it shapes the ways in which policy-makers should understand healthcare systems. They do not exist solely within the realm of the professional sector. Indeed, relying on the viewpoints and agency of sick individuals would provide alternate avenues to formulate health policy around the networks and choices made outside of interactions with professional medicine. Following from Michael Worboys's argument in Chapter 1, policy-makers should use the voices and actions of these individuals to formulate primary care policies, rather than viewing their actions as simply 'secondary care' to biomedicine. Indeed, in today's globalised world, especially in light of the COVID-19 pandemic, networks of non-professional medicine are as active as ever, providing important insight into strategies for addressing this public-health crisis.

## The patient and the biomedical looking glass: following the historiographical precedent

Great War medical historiography written after Porter highlights a shift to incorporate the patient voice. While this work is well known, it is important to reflect on the ways in which military medical historians have approached their research to understand why there is a need to shift beyond the current orthodoxy. As Roger Cooter and John Pickstone note, the history of medicine in the twentieth century is about the history of power in both the abstract (knowledge) and the concrete (doctor and patient experiences).[14] As a consequence, historiography has often focused on the power and authority of the biomedical system, both directly and indirectly.

From the early 1990s, there has been a surge in studies of military medicine and a push to weave this topic into wider historiographies of both medicine and the military. To fuse these once disparate studies, recent historiography highlights how the forces at play within medicine and the military influenced each other to create the modern military medical system.[15] Great War military medicine, these studies argue, is a prime example of Weberian modernity, built on a bureaucratisation and rationalisation of systems – a process occurring in both the Edwardian medical and military worlds.[16] Changes in evacuation and hospital systems, as well as the rise of bureaucratic specialisations such as pathology, bacteriology and sanitation, at once combined biomedical authority and military regimentation.[17] Cooter claims that Great War medicine had its own body politic, formed on the basis of this modern rationalised system.[18] Most medical historians follow suit, arguing that individuals within the military medical bureaucracy understood themselves in relation to their position within this schema, and that therefore they worked as a large, tiered team.[19] At the bottom of the hierarchy dwelled the patient.

Histories aim to understand the fusion of medicine with modern military structures, but they have tended to focus on systematic influence and authority. When discussing patients' approaches to medicine in wartime, these works often unintentionally replicate the military medical blueprint they aim to critique. As stated in the *Lancet* on 16 June 1917:

> In the presence of military discipline it is the individual soldier who carries out the sanitary regime [...] It is here that the battalion medical officer can play his part, for he is brought into intimate personal contact with the men, and on him rests the onus of impressing the elements of sanitation on them in a form which they can understand.[20]

Studies often note that soldiers were responsible for some forms of healthcare, such as manually 'chatting' for lice, using the fingernail and thumbnail to pop the pests. Yet they often focus on the ways in which the medical hierarchy enlisted soldiers to undertake such tasks as part of the broader narrative of medicine as a 'civilising ethos'.[21] Mark Harrison exemplifies this notion documenting how 'authorities embarked on a determined campaign [...] to instil a fear of the louse in British soldiers'.[22] For the medical authorities, through authoritative direction soldiers were capable of medical understanding and thus inclusion within the medical hierarchy.

Numerous studies attempt to unpack the power of the medical system through doctors' experiences and interactions with patients. Research, such as that of Ian R. Whitehead, focuses on doctors' individual efforts to document the systematic differences between military and civilian medicine – how the power of the system pressed on individual doctors. British Army Medical Officers (MOs), especially Regimental Medical Officers (RMOs) who worked in the trenches with the men, owed the majority of their attention and duty to the fighting strength of the army, rather than the individual care of patients.[23] Further, historians note that MOs suffered alongside the men they treated, creating further complexity in the medical narrative.[24] While this focus reveals much about the tension MOs felt between their roles as officer and caregiver, the patient voice becomes lost in the mix.

First World War patient studies have recovered the voices of sick soldiers silenced by more traditional military medical histories and thus draw attention to the inequalities and inherent issues of power within past medical structures (and therefore past medical histories).[25] This framework is not surprising, as patients past and present often have well-developed opinions about the care they receive from the medical profession. In this Great War soldiers were no exception. Joanna Bourke stresses that often military medicine was extremely alienating for its patients.[26] Private Richard Gwinnell of the Gloucestershire Regiment illustrates this point in a bitter anecdote in his diary. Reflecting on the shortcomings of military medicine he recorded:

> One of the men [...] complained all night of pains in the stomach, and had reported sick. The doctor gave him Medicine and Duty [...] During the afternoon the man became worse, and they could not stand his groaning any longer [...] The doctor then condescended to examine the man and afterwards sent them [sic] straight away to the hospital [...] the M.O. at the hospital had said that the man should

have been sent long before and that it was too late to do anything for him.[27]

Studies that rely on voices like Private Gwinnell's often use the patient's view to reveal wider issues in the administration of medicine during the war.[28] As Reid notes, the ordinary soldier was 'the man familiar with wounds and death', the tangible consequences of military and biomedical power.[29] Historians thus use the patient to examine wider trends in the politics, economics and culture of medicine, as such values are built into biomedical knowledge and the biomedical system and thus these scholars attempt to break down concepts of biomedical power and authority.[30] As argued by Carden-Coyne, patients in these settings were not passive victims but 'agents of imagination and cultural creativity'.[31] Yet by examining the manner in which patients navigated or resisted the biomedical system they hold up a mirror to professional practice.

The current historiography, therefore, still relies on the patient's perspective of biomedicine and thus reflects the dominant medical system. It is all the more important, then, to focus on the Great War soldier in a manner that conveys them as unique actors in their own system of medicine, through their subjective viewpoints and actions, rather than in relation to the medical profession.[32]

### Through the biomedical looking glass: the professional's understanding of unhealthy conditions and illness

Most historians accept that Great War soldiers lived under the preventive and therapeutic care of the medical profession. As discipline was an intrinsic component of military life, preventive medicine worked as a form of surveillance as well as care. Hygiene and sanitation formed a component of the 'civilising' ethos handed down from officers to men, as soldiers' wellbeing and civility were intrinsic to the fighting health of the army.[33]

These soldiers, however, were at once patients of biomedicine and practitioners of vernacular medicine. Bourke has noted this dualism, but more recent histories have not since developed it.[34] To comprehend the soldier in this dualistic manner, it is necessary to shift the historical frame with which we examine the patient. This perspective shows that patients are not wholly defined by their interaction with the medical profession. Rather, they are also complementary practitioners, distinctively applying their own unique medical knowledge.

Illness experiences and the meanings that sick individuals divine from them are not based on universal understandings or 'truths', but on local systems of knowledge. Doctor and patient may have markedly divergent understandings of the illness experience due to the differing local and cultural worlds they inhabit.[35] As Arthur Kleinman correctly observes, for doctors, a patient's illness experience and ensuing narrative comprise a 'tale of complaints [that] becomes the text that is to be decoded'.[36] Once decoded this text becomes practitioners' clinical reality; it is the manner in which they define the patient's problem and create attached meaning.[37] For doctors, meaning is often found in the physiological causes and manifestations of disease, with the purpose of locating a preventive management strategy or therapeutic cure.[38] This focus on physiology often comes at the expense of the social, psychological and environmental factors that contribute to illness.[39]

This emphasis on physiology played an intrinsic role in medicine during the Great War, as the 'modern' medical system that doctors worked within envisaged the soldier's body as a 'human motor', a physical mechanism that functioned in a singular manner and thus was rational, efficient and cost-effective for medical services.[40] The army's need for a swift return of soldiers to active service underlay this manifestation of the 'body as machine'. Cooter argues that as all bodies were essentially the same for professionals working in military medicine; they were therefore the same in disease, allowing doctors to deal with bodies in standardised ways, 'like products in a factory'.[41] Hence, unhealthy conditions and the physiological symptoms they produced became routinised and flattened into somewhat singular biomedical explanations.[42]

Writing in 1915, Lieutenant Colonel Percy Samuel Lelean, Assistant Professor of Hygiene at the Royal Army Medical College, described the cause and symptoms of trench foot in clinical terms, with an unsurprising focus on physiology. The determining factor in its onset was 'prolonged contact with cold water', while secondary gangrene occurred due to 'the mechanical obstruction to surface circulation'. Lelean posited that 'protecting the skin from direct contact with water is thus obvious', a physiological response for a physiological abnormality.[43] A rise in popularity of medical plates followed a similar fashion in documenting the disordered body, with the added component of colour illustrations. This trend was another part of the standardised nosology and visual lexicon that was a critical part of the bureaucratic model of military medicine. When illustrating a case history of mustard gas burns, Plate VI of *An Atlas of Gas Poisoning* noted that the burns caused 'inflammation of the buttocks and of the scrotum' and that the physiology appeared as 'a diffuse reddening [...] twenty-four hours after exposure, and this was followed by an outcrop of superficial blisters'.[44] Doctors had to learn to see the same condition by reviewing standardised visual depictions, whether through publications when away from the front line or through the mass of clinical notes that passed through their hands in field ambulances and clearing stations.[45]

Indeed, MO Captain Bruce West of the 3rd Lowland Field Ambulance of the Royal Army Medical Corps (RAMC), working directly with soldiers behind the line, described lice-induced typhus in his diary as a neat set of physical signs and symptoms: 'headache – frontal, tenderness of eyeballs, lassitudes [...] rapid pulse'.[46] Yet Captain West would most likely have experienced similar, if not the same, locations and conditions to the soldiers that he cared for. His account, therefore, conveys the power and importance of biomedical explanations for men of the medical corps. It is likely that these men found familiarity in such explanations, and may have used them as a coping method, despite sharing similar personal experiences to soldiers at the Front.

### Beyond the biomedical looking glass: the patient's understanding of unhealthy conditions and illness

According to Kleinman, practitioners 'are rarely taught that biological processes are known only through socially constructed categories that constrain experience as much as does disordered physiology'.[47] For soldiers, it was through their immediate world and local connections that they understood their health. In this context soldiers created meaning in their experiences of illness by meeting real world resistances such as resource inequality and unpredictable and uncontrollable life problems.[48] The manner in which British soldiers ascribed meaning to experience highlights a local system of knowledge and culture separate from practitioners' observations and ensuing clinical reality.

Soldiers' experiences, as seen in the works of Michael Roper and Jessica Meyer, are often discussed through the history of subjectivities.[49] This framework provides a useful tool to gain insight into the ways that soldiers documented their understandings of health. More recently, histories of emotion have added further nuance to such notions of wellbeing. According to Bourke, the link between emotion, experience and the body is axiomatic: 'the body is never pure soma: it is configured in social, cognitive, and metaphorical worlds'.[50] Hence, soldiers' bodily experiences and understandings of illness were intrinsically linked to their surrounding environment – both social and physical. Barbara H. Rosenwein and Riccardo Cristiani, historians of emotion, further this theory. The body is shaped by the world around it – 'things, people, sounds, and smells' – and incorporates them to form emotional understandings.[51] Hence, the soldier's understanding of illness reaches beyond pure physiology to create new meaning.[52] These shared meanings, derived from the local environment and everyday resistances in soldiers' worlds, meant that they formed a collective vernacular knowledge of health in the trenches.

Historians of emotions argue that writing or speaking about affective experiences is a process known as 'naming emotion'. This practice conveys that the individual is aware of their experiences and is actively seeking to understand and make sense of them in relation to their world.[53] Further, the way individuals create and record the illness experience is a form of healthcare in and of itself, as in the case of patient diaries.[54] Soldiers spoke of fear, disgust, amusement and sadness. Hence, through soldiers' records we see a vernacular medical understanding built on the patient's subjective emotional experiences.

Life in and behind the trenches shaped soldiers' worlds. It also configured their bodies. The duty that soldiers owed to the army fused them to their surrounding conditions, however unpleasant and unhygienic. The sights, sounds and smells that surrounded the soldier affected their experience of illness. As argued by Jonathan Reinarz, we cannot approach the history of the patient without examining the role of the senses.⁵⁵ Soldiers' affective responses revolved around concepts like disgust, fear, endurance and humour. They often felt unable to control their fate and were faced with the possibility of illness that brought discomfort, pain, death and even simply the unknown.⁵⁶ When Captain Samuel Smith of the Cheshire Regiment contracted trench fever he was 'thoroughly disgusted' with himself. He latched onto a description with full disclosure; he had 'a head like a tepid sponge' and feared he was 'rather irritable'.⁵⁷

Yet issues of physical disgust and fear were prominent long before soldiers found themselves in a hospital bed. Environmental determinants, like the trench system, were instrumental in shaping experiences of ill-health at the Front.⁵⁸ When environmental factors gave rise to dysphoric affect it often caused illness.⁵⁹ It was these physical sensations that shaped a shared vernacular understanding of disease among soldiers. Living with fever-spreading lice caused physical sensations of crawling skin that lingered long after the war ended. Lance Corporal Ernest Sheard felt as if he could scratch himself to pieces when he noticed vermin 'creeping about' soldiers wounds and 'wool dressings'.⁶⁰ This concept, known as 'psychic disgust' according to some medical professionals like entomologist Arthur Shipley, caused soldiers to fear lice more than they feared bullets.⁶¹ Corporal William Davies of the Machine Gun Corps described the itch as 'almost maddening', while Private Albert Day of the Gloucestershire Regiment shuddered that 'it felt disgusting'.⁶²

Further, living in the trenches meant living in mud. As Ross Wilson notes, soldiers' senses were limited to earth-packed walls and sandbags.⁶³ When the rain fell and the frost nipped, living in the mud became almost unbearable. Soldiers knew the unstable ground caused trench foot. Private Harold Youngman of the London Rifle Brigade recorded the visceral bodily and emotional experiences of living in the trenches:

> Rain would cause bits and pieces of the trenches to slither away [...] so that we became engulfed in a mass of mud and slime [...] Just imagine how unpleasant it was to descend the steps of a dugout, the steps themselves being nothing but mud, loaded with equipment and rifle, and with boots covered with slime.⁶⁴

Private Aled Parry of the Royal Welch Fusiliers shuddered to recall how terrible it was to be 'up to the middle in mud and cold water'.⁶⁵

Private Archibald Morsley of the Royal Garrison Artillery was afraid of the mud.[66] It was impossible for soldiers to remain dry.[67] Experiences of wet and cold front-line conditions forced soldiers to find meaning in illness and its consequences, likening their trench to a living grave.[68]

Fear not only applied to experiences of the muddy trench systems. Soldiers' intense fear of gas reflected the uncertainty that it produced. Asphyxiating gases that seemed to kill men from the inside and mustard gas that lingered for months on the mud and in the water merely compounded men's fears.[69] Men frequently complained of residual gas in their lungs, the physical sensation causing them to cough persistently.[70] Their bodies, like that of Corporal Alexander Burnett of the Royal Scots Fusiliers, came out 'in big blisters in between the legs, round the bottom and under the arms' when drenched in mustard gas.[71] Some men likened it to gluing 'your flesh up together'.[72] It was not unusual for soldiers to share these stories with their pals, creating a shared emotional narrative born from the adverse physical experience of life in the trenches.

Such shared stories and experiences worked as a form of bonding and understanding, a shared meaning given to health conditions. Ill health not only affected the soldier, but also their immediate networks and social worlds.[73] Soldiers lived and worked together in the trenches. The sights and sounds of their comrades' predicaments were central in soldiers' memories, conveying the importance of affinity between soldiers. Corporal Alfred West of the Monmouthshire Regiment recalled seeing soldiers' feet where the flesh 'burst right open and you could see the bone'.[74] Private Morsley professed that at night in the hospital ward the men with trench foot began to 'cry and shout with pain'.[75] Lance Corporal Sheard witnessed the men's agony first hand, before their feet were even bad enough to warrant being sent out of the line. He recalled at one sick parade:

> The men's feet were now turning a bluey colour and were very tender even to the lightest touch, toes were swollen and covered with a layer of greyish coloured skin [...] all the dirt and wool from the socks [...] was sticking to the sores [...] the aroma in the Aid Post was far from pleasant.[76]

Similar accounts abound about the fear of both asphyxiating gases and mustard gas. Lance Corporal Sheard documented the fear his pal Simons felt. Every time he heard the gas horn sound 'he began shaking like a leaf'.[77] Other men recalled the sounds of men crying with fear, and Private Reg Coldridge of the Devonshire Regiment noted that one man was crying 'cause he couldn't find his gas mask when it was hanging around his neck'.[78]

Soldiers voiced compassion for the effects of their comrades' illness. Corporal West worried because men with trench foot 'couldn't march, you see' – or if they could, somebody had to help carry their kits.[79] The inability to help their comrades placed stress on many men.[80] Captain Samuel Smith felt helplessness, noting that when he saw gassed men he detested only being able to 'sit and watch their agonised struggle to win back the life so foully taken from them'.[81] What most men stressed in their accounts about physical and emotional reactions to poor conditions and illness was its immediacy: 'you can't imagine unless you experienced it'.[82] It is this emphasis on shared lived experience that shaped the way soldiers understood illness both as individuals and as a collective.

Yet, as Coreen McGuire, Jaipreet Virdi and Jenny Hutton also address in Chapter 6, fear and disgust were often countered by an equally strong need to retain agency and control. This vice-hold on restraint manifested as a downplaying of illness experiences.[83] In this manner, soldiers formed a cognitive coping strategy for their fear akin to what Bourke terms 'psychic numbing'.[84] When asked about health and poor conditions in the trenches Corporal George Singleton of the King's Liverpool Regiment stated that 'you were hardened to this kind of thing. It didn't affect you [...] There's an old saying: you can get used to anything, and you got used to that.'[85] For soldiers like Singleton, the daily conditions and ensuing diseases they faced spurred a particular understanding of their lives in and behind the front line; one of endurance.

When making sense of their immediate world, endurance, as a coping mechanism, helped soldiers to shape meaning and retain power over their lives.[86] Often the emphasis of soldiers' accounts did not lie with descriptions of physical discomfort or ailments, but with the endurance they ascribed to them. As argued by Meyer, as well as Carol Acton and Jane Potter, the concept of endurance formed a central part of the 'heroic' narrative of the First World War soldier, providing a somewhat idealised shared story to explain or give meaning to the traumatic experiences of trench life.[87] Further, it worked to counteract the chance of breakdown and to maintain emotional wellbeing; it was a shared form of resilience.[88] Private Gwinnell's account of gas poisoning briefly outlined his physical discomfort, but stressed that he 'still had to track along' and that this was not uncommon; 'there were others in the same plight'.[89] When weather conditions became relentless, often causing foot conditions, Corporal Alfred West recalled grimly how 'you were always [...] over your boots in water [...] it was a survival of the fittest'.[90] Soldiers' attestations to endurance, like Private Gwinnell's and Corporal West's, were a form of agency and a way to create meaning from trauma.

Humour also helped soldiers to understand, moderate and explain adverse health conditions, as well as minimise their experience of illness. It is well documented that humour is a common response to traumatic and stressful situations, as in the case of emergency service personnel.[91] Humour was particularly prevalent in soldiers' discussions of lice. Private Harris recollected the bloodsuckers' persistence, saying that 'they always got their man, like the Canadian mounted police'.[92] Humour was, and is, a heuristic device with which individuals shape meaning from experience, including accounts of illness.[93] As stated by Private Ernest John Blank of the Devonshire Regiment, soldiers would 'say anything for a laugh I suppose in those days'.[94]

Similar to ideas of endurance, humour often revolved around the inescapability of adverse conditions. MO Lieutenant Norman King-Wilson of the 88th Field Ambulance RAMC noted that when trench foot cases increased during wet winters 'one was met not by grumbling or whines, but by jests as "Now I s'pose we'll ave the blinking Nivy sailed up these ere waters [sic]"'.[95] Further, the fact that lice infested most, if not all, men fused a bond of understanding between them, and they often managed collectively through laughter.[96] Sapper George Edward Robinson of the Royal Engineers remembered that the 'first time I had them I said: "what am I to do with all these?" and a guy said: "oh you'll have to pay for those!"'[97] As noted by Bourke, these forms of comic bonding were well established between the men.[98]

Humour also worked to bolster local networks of understanding.[99] Men often wrote comedic poems in the trenches to capture the illness experience. Private Henry Jackson of the 75th Field Ambulance RAMC recalled a section of a friend's poem: 'Although a hundred you may kill, you will find there's hundreds still, for they hide behind one another, and they're good at taking cover.'[100] The humour of Jackson's friend conveys pointed reflection on health and comfort, with soldiers sparing time to creatively express and process their experiences. Further, soldiers published these poems in trench newspapers and informally circulated them from man to man.[101] This jocularity worked as a form of bonding and understanding, a shared vernacular meaning given to health conditions.

Soldiers' lived experiences convey their physical and emotional responses to illness and the meanings they derived from them. Systems of care are shaped and sustained in large part by shared experiences.[102] These experiences took on profound meaning for soldiers and formed for them the basis of a vernacular medical understanding. When we consider these factors, the boundaries of healthcare expand to incorporate a larger world view, one less mediated by biomedicine.

## The patient as practitioner: soldiers' vernacular medical practice

It is not enough simply to explore the inner worlds and experiences of patients. Historians have long used patients' emotions and reactions to reflect on biomedicine, providing powerful evidence to fill spaces that were once silent. By adopting a new model – vernacular medicine – the historian can use these emotions to form a fresh understanding of the patient on their own terms. Patients' understandings and experiences often played into larger narratives driven by the immediate necessities of their life at the Front. Vernacular medical knowledge gave rise to preventive vernacular medical practices.[103]

Soldiers actively used their shared networks to explore and inform each other of their medical techniques, thus engaging in collective practice. Methods spread from soldier to soldier by word of mouth, and they recorded this network in their written accounts. Private Gwinnell recorded one event where he and his battalion comrades conducted an experiment with lice-exterminating powder:

> At last someone told me of some stuff which he declared was THE stuff. It was called trench powder. I [...] sent home for some [...] and [was] determined to test it out at once. Off came my shirt, and I picked out a good specimen. I put it very gently into a small tin,

being careful not to injure it in any way. I then covered it over with plenty of my precious powder, leaving it on a ledge of the trench for 24 hours. We then gathered round, about 20 of us, to see the result [...] All my mates craned their heads forward to see the experiment. The lid came off, and never have I ever seen a more healthy or happy louse. Believe me, it was as lively as a cricket, in perfect condition, and fat as a pig.[104]

Further, not only did soldiers experiment collectively and spread ideas in this informal manner, they also unofficially published techniques and health advice in trench newspapers, circulating their practices among the men. One humorous account in *The Jab*, the newspaper of the Second Rangers, professed, 'perhaps a tip won't bore you! Never go to a medical officer with sore feet – that is unless you want him to give you socks.'[105] Through these networks, men shared ways to alter biomedical techniques, sourced materials and medicine, shared those resources and relied heavily on general improvisation. It is clear from soldiers' documentation of these networks that they were developing their own unique healthcare system.

Although soldiers practised medicine away from medical professionals, many men developed techniques that both built on and reformulated biomedicine. This fusion reveals the importance of perceiving knowledge as not simply a direct consumption from professional to patient, but as a form of power that could be harnessed in a unique manner and altered to suit the immediate environment of the trenches.[106] Soldiers tailored biomedical techniques for their own needs. Adapting MOs' trench foot methods to suit the adverse environment meant that some men, like Private Leonard Davies of the Royal Fusiliers, profited from the waterproof barrier that professionally prescribed whale oil provided. He wore 'two or three pairs of socks' soaking them 'in oil or fat or grease, anything you can get hold of first'.[107] Corporal West placed a large portion of oil into the toe end of his socks, sinking his feet into the viscous liquid before replacing his boots.[108] Lance Corporal Sheard built on existing medical responses to gas attacks. MOs treated gassed men by placing ammonia phials up their nostrils, counteracting and neutralising the noxious chemicals to clear soldiers' airways.[109] Sheard appropriated ammonia phials by breaking them around the corners of the gas-protected quarters, while simultaneously wearing his gas mask. By breaking the ammonia phials, Sheard thought he had a small chance of neutralising the air and avoiding burns and poisoning.[110]

More often, however, soldiers relied on their own ideas aside from biomedicine, putting their faith in the resources available to them through their interpersonal relationships, interaction settings and environment. Local networks bolstered soldier's vernacular medicine beyond adapted professional practice. Soldiers depended on each other in a multitude of ways to maintain their health. When Captain Smith wrote to his sister on 30 July 1917, he mused that she would smile to see his tent:

> It looks like a quack doctor's booth on Blackpool sands [...] the news that I am seedy seems to have got round [sic] among my friends, with the result that they have all very kindly sent me a bottle of their favourite tonic. So I have enough medicine to float a Dreadnought or poison a hippopotamus.[111]

Smith's anecdote about his inherited pharmacy conveys the importance of his local networks in sourcing medical assistance. These bonds of aid between the men coloured their medical practice. Using, re-using and distributing uniforms and associated items to conquer ill health built a system of social care and sharing removed from biomedical authority. Inadequate footwear was the main cause of trench foot. Many men were issued with ill-fitting pairs due to supply problems or they fell into a shocking condition from overuse. Lance Corporal Sheard's toes were 'turned up heavenwards with wearing a size too large'.[112] The battalion cobbler was kept busy as most men could not afford new boots. They enjoyed the mental respite the trip to the shoemaker brought from the stresses of war.[113] Soldiers also found multiple uses for other uniform items. Private Gwinnell documented that 'another man and I shared one [blanket] with a huge hole in it' to keep their feet warm when there were not enough supplies for each soldier.[114]

When bonds in the trenches could not provide for soldiers' practices, men often turned to their wider networks. As argued by Roper, men's lives in the trenches were interdependent with their home lives.[115] Strong links to home were dependent on the soldier's rank, as officers and their families could more likely afford to send new clothes and medical items. For men like Smith, a Captain, the connection between trench and home was consistent. The availability of clean, new uniforms meant less chance of catching diseases spread through contact with the environment. Writing to numerous members of his family he requested a 'vest, pants, collars (15s) and tie' because his underclothing had 'been blown sky high' and '2 or 3 pairs of khaki silk socks' or else 'some black socks'.[116] Lieutenant James H. Butlin of the Dorsetshire Regiment began most letters home thanking his family for parcels or asking for new socks.[117] He boasted that he fashioned a system in which 'with two suits [and pairs of shoes] I can use one for billets and one for the trenches'.[118] Replacement uniforms were an uncommon luxury for men in the 'Other Ranks'. Yet men in the Scottish Regiments who wore kilts sent home for ladies' bloomers in an attempt to protect their genitals against the burning and blistering of mustard gas.[119] It was commoner, as noted by both Private Youngman and Private Gwinnell, for men to source smaller items such as tins of lice exterminating powder.[120]

For most soldiers, it was easier to rely on the provisions and resources available in their immediate environment. This thriftiness highlights the importance of improvisation in soldiers' vernacular medicine. For soldiers, as argued by Meyer, improvisation played a large part of their wider war experience as their immediate environment dictated how they lived day to day.[121] For health maintenance and cleanliness, such improvisation was often a way to deal with the trauma of life in the trenches and was linked to soldiers' understanding of endurance and resilience. As divisional baths were located miles behind the line, makeshift baths were more effective and readily at hand. Lance Corporal Sheard kept his dirty shirt after visiting the baths, 'then had a washing day' using 'an old petrol tin and some boiling water to which had been added plenty of paraffin and soap'.[122] Corporal West noted that when he came out on rest he would 'get an old barrel, cut it in half, and make two baths of it'.[123] Creativity and resourcefulness coloured numerous techniques for keeping their feet dry. Lance Corporal Sheard slept with his boots and tunic as a pillow, relying on his body heat to keep his boots from freezing overnight.[124] Other men whose toes throbbed swaddled their feet in puttees, sandbags or goatskin jackets.[125] Advanced Dressing Station salvage dumps provided cast-off uniforms and equipment from medical and surgical patients deceased or whisked back through the medical chain towards the base hospital.[126] Many secured second-hand boots from the dump and it was not uncommon to find amputated feet left inside.[127] Men fashioned rudimentary gas masks before the introduction of PH helmets and small box respirators.[128] Private Christopher Cockburn of the Northumberland Fusiliers described a makeshift scarf or 'anything you got' soaked in urine tied around the nose and mouth.[129] Corporal West noted a similar prevention based on water-soaked handkerchiefs and another on 'little square pieces of cloth and two tapes'.[130]

Some techniques were tied to soldiers' use of humour in the trenches, conveying the direct link between vernacular understandings and practices. To amuse themselves and to make healthcare a relief from the other aspects of trench life, some men turned to entertaining methods of lice extermination. One jovial practice was turning their shirts inside out – 'uniform tricks' said to confuse the lice. Private Cockburn remembered one man would 'take [his] shirt off and turn it inside out and put it on again. All so that [he] could have a rest before [the lice] could walk around to the other side!'[131] Other amusing methods used rations. A widespread tactic was to 'burn 'em out' with rationed candles or cigarette lighters.[132] This was considered a chief sport.[133] What most recollections of this method note is the auditory sensation, exclaiming that the eggs would pop, crack and burst like fireworks, music to soldiers' ears.[134] Corporal West also recalled his pal used to:

> send out for some pebbles and some [...] powder that made you sneeze [...] and he used to have them [lice and pebbles] in little bags, he said every time they sneezed they bashed their brains out![135]

The most immediate solutions, however, often did not rely on equipment. Some men relied on their knowledge of the physical environment and basic chemistry to prevent gas poisoning. Sapper George Robinson of the Royal Engineers recalled his reaction to mustard gas attacks while out of the line. He climbed a tree as the 'gas was heavier than air' and the effects of the liquid reached only 'seven or eight feet at the most'.[136] In this way, he escaped the attack. Similar practices involved avoiding the water and mud as often as possible. Private Fred Potter of the King's Liverpool Regiment recounted:

> on one occasion two or three of us joined together to stretch our groundsheets from the parapet [...] to the parados [...] and there we were crouching under this thing on the fire step with our feet resting

across the trench on the other side. When the commanding officer came along we got sound berated [sic] for sitting in that fashion because the groundsheets would give away our position. Apparently, standing in wet feet didn't matter![137]

Paradoxically, the adverse physical environment often provided both ailment and aid to soldiers. Men who had holes in their boots 'used to think sometimes the mud caked up on your [boots and] puttees kept out some of the cold'.[138] Private Gwinnell and his pals relied on the physical environment to destroy lice, trying everything from leaving their clothes in the frost overnight, burying their shirts in the mud and weighting their clothing down with rocks in a stream.[139] Corporal West recalled one chap who attested to the efficacy of a specific wall in having a good scratch.[140]

It is evident, then, that soldiers practised their own form of medicine. Soldiers' behaviours, based on shared knowledge and networks, the environment and available tools, shaped a unique healthcare system. Therefore, as the Great War patient had their own understanding of illness and their own practice, the patient was also a practitioner. It is only by understanding the soldier at a remove from biomedicine that this new view of the patient is possible.

## Conclusions

The patient voice in First World War medicine is a less well-known concept than it first appears. Although soldiers had explicit views about the care that they received from the military medical system, exploring their experiences at a remove from biomedicine unveils a fresh approach to the patient voice. While medical professionals viewed their patients' illnesses as physiological ailments to be cured, the patients themselves understood their experiences beyond simply the somatic. Soldiers' local networks and worlds shaped the ways in which they understood their bodies and the experiences they encountered in the trenches. Senses and emotions fuelled powerful understandings of both illness and the environmental factors that stressed ill-health. Soldiers created a shared vernacular knowledge of their illness experiences through moderating factors such as endurance and humour. Further, not only did they understand illness differently from medical professionals, they used their understanding to craft a unique set of practices to cope with the traumas of trench life. They practiced vernacular medicine.

What vernacular medicine lends to the patient voice is not only power outside of the biomedical system, but also a new way to conceive of the patient and what constitutes a healthcare system. In the midst of the COVID-19 pandemic, with many individuals isolated and at the mercy of a plethora of conflicting information, vernacular medicine abounds. Informal medical networks (often found on social-media platforms) present an opportunity for individuals to allay fears and swap information in a similar manner to soldiers' emotional and intellectual networks. Indeed, in this heightened medical climate and with a lack of access to professional materials, examples of vernacular practice proliferate more than ever before. Some well-known concepts include drinking copious amounts of hot water and spending time in the sun or bright light.[141] Likewise, the professional policing of alternative ideas, which in some dangerous cases is necessary, is also increasing.[142] For many, however, vernacular practices and networks are not new and have long been many individuals' 'reality' as the study of Great War soldiers illustrates. For historians of medicine living through COVID-19, fresh approaches to past medical ideas and networks, particularly those that emerged during moments of crisis, are more important than ever before.

For health policy, this chapter conveys the necessity of understanding medicine as a practice undertaken by those outside of the professional sector. When implementing policies surrounding healthcare systems it is, therefore, imperative to acknowledge the existence of multiple systems within one social setting. For policy-makers, the voices of individuals suffering from ill health must be at the core of their work. The local worlds and networks of the sick individual shape the ways in which they both understand their health and how they manage or treat themselves. Policy-makers must look beyond professional medicine to see 'primary care'. As in the case of First World War soldiers, the traumatic experiences of living in the trenches, seen through soldiers' subjective personal accounts, formed bonds of understanding and practice between men. Vernacular medicine helped men cope with their experiences of ill-health, the poor environment and trauma. With this new perspective, the patient voice reveals far more than a reflection of biomedicine.

## Notes

1. Mark Harrison, *The Medical War: British Military Medicine in the First World War* (Oxford: Oxford University Press, 2010).
2. Ana Carden-Coyne, *The Politics of Wounds: Military Patients and Medical Power in the First World War* (Oxford: Oxford University Press, 2014); Fiona Reid, *Medicine in First World War Europe: Soldiers, Medics, Pacifists* (London: Bloomsbury Academic, 2017).
3. Roy Porter, 'The Patient's View: Doing Medical History from Below', *Theory and Society* 14:2 (1985), 175–98, 181–2; Flurin Condrau, 'The Patient's View Meets the Clinical Gaze', *Social History of Medicine* 20:3 (2007), 525–40. This idea is furthered in the first footnote of Arthur Kleinman, *The Illness Narratives: Suffering, Healing and the Human Condition* (New York: Basic Books, 1988), 3–4.
4. Condrau, 'The Patient's View Meets the Clinical Gaze', 525.
5. Jessica Meyer, *Men of War: Masculinity and the First World War in Britain* (Basingstoke: Palgrave, 2009), 9.
6. Reid, *Medicine in First World War Europe*, 21.
7. See Michael Worboys's chapter in this collection.
8. Imperial War Museums (hereafter IWM) Sound Archive, Oral History Recording 578: Percy Webb; P.S. Lelean, *Sanitation in War* (London: J. & A. Churchill, 1915), 110.
9. Arthur Kleinman, *Patients and Healers in the Context of Culture: An Exploration of the Borderland between Anthropology, Medicine, and Psychiatry* (Berkeley: University of California Press, 1980), 72; John W. Reich and Frank J. Infurna, *Perceived Control: Theory, Research and Practice in the First 50 Years* (Oxford: Oxford University Press, 2017), 213.
10. Kleinman, *Patients and Healers in the Context of Culture*, 35.
11. Definition of 'vernacular' according to Collins Dictionary.
12. Kleinman, *Patients and Healers in the Context of Culture*, 26; Edmund Ramsden, 'Science and Medicine in the United States of America', in Mark Jackson (ed.), *A Global History of Medicine* (Oxford: Oxford University Press, 2018), 225–43.
13. Kathryn Shively Meier, *Nature's Civil War: Common Soldiers and the Environment in 1862 Virginia* (Chapel Hill: University of North Carolina Press, 2013). Meier, however, examines 'self-care'. She approaches her study from a military and environmental perspective and therefore does not adopt a medical lens through which to interrogate what it means to practise self-care or the power imbalance in medical history that stops historians from assessing these practices as medicine in their own right.

14 Roger Cooter and John Pickstone, 'Introduction', in Roger Cooter and John Pickstone (eds), *Medicine in the Twentieth Century* (Amsterdam: Harwood Academic Publishers, 2000), xiii–xix.
15 Roger Cooter, 'War and Modern Medicine', in W.F. Bynum and Roy Porter (eds), *Companion Encyclopedia of the History of Medicine*, Vol. II (London: Routledge, 1993), 1536–73.
16 Roger Cooter, 'Medicine and Modernity', in Mark Jackson (ed.), *The Oxford Handbook of the History of Medicine* (Oxford: Oxford University Press, 2011), 100–14, 106; see also Mark Harrison, 'Medicine and the Management of Modern Warfare: An Introduction', in Roger Cooter, Mark Harrison and Steve Sturdy (eds), *Medicine and Modern Warfare* (Atlanta: Rodopi, 1999), 1–22.
17 For studies on these topics see Cay-Rüdiger Prüll, 'Pathology at War 1914–1918: Germany and Britain in Comparison', in Roger Cooter, Mark Harrison and Steve Sturdy (eds), *Medicine and Modern Warfare* (Atlanta: Rodopi, 1999), 131–62; Robert L. Atenstaedt, 'The Response to the Trench Diseases in World War I: A Triumph of Public Health Science', *Public Health* 121:8 (2007), 634–9; Robert L. Atenstaedt, 'Trench Foot: The Medical Response in the First World War 1914–18', *Wilderness & Environmental Medicine* 17:4 (2006), 282–9; Edgar Jones, 'Terror Weapons: The British Experience of Gas and Its Treatment in the First World War', *War in History* 21:3 (2014), 355–75; Edgar Jones and Simon Wessely, *Shell Shock to PTSD: Military Psychiatry from 1900 to the Gulf War* (Hove: Psychology Press, 2005).
18 Roger Cooter and Steve Sturdy, 'Of War, Medicine and Modernity: An Introduction', in Roger Cooter, Mark Harrison and Steve Sturdy (eds), *War, Medicine and Modernity* (Stroud: Sutton, 1998), 1–28.
19 Christopher Lawrence, 'Continuity in Crisis: Medicine, 1914–1945', in W.F. Bynum, Anne Hardy, Stephen Jacyna, Christopher Lawrence and E.M. Tansey, *The Western Medical Tradition: 1800 to 2000* (Cambridge: Cambridge University Press, 2006), 247–404; Harrison, *The Medical War*, 10; Reid, *Medicine in First World War Europe*, 7.
20 Anon., 'Annotations', *Lancet* 189:4894 (16 June 1917), 922.
21 Harrison, *The Medical War*, 123–70.
22 Ibid., 134.
23 Ian R. Whitehead, *Doctors in the Great War* (Barnsley: Leo Cooper, 1999), 223; Ian R. Whitehead, 'The British Medical Officer on the Western Front: The Training of Doctors for War', in Roger Cooter, Mark Harrison and Steve Sturdy (eds), *Medicine and Modern Warfare* (Atlanta: Rodopi, 1999), 163–84; Ian R. Whitehead, 'Not a Doctor's Work? The Role of British Regimental Medical Officers in the Field', in Hugh Cecil and Peter H. Liddle (eds), *Facing Armageddon: The First World War Experienced* (London: Leo Cooper, 1996), 466–74;

Joanna Bourke, 'Wartime', in Roger Cooter and John Pickstone (eds), *Medicine in the Twentieth Century* (Amsterdam: Harwood Academic Publishers, 2000), 589–600.
24 For further research on practitioners as patients see Robert A. Hahn *Sickness and Healing: An Anthropological Perspective* (New Haven: Yale University Press, 1995), 234–61.
25 Some examples include Jeffery S. Reznick, *Healing the Nation: Soldiers and the Culture of Caregiving in Britain during the Great War* (Manchester: Manchester University Press, 2004); Peter Leese, *Traumatic Neurosis and the British Soldiers of the First World War* (London: Palgrave, 2002).
26 Bourke, 'Wartime', 589, 592.
27 IWM Private Papers, Documents 11601: Richard Gwinnell, Diary, 101–2. Further examples include Wellcome Library collections, London (hereafter WL), Herbert Empson, Diary, entry dated 31 January 1916, entry dated 17 February 1917, RAMC/1217: Box 266; IWM Private Papers, Documents 15334: Archibald Morsley, Diary, 44, 107; IWM Private Papers, Documents 14979: F.E. Harris, Diary, 81.
28 Some examples include Emily Mayhew, *Wounded: From Battlefield to Blighty, 1914–1918* (London: Vintage, 2014); Fiona Reid, *Broken Men: Shell Shock, Treatment and Recovery in Britain, 1914–1930* (London: Bloomsbury, 2012).
29 This link to biomedical power comes in the form of rapidly returning men to the front line after wounding or illness. Reid, *Medicine in First World War Europe*, 18.
30 David Cantor, 'The Diseased Body', in Roger Cooter and John Pickstone (eds), *Medicine in the Twentieth Century* (Amsterdam: Harwood Academic Publishers, 2000), 347–66; Carden-Coyne, *The Politics of Wounds*, 3.
31 Carden-Coyne, *The Politics of Wounds*, 4.
32 Lynn M. Thomas, 'Historicising Agency', *Gender & History* 28:2 (2016), 324–39.
33 Harrison, *The Medical War*, 123.
34 Bourke, *Dismembering the Male*; Bourke, 'Wartime', 589–600.
35 This is not always the case. It is dependent on the culture in which the healthcare system resides as to the overlap of patient and practitioner knowledge. See Kleinman, *Patients and Healers in the Context of Cultures*, 205–6; Ludmilla Jordanova, 'The Social Construction of Medical Knowledge', *Social History of Medicine* 8:3 (1995), 361–81.
36 Kleinman, *The Illness Narratives*, 17.
37 Ibid., 52–3.
38 Mark S.R. Jenner and Bertrand O. Taithe, 'The Historiographical Body', in Roger Cooter and John Pickstone (eds), *Medicine in the*

*Twentieth Century* (Amsterdam: Harwood Academic Publishers, 2000), 187–200.
39 Cantor, 'The Diseased Body', 347; Olga Amsterdamska and Anja Hiddinga, 'The Analyzed Body', in Roger Cooter and John Pickstone (eds), *Medicine in the Twentieth Century* (Amsterdam: Harwood Academic Publishers, 2000), 417–34.
40 Cooter, 'Medicine and Modernity', 108; Harrison, *The Medical War*, 3; Cantor, 'The Diseased Body', 349.
41 Cooter, 'Medicine and Modernity', 108.
42 I say somewhat because there is always more than one dialogue occurring within a single context, and in the case of the First World War there was experimentation and the development of theories surrounding war-specific diseases such as trench foot and trench fever. Yet, despite this ongoing conversation, the overarching aim was to locate and apply a central aetiological theory, prevention and treatment for each disease.
43 Lelean, *Sanitation in War*, 24–5.
44 Medical Research Committee, Plate VI, *An Atlas of Gas Poisoning* (France: British Expeditionary Force, 1918).
45 Lorraine Daston and Peter Galison, *Objectivity* (New York: Zone Books, 2007), 309–61.
46 IWM Private Papers, Documents 537: Captain Bruce A. West, Diary, n.d..
47 Kleinman, *The Illness Narratives*, 17; Cantor, 'The Diseased Body', 347.
48 Kleinman, *The Illness Narratives*, 27.
49 Michael Roper, *The Secret Battle: Emotional Survival in the Great War* (Manchester: Manchester University Press, 2009), 7. This concept is explored further in relation to gender in Meyer, *Men of War*.
50 Joanna Bourke, *The Story of Pain: From Prayer to Painkillers* (Oxford: Oxford University Press, 2014), 17, 21.
51 Rosenwein and Cristiani also state that the affective body creates an impression on the surrounding environment too. See Barbara H. Rosenwein and Riccardo Cristiani, *What Is the History of Emotions?* (Cambridge: Polity Press, 2018), 77–80; Ross Wilson, *Landscapes of the Western Front: Materiality During the Great War* (New York: Routledge, 2012), 123–4; Vanda Wilcox, '"Weeping Tears of Blood": Exploring Italian Soldiers' Emotions in the First World War', *Modern Italy* 17:2 (2012), 171–84.
52 This case study, then, also answers the call to 'go beyond abstract discussions of the body and to begin to discuss subjectivity and the self within history', made by Jenner and Taithe in 'The Historiographical Body', 196; see also Wilson, *Landscapes of the Western Front*, 124.

53 Bourke, *The Story of Pain*, 5.
54 Kleinman, *Patients and Healers in the Context of Culture*, 72; Angela Teece and John Baker, 'Thematic Analysis: How Do Patient Diaries Affect Survivors' Psychological Recovery?', *Intensive and Critical Care Nursing* 41 (August 2017), 50–6.
55 Jonathan Reinarz, 'Learning to Use Their Senses: Visitors to Voluntary Hospitals in Eighteenth-Century England', *Journal for Eighteenth-Century Studies* 35:4 (2012), 505–20.
56 Wilson, *The Landscapes of the Western Front*, 128; S.J. Rachman, *Fear and Courage* (New York: W.H. Freeman and Company, 1978), 13.
57 IWM Private Papers, Documents 15947: Samuel H. Smith, Letter to Sister (21 August 1915).
58 Kieran Mitton, *Rebels in a Rotten State: Understanding Atrocity in the Sierra Leone Civil War* (Oxford: Oxford University Press, 2015), 183.
59 Kleinman, *Patients and Healers in the Context of Culture*, 45, 147.
60 IWM Private Papers, Documents 12021: Ernest Sheard, Diary, 415–16.
61 Georgia McWhinney, 'The Lousy Business of War: Lice-Infested Uniforms and British Preventive Medicine in the First World War', in Tristan Moss and Tom Richardson (eds), *Beyond Combat: Australian Military Activity Away from the Battlefield* (Sydney: University of New South Wales Press, 2018), 106–19; A.E. Shipley, 'Insects and War', *British Medical Journal* 2:2803 (19 September 1914), 498.
62 IWM Sound Archive, Oral History Recording 564: William Davies; IWM Sound Archive, Oral History Recording 24854: Albert Day.
63 Wilson, *The Landscapes of the Western Front*, 128.
64 IWM Private Papers, Documents 16008: Harold J. Youngman, Diary, 44.
65 IWM Sound Archive, Oral History Recording 14766: Aled Parry.
66 IWM Private Papers, Documents 15334: Archibald Morsley, Diary, 47.
67 IWM Sound Archive, Oral History Recording 536: Joseph Price.
68 IWM Sound Archive, Oral History Recording 12236: Alfred West.
69 Alexander Watson, *Enduring the Great War: Combat, Morale, and Collapse in the German and British Armies 1914–1918* (Cambridge: Cambridge University Press, 2008), 33.
70 IWM Private Papers, Documents 11601: Richard Gwinnell, Diary, 129.
71 IWM Sound Archive, Oral History Recording 8342: Alexander Burnett; IWM Sound Archive, Oral History Recording 578: Percy Webb; IWM Sound Archive, Oral History Recording 9756: Horace Manton.
72 IWM Sound Archive, Oral History Recording 35804: Percy Francis Aubrey Thomas.

73 Kleinman, *Patients and Healers in the Context of Culture*, 73.
74 IWM Sound Archive, Oral History Recording 12236: Alfred West.
75 IWM Private Papers, Documents 15334: Archibald Morsley, Diary, 44.
76 IWM Private Papers, Documents 12021: Ernest Sheard, Diary, 349.
77 Ibid., 276.
78 IWM Sound Archive, Oral History Recording 24864: Reg Coldridge.
79 IWM Sound Archive, Oral History Recording 12236: Alfred West.
80 IWM Private Papers, Documents 12021: Ernest Sheard, Diary, 276–9.
81 IWM Private Papers, Documents 15947: Samuel H. Smith, Letter to Sister (6 May 1915).
82 IWM Sound Archive, Oral History Recording 18835: John Edward Davis.
83 This phenomenon is also known as 'minimisation' or 'regulating emotion'. See Kleinman, *Patients and Healers in the Context of Culture*, 148; Jan Plamper and Keith Tribe, *History of Emotions: An Introduction* (Oxford: Oxford University Press, 2015), 268.
84 Joanna Bourke, *Fear: A Cultural History* (Virago Press, 2005), 216.
85 IWM Sound Archive, Oral History Recording 24553: George Singleton. Other examples include IWM Private Papers, Documents 14979: F.E. Harris, Diary, 107–8; IWM Private Papers, Documents 16008: Harold J. Youngman, Diary, 40; IWM Sound Archive, Oral History Recording 11045: James Edwin Taylor; IWM Sound Archive, Oral History Recording 8342: Alexander Burnett.
86 Actors discuss resilience strategies within their historical contexts. While First World War soldiers discussed concepts of endurance, in a contemporary setting this is somewhat akin to mindfulness – the ability to control your understanding that life is uncontrollable. For Great War soldiers, endurance was more about carrying on through difficulties (both physical and psychological) rather than more modern concepts about resilience being the ability to 'bounce back'. See Beth Morling, 'The Cultural Context of Control', in John W. Reich and Frank J. Infurna (eds), *Perceived Control: Theory, Research, and Practice in the First 50 Years* (Oxford: Oxford University Press), 71–108.
87 Meyer, *Men of War*, 6; Carol Acton and Jane Potter, '"These Frightful Sights Would Work Havoc with One's Brain": Subjective Experience, Trauma, and Resilience in First World War Writings by Medical Personnel', *Literature and Medicine* 30:1 (Spring 2012), 61–85.
88 Acton and Potter, '"These Frightful Sights Would Work Havoc with One's Brain"', 62.
89 IWM Private Papers, Documents 11601: Richard Gwinnell, Diary, 129.
90 IWM Sound Archive, Oral History Recording 12236: Alfred West.

91 Heidi L. Fritz, Leslie N. Russek and Melissa M. Dillon, 'Humour Use Moderates the Relation of Stressful Life Events with Psychological Distress', *Personality and Social Psychology Bulletin* 43:6 (2017), 845–59; Tricia Scott, 'Expression of Humour by Emergency Personnel Involved in Sudden Deathwork', *Mortality* 12:4 (2007), 350–64.
92 IWM Private Papers, Documents 14979: F.E. Harris, Diary, 107–8.
93 Zsófia Demjén, 'Laughing at Cancer: Humour, Empowerment, Solidarity and Coping Online', *Journal of Pragmatics* 101 (June 2016), 18–30; Pierre Purseigle, 'Mirroring Societies at War: Pictorial Humour in the British and French Popular Press during the First World War', *Journal of European Studies* 31 (September 2001), 289–328; Katherine E. Brown and Elina Penttinen, '"A 'Sucking Chest Wound' Is Nature's Way of Telling You to Slow Down ..." Humour and Laughter in War Time', *Critical Studies on Security* 1:1 (2013), 124–6.
94 IWM Sound Archive, Oral History Recording 24893: Ernest John Blank.
95 IWM Private Papers, Documents 12259: Lieutenant Norman King-Wilson, Diary, 30.
96 IWM Sound Archive, Oral History Recording 9148: Christopher Cockburn.
97 IWM Sound Archive, Oral History Recording 11269: George Edward Robinson. See also IWM Sound Archive, Oral History Recording 24893: Ernest John Blank.
98 Bourke, *Dismembering the Male*, 126.
99 Christie Davies, 'Humour Is Not a Strategy in War', *Journal of European Studies* 31 (September 2001), 395–412.
100 IWM Sound Archive, Oral History Recording 24858: H.D. Jackson.
101 Anon, 'Mud Mud Mud', *The Fifth Glo'ster Gazette: A Chronicle, Serious and Humorous, of the Battalion while Serving with the British* 18 (1 April 1917), 19.
102 Kleinman, *Patients and Healers in the Context of Culture*, 39.
103 McWhinney, 'The Lousy Business of War', 116.
104 IWM Private Papers, Documents 11601: Richard Gwinnell, Diary, 107, original emphasis.
105 The Bore, 'Riflings', *The Jab: The Official Organ of the Second Rangers* 1 (7 April 1916), 5.
106 For other examples of medical exchange and adaption see Michael Worboys's chapter in this collection; Lyn Schumaker, 'History of Medicine in Sub-Saharan Africa', in Mark Jackson (ed.), *A Global History of Medicine* (Oxford: Oxford University Press, 2018), 195–219; Roy MacLeod, 'Colonial Science under the Southern Cross: Archibald Liversidge, FRS, and the Shaping of Anglo-Australian Science', in Benedikt Stuchtey (ed.), *Science Across the European Empires, 1800–1950*

(Oxford: Oxford University Press, 2005), 175–214. For further literature on idea exchange and development see Tony Ballantyne, 'Mobility, Empire, Colonisation', *History Australia* 11:2 (January 2014), 7–37; Julie McIntyre, Rebecca Mitchell, Brendan Boyle and Shaun Ryan, 'We Used to Get and Give a Lot of Help: Networking, Cooperation and Knowledge Flow in the Hunter Valley Wine Cluster', *Australian Economic History Review* 53:3 (2013), 247–67; Tamson Pietsch, 'Between the Nation and the World: J.T. Wilson and Scientific Networks in the Early Twentieth Century', in Brett M. Bennett and Joseph M. Hodge (eds), *Science and Empire: Knowledge and Networks of Science across the British Empire, 1800–1970* (Basingstoke: Palgrave, 2011), 140–59.

107  IWM Sound Archive, Oral History Recording 9343: Leonard Davies.
108  IWM Sound Archive, Oral History Recording 12236: Alfred West.
109  Medical Research Committee, *An Atlas of Gas Poisoning*, 18.
110  IWM Private Papers, Documents 12021: Ernest Sheard, Diary, 276–9.
111  IWM Private Papers, Documents 15947: Samuel H. Smith, Letter to Sister (30 July 1917).
112  IWM Private Papers, Documents 12021: Ernest Sheard, Diary, 195.
113  IWM Private Papers, Documents 3875: Oliver Coleman, Diary entries dated 26 October 1917 and 10 November 1917.
114  IWM Private Papers, Documents 11601: Richard Gwinnell, Diary, 106.
115  Roper, *The Secret Battle*, 6. For further examples of the homefront, medicine, and 'care packages', see Gail Braybon and Penny Summerfield, *Out of the Cage: Women's Experiences in Two World Wars* (London; New York: Pandora Press, 1987); Amy J. Shaw, 'Expanding the Narrative: A First World War with Women, Children, and Grief', *The Canadian Historical Review* 95:3 (2014), 389–406; Ian Willis, 'The Red Cross and the Liverpool Field Hospital, Hope and Despair During 1915', *Health and History* 18:1 (2016), 22–41.
116  IWM Private Papers, Documents 15947: Samuel H. Smith, Letter to Mother and Father (1 May 1915) and Letter to Sister (30 July 1917).
117  For example, see IWM Private Papers, Documents 7915: Lieutenant James H. Butlin, Letter to Sister (7 April 1915), Letter to Mother (11 April 1915), Letter to Sister (4 December 1915).
118  Butlin, Letter to Sister (4 December 1915).
119  IWM Sound Archive, Oral History Recording 9756: Horace Manton.
120  IWM Private Papers, Documents 16008: Harold J. Youngman, Diary, 48; IWM Private Papers, Documents 11601: Richard Gwinnell, Diary, 107.
121  Meyer, *Men of War*, 31–4.

122  IWM Private Papers, Documents 12021: Ernest Sheard, Diary, 195.
123  IWM Sound Archive, Oral History Recording 12236: Alfred West.
124  IWM Private Papers, Documents 12021: Ernest Sheard, Diary, 310.
125  IWM Private Papers, Documents 12259: Lieutenant Norman King-Wilson, Diary, 30, 58–9, 352–3.
126  IWM Private Papers, Documents 3875: Oliver Coleman, Diary entry dated 23 October 1918.
127  Ibid.
128  PH helmets were early gas hoods impregnated with phenate hexamine (PH) to stop the gas reaching the soldier's airways and eyes.
129  IWM Sound Archive, Oral History Recording 9148: Christopher Cockburn.
130  IWM Sound Archive, Oral History Recording 12236: Alfred West.
131  IWM Sound Archive, Oral History Recording 9148: Christopher Cockburn.
132  IWM Sound Archive, Oral History Recording 24854: Albert Day; IWM Sound Archive, Oral History Recording 564: William Davies; IWM Sound Archive, Oral History Recording 379: Fred Potter.
133  IWM Sound Archive, Oral History Recording 14766: Aled Parry.
134  IWM Private Papers, Documents 14979: F.E. Harris, Diary, 107; IWM Sound Archive, Oral History Recording 12236: Alfred West; IWM Sound Archive, Oral History Recording 26870: Ernest Bell.
135  IWM Sound Archive, Oral History Recording 12236: Alfred West.
136  IWM Sound Archive, Oral History Recording 11269: George Edward Robinson.
137  IWM Sound Archive, Oral History Recording 379: Fred Potter.
138  IWM Sound Archive, Oral History Recording 24854: Albert Day.
139  IWM Private Papers, Documents 11601: Richard Gwinnell, Diary, 107.
140  IWM Sound Archive, Oral History Recording 12236: Alfred West.
141  Olga Robinson and Marianna Spring, 'Coronavirus: How Bad Information Goes Viral', *BBC News* (19 March 2020), www.bbc.com/news/blogs-trending-51931394 (accessed 26 June 2020).
142  In Australia, for example, the Therapeutic Goods Administration fined celebrity chef Pete Evans $25,200 for promoting a light machine to fight COVID-19. Amanda Meade, 'Chef Pete Evans Exits Seven's My Kitchen Rules Amid Ratings Slump', *The Guardian* (8 May 2020), www.theguardian.com/tv-and-radio/2020/may/08/pete-evans-mkr-celebrity-chef-leaving-exit-seven-my-kitchen-rules-ratings-slump (accessed 26 June 2020).

# IV

Negotiating stigma and shame

# 8

# 'Dear Dr Kirkpatrick': recovering Irish experiences of VD, 1924–47*

## Lloyd (Meadhbh) Houston

In the growing body of scholarship devoted to the 1913–16 Royal Commission on Venereal Diseases (RCVD) and the state-funded Venereal Diseases (VD) Service to which its findings gave rise in Britain and Ireland, the voices of sufferers, patients and service users are most often conspicuous by their absence.[1] While detailed and nuanced surveys exist of the implementation and administration of the Service at both national and regional levels, by their own admission, such studies can often offer only scant insight into the thoughts, feelings and lived experience of those who suffered from and were treated for VD.[2] As Anne Hanley illustrates in Chapter 9 of the present collection, the archival reasons for this are obvious enough. The materials most readily available to historians – medical publications, local government reports and patient records – seldom, if ever, feature the words of sufferers or, when they do, present them only in mediated form. Meanwhile, as might be expected given the stigma and shame which surrounded VD in the early twentieth century, sufferers were often extremely reluctant to discuss their condition with others or to leave records of their infection, diagnosis or treatment. In this chapter, I discuss a rare exception to the archival vacuum surrounding the voices of VD sufferers in the interwar period: the personal correspondence of Dr Thomas Percy Claude Kirkpatrick, one of twentieth-century Ireland's foremost VD specialists.

Sent to Kirkpatrick by current and former patients, their family members and a range of health professionals between 1924 and 1947, the 120 letters which comprise the Kirkpatrick collection offer an unparalleled insight into the medical, social and emotional experiences of VD sufferers and those who supported them during a formative period in the development of state welfare provision in Britain and Ireland. In the process, they contradict a range of common assumptions about the levels of knowledge, agency and self-understanding that VD sufferers enjoyed in their engagement with the individuals and institutions who treated them. They reveal the ways in which former and current patients could strategically perform their gender, age and class identities in their communications with health professionals to solicit aid, advice and support. They illustrate the transformative effect that treatment for VD could have on an individual's capacity to understand, monitor and describe their body in a period in which 'profound and widespread ignorance over sexual matters' was the norm.[3] They reveal some of the paradoxical ways in which stigmatising illnesses could foster deep and wide-ranging bonds of trust between patients and their physicians. They show how, amid the mixed welfare economies of interwar Ireland and Britain, individuals from a range of socio-economic backgrounds could leverage state-funded VD services to achieve their desired social and healthcare outcomes. Above all, they afford a rare and unusually direct view into the intimate lives of Irish people and their attitudes towards sexuality, sexual health and medical authority during a period of significant social and political upheaval.

In my exploration of these aspects of Kirkpatrick's correspondence, I adopt an analytical framework that combines close-reading techniques with aspects of both regional and four-nations history perspectives.[4] Linguistic features such as lexicon, register and tone can offer a valuable insight into the self-understanding of VD sufferers and the strategies of self-presentation they adopted when engaging with medical professionals such as Kirkpatrick. The language and imagery through which sufferers and their loved ones sought to describe their symptoms and experiences offer both an index of the kinds of information – medical or otherwise – to which they had access and a record of their emotional response to illness and its aftermath. Close textual analysis is also a useful means by which to explore the nuances of the doctor–patient relationship and the complex power dynamics which determined it. By attending closely to the linguistic choices made by VD sufferers and those who cared for them when addressing Kirkpatrick, I aim to offer not only a vivid account of the experiences of individuals living with a stigmatising illness in interwar Ireland, but a fuller sense of the ways in which they exerted agency over their treatment and care.

A sensitivity to regional context is particularly necessary in the case of VD sufferers in the interwar period, because, as an early and radical step towards an as yet largely untried model of public-health provision, the Local Government Board (LGB) VD Service was far from uniform in its implementation across Britain and Ireland. Thus, for example, where doctors in Rochdale might have paid little attention to 'gendered difference' in infection rates and sexual behaviours, doctors in nearby Liverpool, with its transient male seafaring population, retained a tacit belief in 'men's need for sexual release'.[5] This potential for idiosyncrasy was compounded by the shifting political situation in Ireland, where the scheme was adopted under British rule, implemented during the upheavals of the War of Independence (1919–21) and became a focal point for government infighting during the uneasy period of state-formation that followed the Civil War (1922–23).[6] As Susannah Riordan notes, the introduction of the VD Service in Ireland was impeded by 'legislative delay', 'the disarray of local government after 1919' and, in contrast to the situation in England and Wales, the Irish government's willingness to allow the effects of local government health cuts to fall 'almost entirely' on VD schemes.[7] This meant that by the time the Free State was established in 1922, only four local authority VD services were up and running, served by two centres in Dublin hospitals (St Patrick Dun's and Dr Steevens').[8] In such an atypical context, a four-nations approach is necessary to identify the points of continuity and discontinuity which existed between the experiences of VD sufferers in Ireland and those of their English, Welsh and Scottish counterparts.

A balance between a regional and a four-nations perspective is similarly important when addressing the history of sexuality in Ireland. Until relatively recently, historians and sociologists have offered accounts of early twentieth-century Irish sexuality in which repression, shame and sin have been the presiding themes.[9] In a range of influential monographs and essays, Tom Inglis has emphasised the 'moral monopoly' of the Catholic Church in Irish institutions of health, medicine and welfare, asserting that, in post-independence Ireland, the 'Irish body' came to be shaped according to the template established by a 'normative, particularly sexual, Catholic social order' from which 'alternative or resistant voices were relatively absent' and in which 'transgressions were limited'.[10] This perspective has been echoed by figures such as James M. Smith, who frames Ireland's institutions of state and ecclesiastical welfare provision as interlocking components of a sexual 'containment culture'.[11] As Diarmaid Ferriter has argued, while the Catholic Church's influence in sexual matters in Ireland was undoubtedly widespread, conservative and sometimes abusive, to reduce the field of Irish sexuality to the univocal Catholic hegemony presented by Inglis and Smith risks artificially homogenising and exceptionalising the experiences of Irish people, ignoring the extent to which the sexual history of Ireland could be 'just as complicated and multilayered as the sexual history of many other countries'.[12] By transcribing the 'alternative and resistant voices' preserved in these letters (particularly those of women), detailing a number of common transgressions (infidelity, pre-marital sex, separation) and identifying the ways in which Irish VD sufferers sought to influence their treatment and care, I hope to contribute to this more complex and multi-layered image of twentieth-century Irish sexuality.

## Kirkpatrick and his practice

Thomas Percy Claude Kirkpatrick (1864–1959) lived and worked during one of the most tumultuous periods of change in Irish civic, political and social history, witnessing the First World War (1914–18), the Easter Rising (1916), the War of Independence, partition and the Anglo-Irish Treaty (1921), the Civil War, the establishment of Éire (1937) and the Republic of Ireland Act (1948). During a long and prestigious medical career, he served as the anaesthetist and, later, visiting-physician at Dr Steevens' Hospital, Dublin, Registrar for the Royal College of the Physicians of Ireland (1910–54) and General Secretary for the Royal Academy of Medicine in Ireland.[13] He was also an enthusiastic amateur historian and bibliographer, publishing monographs on a range of prominent figures and institutions in Irish medicine and print culture.[14] Unusually for a period in which stigmatising illnesses were largely confined to the periphery of respectable medical practice, Kirkpatrick's passion, both professionally and academically, was VD. Both his published output and private holdings of pamphlets, journal articles and circulars reveal Kirkpatrick's consistent efforts to identify and publicise best practice in the field of sexual health.[15] The *Dublin* and *Irish Journal of Medical Science* contain numerous articles, notes and testimonials from Kirkpatrick on the treatment, impact and history of VD, with a particular focus on syphilis. While by no means radical in their social agenda, they reveal Kirkpatrick to have been liberal in outlook, averse to moralising and keen to embrace the pragmatic spirit of the RCVD and the LGB Regulations to which its Report gave rise.[16] Though convinced that only the eradication of commercial sex could entirely curtail the spread of VD, Kirkpatrick was circumspect in his appraisal of regulationist strategies, noting the shortcomings of the Contagious Diseases Acts (1864, 1866 and 1869) and emphasising the need to hold the male clients of sex workers equally responsible for the transmission of infection.[17] For Kirkpatrick, VD was a public-health issue which should be met with the most advanced treatment possible, pursued to the point of total cure, made freely and discretely available to the public by the state.[18] These published reflections were rooted in his experiences of diagnosing and treating venereal infection in his private practice at 11 Fitzwilliam Place on Dublin's Southside, at the Westmoreland Lock Hospital on Townsend Street and through the sexual-health clinic he oversaw at Dr Steevens' Hospital on Steevens' Lane.

Established near Kilmainham in west Dublin in 1733, Dr Steevens' was one of the capital's four voluntary hospitals. Alongside the Westmoreland Lock (founded in 1792), the hospital served as Dublin's major institution for the treatment of VD patients throughout the eighteenth and nineteenth centuries.[19] As a result of this heritage and in accordance with the 1916–17 LGB Ireland (LGBI) Regulations, the hospital became the designated centre for the treatment of venereal infection for the Dublin county borough and Counties Kildare and Wicklow, in 1919.[20] In a 1923 article in the *Irish Medical Journal*, Kirkpatrick described how the centre's clinic and wards were organised:

> The Centre was put in the charge of my colleague, Mr Arthur Chance and of myself and each of us had had two morning sessions of two hours each week and one joint session of two hours. Soon, however, it was found that this time was quite insufficient to deal with the

number of patients who attended and two evening sessions and four morning sessions were started. The two evening sessions and two of the morning sessions were for men and the remaining two morning sessions were women and children. The expenses of the Centre were borne entirely by the Corporation and the Government. A separate apartment in the dispensary of the hospital was fitted up for the accommodation of the Centre and two wards, containing fifteen beds for men and ten beds for women, were set apart for the patients of the clinic. Two trained orderlies were put in charge of the men's ward and a trained nurse in charge of the women's ward.[21]

As Kirkpatrick noted, in line with the LGBI Regulations and in contrast with the majority of contemporary medical treatment, this service was paid for by the state and local authorities.[22] As a result, Kirkpatrick's clinic served a wide and varied client-base, many of whom remained in contact with their physician long after their treatment had come to an end. This diversity is reflected in the variety of correspondence gathered in the Kirkpatrick collection.

## The Kirkpatrick collection

Held at the Library of the Royal College of Physicians of Ireland in two uncatalogued files compiled by Kirkpatrick himself, Kirkpatrick's correspondence comprises 120 letters from 80 individuals sent between March 1924 and October 1947.[23]

As Figure 8.1 shows, the majority of the letters contained within the Kirkpatrick collection were sent between 1924 and 1927, with a sharp decline in 1928 and small spikes in 1930–31 and 1935. While the present chapter will necessarily focus primarily on these periods of activity, it is worth interrogating briefly what might account for the varied distribution of the letters. Though it is not immediately apparent from the files themselves whether a principle of selection governed which letters were retained, Kirkpatrick's tendency towards assiduous record-keeping and archiving suggest that as much material would have been preserved as possible.[24] This intuition appears to be borne out by the absence of any conspicuous gaps or breaks in the chains of correspondence which the files contain. Likewise, while the majority of the correspondence paints a picture of Kirkpatrick as a generous, compassionate and industrious professional with a sincere concern for the wellbeing of current and former patients, the presence of a handful of letters which criticise Kirkpatrick and his conduct suggest that he did not seek to sanitise the collection for posterity's sake.[25] If Kirkpatrick's record-keeping does not appear to have been responsible for these peaks and troughs in correspondence, nor do fluctuations in contemporary rates of infection. While recorded cases of VD in the Free State and Éire progressively fell by roughly a third between 1924 and 1939, this steady decline does not mirror the sharp drop in Kirkpatrick's correspondence from 1928 onwards.[26] Meanwhile, absolutely no correlation seems to exist between the rate of Kirkpatrick's correspondence and reported infection rates from 1939 to 1945, during which time the number of recorded cases doubled.[27] It is tempting to attribute the concentration of correspondence for the years 1924–27 to the operations of the Interdepartmental Committee of Inquiry Regarding Venereal Disease (ICVD), which was constituted in December 1924 and reported in February 1926. It is possible that the increased official attention being paid to Irish sexual health in this period may have prompted Kirkpatrick to be particularly scrupulous in retaining material relating to VD from his practice. However, in the absence of evidence that Kirkpatrick contributed directly to the Committee's investigations or Report, the overlap in dates must remain only a

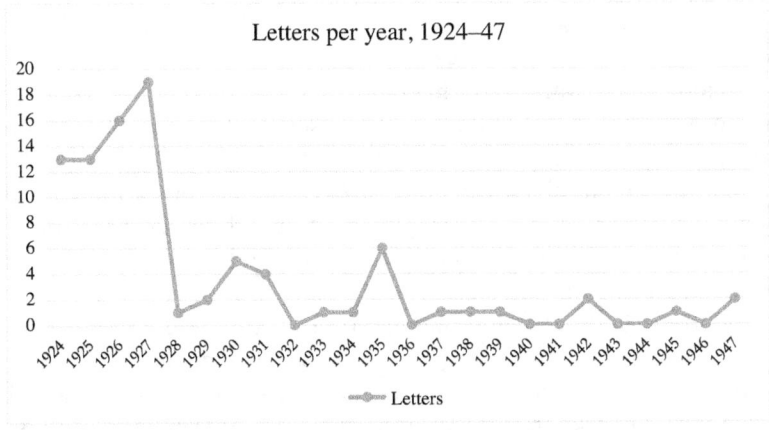

8.1 Graph showing letters sent to Dr T.P.C. Kirkpatrick per year for the period 1924–47

suggestive coincidence. Likewise, while one might note that the spike in correspondence in 1935 coincides with the passage of the revised Criminal Law Amendment Act – raising the age of consent and prohibiting the sale and distribution of contraception in the Free State – there appears to be no meaningful relationship between the letters for this period (all but one of which were sent by former patients by then residing overseas) and the legislation or the debates it generated.[28]

The surviving letters and their subjects can be broken down in a number of ways that reflect the make-up of Kirkpatrick's case-load and the variety of administrative, social and pastoral roles his correspondents expected him to fulfil. Of the seventy-nine individuals who wrote to Kirkpatrick, sixty-four were current or former patients, seven were relatives of patients (four parents, one child, one sibling, one spouse), six were medical professionals (five male, one female), one represented a welfare institution (the Legion of Mary Catholic Girls' Hostel on Harcourt Street, Dublin) and one wrote on behalf of a business (the Dublin office of Prudential Insurance, Ltd). As these figures suggest, in contrast to the institutionally dominated landscape mapped in much Irish and British medical historiography, these letters offer a rare and consistent insight into the attitudes and experiences of patients, service users and the general public concerning sexual health – albeit one that necessarily excludes the 'non-patient' perspectives charted by Michael Worboys in Chapter 1. These individuals likewise appear to have hailed from a diverse array of socio-economic backgrounds, ranging from severe poverty to middle-class comfort. While adjudications of class are difficult to make with any certainty in the absence of more information concerning the background of Kirkpatrick's correspondents, on the basis of contextual measures (orthography, lexicon, grammatical style, address, references to employment or lack thereof) the socio-economic make-up of Kirkpatrick's correspondents seems to break down as shown in Table 8.1.

More verifiably, twenty-one letters from twelve correspondents (a roughly equal proportion to those seeking medical advice or referral) make direct reference to financial hardship or appeal for charity from Kirkpatrick, indicating that a sizeable portion of those contacting him lived in a state of economic precarity (a situation no doubt exacerbated by both the Great Depression and, from 1932,

Table 8.1 Breakdown of Dr T.P.C. Kirkpatrick's correspondents by class

| Class | No. of Correspondents |
| --- | --- |
| Working-class | 29 |
| Lower middle-class | 33 |
| Middle-class | 17 |

Table 8.2 Breakdown of letters to Dr T.P.C. Kirkpatrick by subject

| Subject of Letter | Number of Letters |
| --- | --- |
| Male | 15 |
| Female | 88 |
| Relationship/Couple | 11 |
| Child/Children | 13 |

Ireland's 'Economic War' with England).[29] As Claire Martin notes, sexuality (and, one might add, illness) never play out 'in a socioeconomic vacuum' and the ways in which class factors influenced how these individuals experienced the ramifications of VD and navigated the mixed healthcare economy of the Free State and Éire will be a consistent focus of this chapter.[30]

A no less significant factor in shaping the ways in which those who wrote to Kirkpatrick experienced sexuality, sexual health and the VD Service is, of course, gender. Of Kirkpatrick's seventy-nine correspondents, fourteen were male, fifty-six were female and nine do not identify their gender. As Table 8.2 shows, a similar gender ratio is found when the letters are broken down by the identity of the individuals they concern.

This gender imbalance, in which women outnumber men by a ratio of almost five to one, stands in stark contrast to the structure of Kirkpatrick's clinics at Steevens' – two evening sessions and a two-hour morning session for men, with only a single two-hour morning session for women and children – and the attendance rates they reported, as shown in Table 8.3.[31]

The disparity is at least in part a by-product of the fact that Kirkpatrick had sole responsibility for the women's VD ward at

Table 8.3 VD clinic attendance figures for Dr Steevens' Hospital, 1919–24

| Year | Male Patients | Female Patients | TOTAL |
| --- | --- | --- | --- |
| 1919 | 794 | 110 | 904 |
| 1920 | 968 | 178 | 1146 |
| 1921 | 852 | 242 | 1094 |
| 1922 | 865 | 213 | 1078 |
| TOTAL | 3479 | 743 | 4222 |

Steevens', a setting more conducive to feelings of trust, intimacy and gratitude than the less personal outpatient clinic.[32] Nevertheless, this fact does not seem fully sufficient to account for the disparity (many of his female correspondents appear to be outpatients and only a handful make direct reference to the ward). Likewise, while it is true that the Westmoreland Lock had excluded male patients since 1820, only six letters are addressed by patients to the hospital and only a handful of others mention it, suggesting that patients from the women-only institution do not make up a substantial portion of Kirkpatrick's correspondents.[33] Instead, the imbalance seems to suggest differences in the ways in which men and women engaged with Kirkpatrick and the networks of diagnosis, treatment and care with which he was connected.

### 'Yours fraternally': the gendered politics of patienthood

The distinctions in the register, tone and content of letters from Kirkpatrick's male and female patients are often noticeable. In claiming this, I do not wish to reinforce staid gender dichotomies, nor to reify early twentieth-century stereotypes of men as active and worldly sexual agents and women as the passive and ignorant objects of their attentions. Rather, I wish to highlight the ways in which male and female patients alike seem to have played on gendered social codes for strategic ends in their engagement with Kirkpatrick and the ways in which these codes were further inflected by the age and socio-economic background of the correspondents in question. At the almost comically stereotype-reinforcing end of the spectrum, a middle-class Wexford man afflicted with cramp explained how he sought liquid relief for his ailment.

> Dear Sir
> You will excuse me in taking the liberty in writing to you but I think it best to let you know that on a few occasions I took cramp in my stomach & I had to take a few drops of whiskey & some stout[.] I would be very thankful to you if you would kindly let me know if it would be injurious to my complaint if I was to continue to take a drop of stout or whiskey now and again as I am fond of some.
>     Thanking you in anticipation
>     I am sir
>     Yours Fraternally
>     [Mr R.][34]

As the bibulous correspondent's cordial tone and pointedly familiar sign-off make clear, Kirkpatrick's male patients could exploit both his good nature and the codes of middle-class homosocial intimacy – and the culture of communal, rounds-based drinking with which those codes were synonymous – to reformulate their treatment along more convivial lines.[35] This assumption of a shared 'fraternal' code is particularly apparent in the author's shift from an apparently medical justification for his drinking to a plea based on personal preference and the understanding with which he anticipated both arguments would be received.[36] In another, less jocular letter, a male patient by then living in Ottawa, Canada, invoked a different kind of masculine 'understanding' when he insistently asked whether a complete cure for his condition was actually possible:

> In your letter you mentioned that I did not say how I felt when writing[.] Well, I must say – I do not feel any ill effects. I suppose that is the worst of this business. It is hard to know when one is completely cured or *is it even possible to effect a complete cure*? Could you give me your opinion on the latter[?] As a doctor I assume you are sufficiently broadminded to understand human failings and that we all do d–ed foolish things which we have reason to regret in after life.
>     Now I have come to Ottowa [sic] since I came back (in fact I am writing this from Ottowa [sic]) and have gone to see a doctor who was recommended by the house surgeon in one of the hosps [sic] here as a man who specialised in V.D. cases and he has decided after reading your report to give me another course and has already given

me one injection. There are V.D. clinics here but they are under Government supervision and he advised me not to touch them so I expect he is advising me for the best. I am enclosing stamp [sic] addressed envelope for reply as I want you to tell me frankly what you think of my chances and enclose bill for amnt [sic] of fee.[37]

At the level of patient experience, the letter demonstrates the profound anxiety that VD could inspire in its sufferers, even after treatment and in the apparent absence of physical symptoms. Indeed, the author's apparent insistence that an unspecified youthful indiscretion had left him incurably tainted may offer an example of the sorts of syphilophobic panic charted by Hanley in Chapter 9.[38] At the level of gender and class, the interplay of the author's obvious anxiety, betrayed in the underlined question, his performatively off-hand rationality and his appeals to Kirkpatrick's 'broadminded', professional and implicitly male understanding all suggest an anxious desire to seek reassurance and honesty through the circuits of middle-class homosocial masculinity. The author's shift to the plural first person and his use of a mild expletive when discussing the 'd–ed foolish things' that '*we* all do' in youth are particularly telling in this regard, situating his conduct and anxieties within an implicitly shared body of worldly male experience.[39] This network of well-educated masculine understanding is further extended in the anecdote of the Canadian venereologist with which the letter concludes and the classist distrust of public-health provision it reflects.[40]

The feminine correlative of this strategically signalled masculinity is most visible in letters sent by Kirkpatrick's older female correspondents. An almost exaggeratedly guileless example of this phenomenon is given in a pair of letters and a Christmas card from a working-class woman who affectionately referred to Kirkpatrick as 'Dr Understanding Heart', identified herself as 'Noleen's Mammy' and signed her missives with a trio of kisses.[41] However, beneath this borderline flirtatious performance of matriarchal affection, there is a very real sense of trust, comfort and emotional dependency that becomes particularly apparent in the regular descriptions she offered of her increasingly poor health. In a letter sent from an address in Brixton, London in mid-September 1935, she discussed her family's move to England and the various forms of employment her children had sought. However, the majority of the letter is given over to a forthright and increasingly distressed account of receiving radiotherapy at the Marie Curie Hospital for Cancer and Allied Diseases in Hampstead:

> Well you will be surprised to here [sic] I am at the Marie Curie Hospital it was the only one I knew. I told you about being in it in 1932 & it was here they stopped my courses as I had hemmorage [sic] but if I had known they were going to do so I would not have let them. As I went to another Dr. [sic] when I came here and he said he thought the lumps in the groin were the result of the Raydum [radium]. anyway [sic] they said here at the Marie Curie that it would be ExRay [x-ray] treatment this time and all I had to do was lie on a couch and go to sleep.[42]

The letter is affecting in the sense it gives of the author's investment in Kirkpatrick as one of the few figures sufficiently medically (and, perhaps, emotionally) qualified to understand her experiences, as evidenced by her amusing reflections on her family's rough-and-ready approach to good health and her more poignant remarks concerning her isolation:

> Im [sic] here all on my own ad and [sic] don't know what to do[.] they won't understand if I write home as you know their cure was a good swim and a long walk, but I know you will understand every thing [sic] and if you can at all I know you will help me.[43]

The imagery and lexicon through which the woman evoked the pain caused by her treatment is also striking, drawing on both relatively common-place similes ('like a knife [...] cutting all down the right side'), morbid evocations of lethargy that blur the affective and the somatic ('like dead with my eyes open') and a description of the pain of radiotherapy that she appears to have felt, which could only be evoked through the pointedly feminine embodied experience of birth pangs:

> It was just like childbirth pains nothing else would describe it to you. I lay there one hour in the morning & one hour in the evening. So that was like having 2 Babies each day and all night.[44]

The author evidently set huge store by Kirkpatrick's medical knowledge and appeared to call on him for medical advice.[45] This faith was undoubtedly inflected by a patriarchal investment in Kirkpatrick's masculine authority compared to what she perceived as the more dubious credentials of the female staff of the Marie Curie:

> I dont [sic] think they are real Drs [sic] here. I think they call them Radiologists or something but you will understand what I mean[.] they are all women not one gentleman Dr. [sic].[46]

However, as her affectionate soubriquet for Kirkpatrick suggests, the form of support sought in this letter was emotional at least as much as it was medical and the opportunity to describe the painful and disorienting experience of the treatment she had undergone and to feel that she had been listened to and understood (a word whose cognates recur throughout the letter) seems to have been at least as cathartic and valuable as any practical advice Kirkpatrick may have been able to offer. In this sense, letters such as those from 'Noleen's Mammy' seem to bear out arguments about the centrality of emotions (both those of the patient and the physician) to the therapeutic encounter made by the 'Surgery and Emotion' project.[47] This is particularly clear given that, while obviously gynaecological and, by extension, potentially stigmatising in nature, the condition (presumably cervical cancer) and the experiences she described in the letter do not appear to relate directly to venereal infection. Her tendency to identify herself as 'Noleen's Mammy' suggests that she was either the mother of one of his former patients or, more likely, that Kirkpatrick was involved in treating her for a condition which, in turn, affected her daughter.[48] As such, it indicates the ways in which, under the smoke-screen of a deliberately light-hearted, blithe and uneducated 'Irish Mammy' persona, older, working-class women could continue to confide in Kirkpatrick experiences and anxieties that were otherwise inexpressible in their social milieu, long after his formal involvement with them or their relatives had come to an end.

This dynamic was not confined to working-class women. One of the most thoroughgoing examples of the extent and duration of the emotional support female patients found in Kirkpatrick comes in the case of E.M., a middle-class woman whose correspondence with Kirkpatrick spanned almost two decades. Her first letter, written when she was fifty-two, is one of the most emotionally direct in the collection, reflecting both the openness with which Kirkpatrick's patients felt able to express themselves to him and the hopelessness, desperation and despair which VD could inspire in its sufferers:

> I wish to thank you very much for your great kindness to me, I was very comfortable here the Matron, Nurse [Cor.] did all in their power to make me happy, the only good turn you can do for me now[:] *pray* for me *to die.*⁴⁹

Any such prayers went unanswered. A year later, E.M.'s daughter wrote from the married quarters of the 1ˢᵗ Battalion York and Lancers in Bordon, East Hampshire, describing her mother's poor health and requesting a prescription. Her letter concluded by noting that:

> She wishes to be remembered to the Matron and Nurse [Con.] and Nurse [Cor.]. I think my mother is fretting after you all. I think you must have made a pet of her. I am sorry to say I cant [sic] get any good of her.⁵⁰

The young woman's characterisation of E.M. as fretful for Kirkpatrick and his colleagues and 'a pet' of the staff at Steevens' plays on multiple codes of femininity to position her simultaneously as a fussing matriarch and a doting child, in both cases emphasising her affection for and emotional dependence on the hospital and Kirkpatrick's care. It is significant that in the cases of E.M. and 'Noleen's Mammy' this dependence persisted even when both women were resident in England and had ready access to medical care.⁵¹

An apparent exception to this pattern of strategically performed femininity were the young, working-class and lower middle-class women who wrote to Kirkpatrick, who tended to articulate both their feelings and symptoms in a more direct and straight-forward manner than the chummy but reticent men or playfully maternal 'Irish mammies' discussed above. In one unguarded example, K.C., a thirty-one-year-old woman from Portarlington, County Laois, sent Kirkpatrick a string of increasingly distressed letters in which she implored him for advice following a recurrence of what we might diagnose today as Pelvic Inflammatory Disease, which may or may not have arisen from a venereal infection. In her first letter, she explained that, despite having had 'hopes of been [sic] completely cured' of her ailment through a prolonged hospital stay under Kirkpatrick's care, her symptoms ('that peculiar feel [sic] around my abdomen & sides') had not abated, though her 'monthly periods' had returned since she was discharged.⁵² She proceeded to describe how she had 'made a change of lodgings', 'got new underclothes', 'disinfected everything' in her possession and kept herself 'scrupulously clean' in an effort to minimise her risk of reinfection since her return home.[53] However, she noted that, despite these precautions, she remained 'afraid to walk distance', 'dreading that the discharge might return' and implored Kirkpatrick to instruct her as to whether 'further douches and injections' might be necessary at his earliest convenience.[54] As a record of patient experience, K.C.'s letters highlight the intense anxieties around hygiene and persistent fears of lingering infection to which VD and gynaecological issues could give rise in sufferers.[55] In multiple letters, she records her insistent desire 'to get thoroughly & completely *rid of it* [her condition]', to 'have no trace whatever of it left' and 'to destroy all traces of this disease', 'no matter *how long*' she has to remain under treatment.[56] These letters also offer a suggestive insight into the ways in which the experience of being treated for sexual-health problems could transform patients' understanding of and capacity to communicate about their bodies. As K.C.'s directness regarding underwear and menstruation and her references to disinfection, discharge and douches in her first letter suggest, she was not at all squeamish in discussing her gynaecological issues with Kirkpatrick, viewing them as a medical problem requiring therapeutic intervention which should be discussed in a largely clinical vocabulary. This frankness is even more apparent in a subsequent letter, in which she described an episode of acute pain and discharge she had experienced:

> I went for a walk of about a mile only today, when the discharge came on just as it did f [sic] before I went to Steevens [sic], quite a lot & I felt so scalded I thought I'd never get back quickly enough, now after my having Hospital treatment & doing my very utmost to try rid [sic] myself of this illness it makes me feel disheartened that I don't know what to do. – & the feeling around my abdomen & sides makes me believe I am still affected with that complaint, would you advise me continue [sic] daily the douches? I could do so myself, I wonder without your advice if they'd be sufficient.[57]

Given the presumably public nature of the attack (in a separate letter K.C.'s sister noted that it occurred during a trip into town), her sensations of shame and vulnerability during the flare-up and her depression and frustration in its aftermath are unsurprising.[58] What is perhaps more unexpected is the clarity, confidence and relative technical proficiency with which she described her symptoms and the processes of self-monitoring and self-diagnosis this proficiency appears to have facilitated. For all the author's professions of ignorance and doubts as to the efficacy of further self-administered treatment, the confidence with which she reached these conclusions is striking and reflects an underlying feeling of self-possession and an awareness of her condition that stands in contrast to the much-discussed culture of ignorance and cultivated 'innocence' that surrounded women's sexual and reproductive knowledge in early twentieth-century Ireland and Britain.[59] If, as Simon Szreter and Kate Fisher note, 'innocence became a strategy and identity' for young working-class women in the interwar period, letters like those from K.C. suggest that young, female VD sufferers were obliged (or found it efficacious) to abandon this strategy in the interest of their health.[60]

The source of K.C.'s vocabulary and knowledge appears to have been Kirkpatrick, whom K.C. credited with introducing her to terms like 'inflammation'.[61] Nor was this increased knowledge and forthrightness confined to K.C. herself. K.C.'s sister, who wrote to Kirkpatrick expressing her concerns about the same incident, was no less direct in describing the recurrence of 'thick yellow' discharge and 'blood' precipitated by K.C.'s walk to town.[62] As this letter suggests, the experience of caring for and living intimately with VD sufferers could serve as an impromptu education in sexual health for all involved:

> Am I writing you too early re. my Sister's 'Blood Test' of October the 30th [?] if so it's because I am anxious re. her health. I have been seeing her daily for the past week and she still complains of that dragging feeling and weakness round abdomen and sides [sic]. After she Visiting [sic] you on that date she told me she intended following your advice 'To fight in future against this illness.' [...] I am very worried about her – besides as she has always led *a clean life* and I have intimate knowledge of it.[63]

Whatever the accuracy of T.C.'s claims concerning her sister's 'clean life', the fact that the sisters appear to have discussed both K.C.'s sexual history, her blood test (presumably a Wassermann reaction) and Kirkpatrick's advice on how to 'fight in future against [her] illness' indicates the ways in which those who had received treatment for venereal infection and those who were involved in their care were obliged to confront topics and share knowledge otherwise deemed taboo. Furthermore, as these examples make clear, while the disproportionately small number of male-authored and male-centred letters does not, necessarily, suggest that men were more coy in sexual matters or less concerned with their treatment, the robust cohort of female correspondents and wide array of female-centred correspondence Kirkpatrick received undoubtedly reflects a willingness and ability on the part of Irish women to speak frankly and knowledgably about sex and sexual health in a period more often noted for its repression and silences than its frankness and pragmatism. More particularly, given the culture of silence and the sexual double-standard that confronted female VD sufferers in this period, it suggests the ways in which women who had already received treatment occupied a unique position of knowledge and experience concerning their conditions and their physiology.[64]

## '[I]ts [sic] in *you* my faith *is placed*': stigmatising illness and confession

Beyond its forthright tone and technical vocabulary, a significant feature of K.C.'s correspondence with Kirkpatrick is the clear sense it gives of the trust the author placed in him compared to other medical professionals:

> I hate troubling you again Dr [sic] after your treating me & I daresay you hoped it was gone from me alas, I don't want approaching [sic] other Drs [sic] again re. this, reason I am writing you [sic], & I can't turn for advice anywhere.[65]

Her remarks record a number of related aspects of patient experience which may have combined to inspire her profound reliance on Kirkpatrick. First, they suggest the chronic lack of access to information, expert opinion and co-ordinated after-care which confronted VD sufferers in this period, even after having undergone treatment. While K.C. had emerged from her initial hospitalisation with the ability to describe her symptoms with clarity and confidence, it is clear that, beyond Kirkpatrick, she had no clear sense of where to look for further advice or treatment – a fact which had serious negative ramifications for her physical and mental health. Second, they reflect a more general reluctance to disclose her condition and describe her symptoms to other medical professionals. This reticence may have had a number of causes. On the one hand, it attests to the emotional cost that attended disclosing one's condition and recounting one's medical history as a sufferer of a stigmatising condition such as VD, even in a clinical context. On the other hand, it betrays a profound lack of faith in the distribution of expertise and experience regarding the diagnosis and treatment of VD and gynaecological issues among Irish physicians in the period. Hanley has emphasised the 'often haphazard and opportunistic way' in which knowledge of VD was circulated in early twentieth-century English undergraduate medical training.[66] This imbalance was even more pronounced in Ireland, where, as has been seen, centres for the treatment of VD (and, thus, wards where students might observe patients) were almost exclusively confined to Dublin.[67] Diarmaid Ferriter notes that, while grants were available to provide GPs outside the counties covered by the designated centres with salvarsan treatment, Wassermann testing facilities and appropriate training, these funds went virtually untouched.[68] In the case of K.C., while her letter mentions a local physician whom she appears to have trusted to administer any treatment Kirkpatrick recommended, it is clear that this trust did not extend to having him decide on the course of treatment itself.[69] K.C.'s simultaneous conviction that she did not want to approach another doctor and that she couldn't 'turn for advice anywhere' suggests that both the emotional and practical factors listed above may have influenced her actions. In either case, it is clear from her use of the word '*again*' that her reluctance was based on previous negative experiences, to which Kirkpatrick's care compared favourably.[70]

In contrast to the less effusive tone of the letters Kirkpatrick received from men, this investment in Kirkpatrick as a uniquely privileged interlocutor on medical and sexual topics is a constant refrain in the collection's female-authored correspondence. For example, in October 1925, B.D., a young mother from Rathronan near Naas, wrote to inform Kirkpatrick how, when a female GP had sought to have her sixteen-month-old daughter admitted to another hospital, she vociferously objected:

> I up & told her that I would not let her go in to any hospital in Ireland except Stevens [sic] as I was there myself & went in a bad case (not telling her wat [sic]) & that now I am better than ever owing to you & Sister [C.].[71]

She concludes her letter with an effusive endorsement of Kirkpatrick and his practice:

> I have no discharge or no trouble with the womb since I was there [at Steevens'], & I have no faith in any other Hospital only yours, no matter if she was to get me under the greatest in the world, you are the Doctor who cured me when three others failed & *its* [sic] in *you* my faith *is placed*.[72]

The young woman's deliberate efforts to conceal the reason for her stay in Steevens' from a female health professional stands in stark contrast to the frank tone in which she was prepared to discuss her sexual health with Kirkpatrick. It also contradicts a growing perception in Britain that women doctors were a boon to VD clinics because they would help female patients to feel less self-conscious when discussing their condition and being examined.[73] The author's coyness may have stemmed from a desire to avoid disclosing a potentially stigmatising piece of information unnecessarily (she was discussing her daughter's health, not her own, with the female doctor). However, it also appears to reflect a wider distrust of the medical profession born of previous negative experiences. In the context of such suspicion and hostility, the almost beatific regard in which B.D. held Kirkpatrick and Dr Steevens' Hospital is striking. While it would be dangerous to read too deeply into the lexical choices made in what appears to be a relatively off-the-cuff piece of personal correspondence, the young woman's repeated insistence on the 'faith' she placed in Kirkpatrick positions him as a figure of almost ecclesiastical authority. This tendency to treat Kirkpatrick as a sort of father-confessor is notably common in the collection's female-authored correspondence, a fact perhaps unsurprising in a nation whose female population was over 93 per cent Catholic in 1936.[74] Such a pattern obviously corresponds with Foucault's infamous characterisation of the post-Enlightenment therapeutic encounter as a mode of secular confession, but seems to go beyond even his somewhat allegorical understanding of this phenomenon.[75] As David Barnard has influentially argued, whether or not physicians consider themselves to serve a priestly function, it is often a role in which they find themselves cast by their patients:

> Physicians are not priests. They have their own work to do. At the same time, their medical work has three aspects that make inevitable

their assumption of some form of priestly role. First, the nature of illness is such that patients present themselves with existential – and not only biophysical – distress and pin on the physician intense existential hopes. Second, the treatment relationship itself, with its demands on the physician's personal qualities of care and concern, is a critical mode of therapy. Third, medical work is value-laden in both its individual and social contexts.[76]

Where Kirkpatrick's male correspondents appear to have engaged with him first and foremost as a man, 'broadminded' in outlook and 'fraternal' in attitude (albeit while investing with many of the same 'existential hopes' as their female counterparts), his female correspondents were more explicit in treating him as a figure to whom a wide range of perceived transgressions could be confessed and from whom an array of social interventions could be sought.

In an emotionally charged follow-up to her initial letter concerning her daughter's admission to Steevens', the young mother quoted above updated him about a relapse of symptoms ('discharge', 'headaches', 'nerve pains' and sleeplessness) arising from an illness contracted several years earlier:

> [A] line to let you know there is a slight discharge coming from me. & as the trouble I had over two years ago was my own fault and my husband was not aware of it I am nervous over it at present.[77]

She arranged to call on Kirkpatrick at Steevens' the following week and explained that she should be able to remain an in-patient if he deemed it necessary as her baby was 'not at home' (such a trip 'would nearly be impossible' if she were).[78] Alongside this medical discussion, the young woman also opened up to Kirkpatrick about her 'great sorrow' over her recently deceased sister, 'who met such a death' the she could not bring herself to recount it and enclosed a 'bit of paper' (presumably a press clipping) that reported on the trial of an unnamed man who appears to have been imprisoned in connection with the death.[79] The letter concludes with an expression of gratitude to Kirkpatrick for his understanding ('it is because you have been so kind to me that I am telling you so much') and an expression of shame at her previous conduct and its impact on her health ('it was all through my own dirt that I was like I was').[80] The young woman's sense of the confessional dynamics of her correspondence with Kirkpatrick seems to be reflected in the letter's references to 'fault', 'dirt' and 'nervous' feelings, all of which evoke the 'thematic of sin' and Catholic guilt traditionally synonymous with discussions of Irish sexuality.[81] This guilt seems to be related to the fact that the young woman contracted her illness through pre- or extra-marital sex, a fact suggested by her eagerness to maintain her husband's ignorance of her 'trouble' and its cause. As this example indicates, where female patients are concerned, Kirkpatrick's caseload could feel less like a practice than a ministry. However, it is important to acknowledge the limits of this analogy and of the 'thematic of sin' as the principle paradigm through which to interpret this young woman's case. One might note, for example, that the young's woman's guilt and anxiety seem to have been prompted less by the fact of having contracted an infection in itself, than by the practical demands of childcare, the emotional strain of a recent (and seemingly violent) bereavement and the obligation to deceive her spouse. Indeed, the very fact that the young woman was so willing to express her distress to Kirkpatrick in such relatively straightforward terms bespeaks a pragmatic engagement with the realities of sexuality and sexual health that seems to belie narratives of thoroughgoing silence and repression. Likewise, while it is tempting to find in this zealous devotion to Kirkpatrick and Dr Steevens' Hospital evidence of an uncritical deference to institutional authority comparable to that apparently enjoyed by the Catholic Church in this period, it is worth bearing in mind the woman's mistrust of her female GP, her vociferous refusal to 'go in to any hospital in Ireland' except Steevens' and, crucially, the fact that her wishes ultimately appear to have been granted.[82] Whatever the cultural dynamics informing the young woman's sense of her relationship to Kirkpatrick, her letters seem to suggest a paradox in the nature of the patient testimony surrounding stigmatising illnesses such as VD in this period: the very impossibility of discussing such illnesses publicly made patients particularly voluble when discussing their experiences with an apparently neutral, understanding and institutionally sanctioned figure such as Kirkpatrick.

### 'I am living unhappy with him': divorce and separation

This dynamic, which determined many of the social interventions Kirkpatrick was called on to make by his patients, is further illustrated in a letter from a Mrs A.B., a working-class or lower middle-class former patient from Athlone who asked him for testimony confirming that she had been treated for venereal infection. She explained that she was seeking this certification as she was 'taking steps to obtain a separation' from her husband, with whom she was 'living unhappy' and with whom 'things [were] not right'.[83] She promised to come to see Kirkpatrick as soon as matters were 'fixed up' and asked him to remember her to one of the nurses on her former ward at Steevens' as she 'would love it if Nurse was near' to 'tell her all [her] troubles'.[84] Several things are striking about the letter, particularly in an Irish context. The first is the insight it offers into the fraught field of divorce and separation in early twentieth-century Ireland. While it is true that, prior to the 1937 Constitution, divorce *a vinculo matrimonii* (from the tie of marriage) was technically available in Ireland, as a range of commentators have shown, in reality, the legal dissolution of marriages was a rarity.[85] Though the 1857 Divorce and Matrimonial Causes Act had transferred jurisdiction for divorce in England and Wales from Westminster to the courts – obviating the costly, time-consuming and often embarrassing necessity to petition parliament – the Act was never extended to Ireland. As such, where over a hundred petitions for dissolution or nullity were submitted in England between 1857 and 1910 (over forty by women), only thirty-nine Irish divorces were obtained in the same period (all by Protestants).[86] While the transfer of powers from Westminster following Irish Independence in 1922 left the possibility of divorce by private bill in the Irish Seanad (Senate) open, the Cosgrave government's pragmatic efforts to navigate the difficulties of squaring the broadly secular 1922 Constitution – which prohibited any legislation that would discriminate between religions – with the demands of a Catholic hierarchy keen to see divorce explicitly prohibited ultimately resulted in an unhappy work-around which effectively rendered divorce impossible in the Free State.[87] Yet, as David Fitzpatrick has noted and the case of Mrs A.B. illustrates, if divorce was scarcely known in Ireland, 'separation in many guises was ubiquitous'.[88] While the nature of the separation sought by Mrs A.B. is unclear, given the circumstances suggested in her letter, a High Court decree of civil separation without right of remarriage – *divortium a mensa et thoro* (divorce from table and bed) – based on spousal cruelty would seem the most plausible line of recourse for her to have pursued.[89]

The circumstances faced by Mrs A.B. and other women infected with VD by an unfaithful or deceitful spouse who sought a legal remedy were distressing on a range of levels. Most obviously, there was the experience of infection itself and the pain, stigma and practical problems it entailed. These must have been particularly difficult to face in an 'unhappy' living situation such as the one to which Mrs A.B. alludes. Second, there was the source of that infection, knowingly or unknowingly transmitted to the patient by a spouse who had committed adultery or misled them concerning their pre-marital sexual history. While it is unclear in what way things were 'not right' between Mrs A.B. and her husband, it may be assumed that at least part of their troubles arose from the feelings of betrayal and violation such a situation might be expected to have inspired. Third, there were the legal barriers and social stigma surrounding separation and divorce discussed above. Indeed, such legal difficulties ran deeper than Mrs A.B. perhaps even realised. Her request to Kirkpatrick was made at the height of an ongoing dispute between the recently founded British Ministry for Health and the Lord Chancellor's Office over whether the confidentiality of patient records recommended by the RCVD Report and prescribed by the 1917 LGB Regulations should be respected in civil court cases.[90] Matters first came to a head in 1920, when Clara Garner subpoenaed Dr Saloman Kandinsky of the Westminster Hospital to confirm that she had been infected with syphilis as evidence of her husband's adultery and cruelty. Kandinsky was reluctant to breach the pledge of secrecy to which the government's VD scheme enjoined him and lodged a protest to that effect with the judge, Alfred McArdie, who in turn disregarded Kandinsky's objections and compelled him to testify. The case and the dispute to which it gave rise were widely reported in the press, particularly by the London *Times*.[91] Though the Irish legal system notionally became independent of its British counterpart with the establishment of the Free State, the VD Service through which Mrs A.B. had been treated had been set up in line with LGBI Regulations devised before Independence and, as such, might be expected to generate similar conflicts of interest for Irish medical professionals called on to give evidence in court. While the debate ultimately centred more on the difficulties faced by physicians subpoenaed to give evidence against a patient without that patient's consent, it nevertheless serves as a reminder of the ways in which female VD sufferers who sought separations were obliged to forego their privacy and confidentiality and, in Ireland, to do so without even the eventual possibility of remarriage.

In such a context, the tone of the letter is, in itself, telling. Despite the personal and legal difficulties outlined above, Mrs A.B. communicates her request in a matter-of-fact tone that reflects only her strong and straightforward desire to separate from her husband. While she notes that she is 'sorry to have to admit' that she is 'living unhappy with him', this remark seems to indicate regret at the failure of the marriage and the circumstances that have prompted it, rather than a sense of shame or stigma around the process of separation itself. In this sense, the letter (as with so many others in the collection) seems to put pressure on Tom Inglis's assertion that transgressions of the normative Catholic social and sexual order were 'limited' in twentieth-century Ireland, suggesting instead that the normative Catholic order and the Irish legal system had a tendency to render those transgressions less socially and institutionally legible than in Britain or Europe.[92] Furthermore, in the range of pastoral functions it reveals Kirkpatrick's clinic to have played for its author ('I would love if Nurse was near that I could tell her all my troubles'), the letter reveals the extent to which the stigma of venereal infection and the marital difficulties to which it could give rise may have prompted patients to rely more heavily on medical professionals for emotional support than in other clinical contexts. This reliance only appears to have been sharpened in early twentieth-century Ireland, where the greater social and legal barriers to divorce and the absence of meaningful public-health campaigns to destigmatise VD and its 'innocent victims' left women infected by their spouses more vulnerable than their British counterparts.

## 'I have not a p[enny] to bless myself': fees, charity and welfare

Another facet of Kirkpatrick's secular ministry is reflected in the large number of letters which make direct reference to poverty or appeal for charity. As mentioned above, in almost 20 per cent of letters patients apologise to Kirkpatrick for failing to settle bills, ask for discounts on treatment, seek to borrow money or entreat him to intervene on their behalf with various institutions of state or charitable welfare. In one, a former male patient asked Kirkpatrick to write on his behalf to the local Board of Guardians to state that 'a new set of teeth would be an advantage to [him] in seeking employment':

> My reason for this request is that if medical proof be forthcoming the local Board of Guardians will, I have reason to believe, defray some if not all the expenses[.][93]

Though Kirkpatrick responded in the affirmative, the request was unsuccessful. In light of the refusal, the correspondent noted that, despite having 'felt very strong for some time after coming out of Hospital', his eyes were now 'very weak and sore' and he would be 'very thankful' if he could be readmitted to Steevens' for further treatment.[94] As this example suggests, many of Kirkpatrick's patients possessed a sense of the increasingly joined-up nature of welfare provision within the Free State and sought to leverage its different institutions to achieve the healthcare outcomes and social advancement they desired.[95] This strategic engagement with welfare provision is also reflected in the correspondent's change of argumentative tack following the failure of his petition for false teeth – as his second letter seems to imply, if the state would not provide him with the support he needed to seek employment, then he would instead have it provide him with hospital accommodation.

In other letters, patients emphasise to Kirkpatrick the costs arising from their complaints and petition him for reductions and credit. One former patient writing from Birkenhead, Cheshire spoke for many when she insisted that she had 'not a p[enny] to bless' herself (though her claim not to have had 'a *meal* in over a fortnight' also illustrates some of the hyperbole that could attend such claims).[96] Another letter records the distress of a father from Bealistown, Ballycullane whose daughter was suffering from mouth problems. He asked Kirkpatrick about the hospital's fee structure and explained that he would only be able to make a small contribution as he has had to pay £46 per annum (approximately £2,747 in 2018) for his wife's care at Wexford County Lunatic Asylum (later St Senan's Psychiatric Hospital) in Enniscorthy for almost thirty years:[97]

> She is a softy Poore [sic] little girl Oh she is after suffering a lot with her mouth. I suppose it will hardly ever by cured now its [sic] gone so far[.] Please let me no [sic] will their [sic] be anything to be paid for

her in this hospital[?] I would not be able to pay much I am paying for her mother at eniscorthy [sic] asylum Nearly 30 years. I have to pay £46 per year. And I am not able to pay any more. if [sic] she cannot be Kept free I would do my best to pay a Small thing weekly or monthly: it would be a very Small thing I could pay: pleas [sic] drop me a line and let me Know how She is getting on Dr. Kirkpatrick.[98]

At the same time as offering a sincere manifestation of paternal concern and affection, the correspondent's characterisation of his daughter as a 'softy' and his emphasis on the protracted nature of her suffering may reflect an effort to play on Kirkpatrick's sympathies to ensure that his daughter received favourable (and discounted) treatment. A subsequent letter reveals this emotional leverage to have had the desired effect, with Kirkpatrick appearing to have secured the girl free admission and treatment, for which her father thanked him profusely. As a mark of gratitude and perhaps as a matter of pride, the father informed Kirkpatrick that he would be sending a postal order of £1 (£60 in 2018) 'as a Subscription to the Hospital' and implored him not to 'let her home' until he is 'right Satisfied' of her full recovery.[99]

Such requests were not always communicated so ingratiatingly. One of the most confrontational and assertive letters in the collection concerns Mrs B., a working-class female patient, who chastised Kirkpatrick for having discharged her too early and demanded to be readmitted to hospital. Mrs B. claimed that she was 'not half cured' when she was sent home and that she remained bed-ridden and in 'great pain'.[100] In petitioning Kirkpatrick, she repeatedly invoked his sense of fair play, claiming that he had treated her unfavourably compared to her other, less deserving wardmates:

> [Y]ou know well it wasnt [sic] fair for to send me home you have patients in your ward for the past 7 months and nothing wrong with them if there was they wouldnt [sic] be able to work. I was the only patient in it that was in pain so it wasnt [sic] fair to send me home[.][101]

In a final act of emotional and professional leveraging, Mrs B. unfavourably compared Kirkpatrick to Dr Bethel Solomons (former Master of the Rotunda maternity hospital and Kirkpatrick's colleague at Steevens') who had operated on her in Carlow, whom she claimed would 'never send [patients] home without learning that they are all right'.[102] She underscored this professional harangue with a threat:

if Kirkpatrick did not 'do justice' to her complaint, there 'would be more about it at the Carlow Board'.[103] The letter is a strikingly clear example of how a VD sufferer could exert agency over their care by both formal and informal means. However, while unusually pugnacious in tone (it is unlike almost any other item in the collection in this regard), the letter is, in many ways, simply a particularly extreme example of many of the strategies discussed above. Mrs B. presents herself as more vulnerable and hard-done-by than what she considers to be her better-off peers, exploits Kirkpatrick's personal sympathies and professional pride and, when faced with a set-back in her engagement with one wing of the Irish welfare state, seeks to instrumentalise another to help improve her situation.

Beyond suggesting that Kirkpatrick was both unstinting in his generosity and something of a soft touch, examples such as these throw into sharp relief the ways in which Irish people in often straitened financial circumstances navigated (and, as far as possible, exploited) the emergent welfare state to maximise their access to care and support. The tendency of former patients to present their pleas for readmission to the state-funded VD ward at Steevens' in strategic conjunction with professions of poverty and destitution highlight the tacit and more explicit forms of agency that service users sought to exert in leveraging access to the (relative) comforts state medicine could afford. In particular, these letters suggest the extent to which the LGBI's VD Regulations and the reforms to which they gave rise present a significant and valuable case-study for historians and sociologists interested in the operation of welfare in Ireland in the transitional period between Independence and the passage of the long-gestated 1952 Social Welfare Act.

## 'Almost unknown in Ireland': locating VD

An important consideration in any such analysis of the operation of the emergent Irish welfare state in the domain of sexual health is the intense and long-standing politicisation of the question of the geographical and social origins of VD in Ireland. Since the late nineteenth century, advanced nationalist anti-enlisting propaganda had vilified the British military garrison in Ireland as a source of sexual corruption and contagion.[104] In a 1906 polemic published in the republican journal *Sinn Féin*, Oliver St John Gogarty (an Ear, Nose and Throat specialist and the model for James Joyce's Buck Mulligan) claimed that, by its own statistical admission, the British army constituted 'a body of men [...] more than half leprous with venereal excess'.¹⁰⁵ In their inaugural February 1918 *Public Health Circular*, the Sinn Féin Public Health Committee emphasised what they presented as the eschatological threat that the demobilisation of Irish soldiers serving in the British armed forces would pose to the health of rural Ireland in the wake of the Great War:

> In the normal course of events, 100,000 Irishmen serving in the British army will come back to Ireland at the war's end. At the very lowest estimate, 15,000 of that number will return affected with this disease – the actually number we believe will be much more. With the return to civil life of a large proportion of these, this infection will extend its ravages even to the rural districts.¹⁰⁶

The authors of the *Circular* insisted that VD was 'almost unknown in Ireland outside the British military centres' and that, as their 'blood [had] no immunity against it', the Irish were singularly susceptible to infection.¹⁰⁷ Even in less openly partisan settings, a perception existed that VD in Ireland was essentially an urban problem, concentrated near British garrisons, which had not affected the agrarian west of the country. Presenting evidence to the RCVD in 1914, the Chief Medical Inspector for the LGBI, Dr Brian O'Brien, asserted that syphilis was virtually unknown in the nation's smaller towns and villages. He attributed this 'splendid result' to the fact that there was 'very little immorality' in rural Ireland.¹⁰⁸ A handful of letters in the Kirkpatrick collection are undeniably inflected by this narrative and the urban-rural geography of purity on which it was predicated. One, sent by an older male physician in Carrickmacross, County Monaghan, in November 1926, asked Kirkpatrick to admit a patient of his to hospital for treatment. McKenna described her as a 'little country girl' – the 'daughter of a small farmer' – who had contracted gonorrhoea 'from a town lad at a country dance' who, she said, 'took advantage of her'.¹⁰⁹ He asked Kirkpatrick to handle the matter 'with little fuss', as it was 'a pity on her' and he did not see 'what else can be done with her'.¹¹⁰ The details of the case are, of course, irrecoverable. It is impossible to determine whether the phrase 'took advantage of her' was intended as an indication of the young woman's naiveté or as a euphemism for sexual assault.[111] Nor is it possible to recover a sense of whether the young woman in question presented this narrative to the doctor in an effort to mitigate the social stigma of pre-marital sex in 1920s Ireland. What is undeniable is that, in a manner consonant with the geography of purity sketched by Dr O'Brien and Sinn Féin, the doctor framed the narrative in terms of a dichotomy between the knowing and corrupting masculine sexual licence of the town and the feminine innocence and purity of the countryside.

However, as Table 8.4 shows, around 13 per cent of letters with identifiable addresses or postmarks in the Kirkpatrick collection came from rural correspondents in towns or villages such as Rossgeir in County Donegal (population seventy-four), Ballycullane in County Wexford (population ninety-six) and Kilmeague in County Kildare (population ninety) and feature sufferers who discussed their symptoms with the same familiarity and frankness as their urban counterparts.[112] While any statistical conclusions reached from such a small sample dispersed across such a long period should be treated with due circumspection, the robust cohort of rural correspondents who feature in the Kirkpatrick collection puts pressure on O'Brien's rosy image of a sexually continent country population. In this sense, the geographical and social make-up of Kirkpatrick's correspondence comes much closer to the findings of the 1926 Report of the ICVD, which concluded that 'contrary to popularly held opinion', VD was 'widespread throughout the country' with 'no considerable area entirely free' from infection and that its primary vector was neither sex work nor the military.[113]

Table 8.4 Breakdown of letters to Dr T.P.C. Kirkpatrick by size of settlement

| Location | Number of Letters |
| --- | --- |
| Urban | 58 |
| Suburban | 3 |
| Town | 23 |
| Village | 13 |

## Conclusions

As these letters suggest, the experiences of VD sufferers in Ireland in the interwar period were seldom uniform and were often far removed from received notions of the Irish as an infamously repressed or implausibly 'pure-minded' people. They were also often closer in kind to those of their English, Welsh and Scottish counterparts than has sometimes been acknowledged. The VD sufferers who wrote to Kirkpatrick discussed their conditions with confidence, self-possession and very little squeamishness and in a manner that suggests that diagnosis and treatment had provided them with a vocabulary and knowledge unusual for members of the general public at the time. Sufferers placed substantial trust in Kirkpatrick, setting apparently equal store by his medical expertise and his capacity for generosity, sympathy and understanding, in ways that suggest that they found these aspects of the clinical encounter virtually inseparable. However, they did not do so passively or out of blind deference to medical authority. Kirkpatrick's patients complained about other patients, about other physicians and about him. They strategically emphasised aspects of their gender, class and age to shape Kirkpatrick's perception of them and to garner practical aid and pastoral support. They played on Kirkpatrick's emotions, his professional pride and his charitable disposition and, through his influence and standing, sought to leverage an emerging network of state welfare provision to achieve personally advantageous medical and social outcomes. In the process, they left behind a rich archive of personal testimony and lived experience the surface of which this chapter has only scratched.

In discussing these letters, I have sought to emphasise their value as a resource for historians of medicine, gender, sexuality and welfare in Ireland and Britain and to do justice to the voices they contain. However, the Kirkpatrick collection, and the insights it offers into ordinary Irish people's experiences of sexual ill-health and the institutions through which it was diagnosed, treated and regulated during a formative moment in the history of British and Irish state welfare, also provide an important point of reference for those seeking to promote good sexual health in the present day. At a moment in which the governments of Ireland and Britain are both seeking to integrate heterogenous local sexual-health services into a wider national strategy and address regional inequities in access and outcomes, historiography which combines a regional focus with a four-nations perspective, as I have sought to do in this chapter, can offer vital insights into the interplay of local, national and transnational forces which shaped existing services and the challenges they face to this day.[114] Moreover, historiography which attends in granular detail to ordinary individuals' experiences of sexual ill-health, the aims they pursued in engaging with services, and the strategies they adopted to obviate what they experienced as the shortcomings of those services, can offer health professionals and policy-makers an insight into needs as yet unmet in existing provision. This is particularly the case where vulnerable, marginalised or understudied population groups are concerned. The letters surveyed in this chapter reveal the extent to which sufferers regularly felt it necessary, or, at least, advantageous to offer strategic performances of aspects of their identity in order to secure beneficial outcomes in their engagement with Ireland's emergent welfare state. A greater understanding of the social codes which trans people, migrants and other marginalised populations are obliged to navigate in order to access, or feel able to access, effective advice, support and treatment may yield valuable insights into how to address the low levels of uptake of sexual-health services that currently exist in these groups.[115] If, as Hanley suggests in the next chapter, the challenges facing sexual-health services in the 2020s (disease prevalence, lack of information, inequality of access and outcome) closely resemble those of the 1920s, then letters such as the ones surveyed in this chapter afford a vital insight into the ramifications of those challenges for ordinary people and their physical, emotional and social wellbeing. Like Kirkpatrick in his decades-long correspondence with his patients and their loved-ones, where the voices of these individuals are available to us, we must learn to listen to and engage with them, both on their own terms, and as the basis for reflection on how best to meet the needs of sufferers in the present day.

## Notes

* I am indebted to Harriet Wheelock at the Royal College of Physicians of Ireland for her generosity, patience and insight while I researched

this chapter. I am also grateful to David Dwan, Isabella MacPherson, Diane Urquhart, the judges and attendees of the 2018 RCPI Kirkpatrick History of Medicine Award and the editors of this collection for their comments on versions of the material presented here. My thanks also to Claire Martin for access to her unpublished thesis.

1  David Evans, 'Tackling the "Hideous Scourge": The Creation of the Venereal Disease Treatment Centres in Early Twentieth-Century Britain', *Social History of Medicine* 5:3 (1992), 413–33; Roger Davidson, '"A Scourge to Be Firmly Gripped": The Campaign for VD Controls in Interwar Scotland', *Social History of Medicine* 6:2 (1993), 213–35; Roger Davidson, *Dangerous Liaisons: A Social History of Venereal Diseases in Twentieth-Century Scotland* (Amsterdam: Rodopi, 2000); Angus H. Ferguson, *Should a Doctor Tell? The Evolution of Medical Confidentiality in Britain* (Farnham, Surrey: Ashgate, 2013), chapters 4 and 7; Simon Szreter, 'The Prevalence of Syphilis in England and Wales on the Eve of the Great War: Re-Visiting the Estimates of the Royal Commission on Venereal Diseases 1913–1916', *Social History of Medicine* 27:3 (2014), 508–29; Anne Hanley, *Medicine, Knowledge and Venereal Diseases in England, 1886–1916* (Basingstoke: Palgrave, 2017), chapter 5; Anne Hanley, '"Sex Prejudice" and Professional Identity: Women Doctors and their Patients in Britain's Interwar VD Service', *Journal of Social History*, 54:2 (2020), 569–98.

2  Roger Davidson, '"Searching for Mary, Glasgow": Contact Tracing for Sexually Transmitted Diseases in Twentieth-Century Scotland', *Social History of Medicine* 9:2 (1996), 195–214; Elaine Thomson, 'Between Separate Spheres: Women, Moral Hygiene and the Edinburgh Hospital for Women and Children', in Steve Sturdy (ed.), *Medicine, Health and the Public Sphere in Britain, 1600–2000* (London: Routledge, 2002), 107–22; Philip Howell, 'Venereal Disease and the Politics of Prostitution in the Irish Free State', *Irish Historical Studies* 33:131 (May 2003), 320–41; Susan Lemar, '"The Liberty to Spread Disaster": Campaigning for Compulsion in the Control of Venereal Diseases in Edinburgh in the 1920s', *Social History of Medicine* 19:1 (2006), 73–86; Pamela Cox, 'Compulsion, Voluntarism and Venereal Disease: Governing Sexual Health in England after the Contagious Diseases Acts', *Journal of British Studies* 46:1 (January 2007), 91–115; Susannah Riordan, 'Venereal Disease in the Irish Free State: The Politics of Public Health', *Irish Historical Studies* 35:139 (2007), 345–64; Philip Howell, 'The Politics of Prostitution and the Politics of Public Health in the Irish Free State: A Response to Susannah Riordan', *Irish Historical Studies* 35:140 (2007), 541–52; Leanne McCormick, *Regulating Sexuality: Women in Twentieth-Century Northern Ireland*

(Manchester: Manchester University Press, 2009), chapter 4; Susannah Riordan, '"A Probable Source of Infection": The Limitations of Venereal Disease Policy, 1943–1951', in Margaret H. Preston and Margaret Ó hÓgartaigh (eds), *Gender and Medicine in Ireland, 1700–1950* (Syracuse, New York: Syracuse University Press, 2012), 203–20; Leanne McCormick, 'Prophylactics and Prejudice: Venereal Diseases in Northern Ireland During the Second World War', in Margaret H. Preston and Margaret Ó hÓgartaigh (eds), *Gender and Medicine in Ireland, 1700–1950* (Syracuse, New York: Syracuse University Press, 2012), 221–34; Francesca Patricia Moore, '"A Mistaken Policy of Secretiveness": Venereal Disease and Changing Heterosexual Morality in Lancashire, UK, 1920–1935', *Historical Geography* 43 (2015), 37–56; Samantha Caslin, 'Transience, Class and Gender in Interwar Sexual Health Policy: The Case of the Liverpool VD Scheme', *Social History of Medicine* 32:3 (2019), 544–64.

3 Simon Szreter and Kate Fisher, *Sex Before the Sexual Revolution: Intimate Life in England, 1918–1963* (Cambridge: Cambridge University Press, 2010), 65.

4 For recent studies which exemplify a regional history approach to the histories of medicine and sexuality, see Lucinda McCray Beier, '"We Were Green as Grass": Learning about Sex and Reproduction in Three Working-Class Lancashire Communities, 1900–1970', *Social History of Medicine* 16:3 (2003), 461–80; Lucinda McCray Beier, *For Their Own Good: The Transformation of English Working-Class Health Culture, 1880–1970* (Columbus: Ohio State University Press, 2008); Szreter and Fisher, *Sex Before the Sexual Revolution*; Claire Martin, 'Bodies of Knowledge: Science, Popular Culture and Working-Class Women's Experience of the Life Cycle in Yorkshire, c.1900–1940' (unpublished PhD Thesis, University of Leeds, 2018). For accounts of the nature and utility of a four-nations approach to Britain and Ireland, see Raphael Samuel, 'British Dimensions: "Four Nations History"', *History Workshop Journal* 40:1 (1995), iii–xxii; Naomi Lloyd-Jones and Margaret M. Scull, 'A New Plea for an Old Subject? Four Nations History for the Modern Period', in Naomi Lloyd-Jones and Margaret M. Scull (eds), *Four Nations Approaches to Modern 'British' History: A (Dis)United Kingdom?* (Basingstoke: Palgrave, 2018), 3–31. For examples of such an approach in the context of the social history of medicine, see Donnacha Seán Lucey and Virginia Crossman (eds), *Healthcare in Ireland and Britain from 1850: Voluntary, Regional and Comparative Perspectives* (London: School of Advanced Study, University of London, Institute of Historical Research, 2014).

5 Moore, '"A Mistaken Policy of Secretiveness"', 41; Caslin, 'Transience, Class and Gender in Interwar Sexual Health Policy', 3.

6  Howell, 'Venereal Disease and the Politics of Prostitution'; Riordan, 'Venereal Disease in the Irish Free State'; Howell, 'A Response to Susannah Riordan'.
7  Riordan, 'Venereal Disease in the Irish Free State', 347.
8  Riordan records that between 1926 and 1951, VD schemes were introduced in the county boroughs of Cork, Limerick and Waterford and in all counties except Cork, Donegal, Dublin, Kilkenny, Mayo, Meath, Sligo, the North Riding of Tipperary and Waterford. However, she also notes that, notwithstanding an extension of the therapeutic preparations available to GPs in 1948, the Department of Local Government and Public Health remained 'remarkably resistant to change' in the treatment of VD. Riordan, 'Venereal Disease in the Irish Free State', 347; Riordan, '"A Probable Source of Infection"', 205.
9  Tom Inglis, 'Foucault, Bourdieu and the Field of Irish Sexuality', *Irish Journal of Sociology* 7:1 (1997), 5–28; Tom Inglis, 'Origins and Legacies of Irish Prudery: Sexuality and Social Control in Modern Ireland', *Éire-Ireland* 40:3 (2005), 9–37; Sandra McAvoy, 'Sex and the Single Girl: Ireland 1922–1949', in Chichi Aniagolu (ed.), *In From the Shadows: The UL Women's Studies Collection* Vol. III (Limerick: Women's Studies, Department of Government and Society, University of Limerick, 1997), 55–67; Chrystel Hug, *The Politics of Sexual Morality in Ireland* (Basingstoke: Palgrave, 1998); Finola Kennedy, 'The Suppression of the Carrigan Report: A Historical Perspective on Child Abuse', *Studies: An Irish Quarterly Review* 89:356 (2000), 354–63; Mark Finnane, 'The Carrigan Committee of 1930–31 and the "Moral Condition of the Saorstát"', *Irish Historical Studies* 32:128 (2001), 519–36; James M. Smith, 'The Politics of Sexual Knowledge: The Origins of Ireland's Sexual Containment Culture and the Carrigan Report (1931)', *Journal of the History of Sexuality* 13:2 (2004), 208–33.
10 Tom Inglis, *Moral Monopoly: The Rise and Fall of the Catholic Church in Modern Ireland*, 2nd edition (Dublin: University College Dublin Press, 1998); Tom Inglis, 'The Irish Body', in Tom Inglis (ed.), *Are the Irish Different?* (Manchester: Manchester University Press, 2014), 88–98, 90; Inglis, 'Foucault, Bourdieu and the Field of Irish Sexuality', 12.
11 James M. Smith, *Ireland's Magdalen Laundries and the Nation's Architecture of Containment* (Manchester: Manchester University Press, 2008), 5.
12 Diarmaid Ferriter, *Occasions of Sin: Sex and Society in Modern Ireland* (London: Profile Books, 2009), 2.
13 J.B. Lyons, 'Kirkpatrick, Thomas Percy Claude', in James McGuire and James Quinn (eds), *Dictionary of Irish Biography* (Cambridge:

Cambridge University Press, 2009), https://dib.cambridge.org/view ReadPage.do?articleId=a4583 (accessed 25 February 2021).

14  For a catalogue of Kirkpatrick's published medical and historical output, see F.S. Bourke, 'Chronological Handlist of Dr Kirkpatrick's Published Work', *Irish Journal of Medical Science*, 344 (1954), 371–4.

15  These materials are held in Royal College of Physicians of Ireland, TPCK/2/5/1–8. For a discussion of the methods by which professional knowledge concerning the diagnosis and treatment of venereal diseases circulated in the United Kingdom in the late nineteenth and early twentieth centuries, see Hanley, *Medicine, Knowledge and Venereal Diseases*.

16  For an account of the Commission's findings and their implementation, see Evans, 'Tackling the "Hideous Scourge"'.

17  Thomas Percy Claude Kirkpatrick, 'Syphilis and the State', *Dublin Journal of Medical Science* XLV:558 (1 June 1918), 356–7. For competing accounts of the political stakes of regulationism in Free State public-health policy in the late 1920s, see Howell, 'Venereal Disease and the Politics of Prostitution'; Riordan, 'Venereal Disease in the Irish Free State'; Howell, 'A Response to Susannah Riordan'.

18  Thomas Percy Claude Kirkpatrick, 'The Treatment of Syphilis', *Dublin Journal of Medical Science* XLV:557 (1 May 1918), 273–80.

19  Thomas Percy Claude Kirkpatrick, *The History of Doctor Steevens' Hospital, Dublin, 1720–1920* (Dublin: Ponsonby and Gibbs, 1924), 153, 167–70.

20  Ibid., 329; *Annual Report of the Local Government Board Ireland 1916–17* [Cd. 8765.] (Dublin: His Majesty's Stationer's Office, 1917), xlix–l.

21  Thomas Percy Claude Kirkpatrick, 'The Work of a Venereal Disease Treatment Centre', *Irish Journal of Medical Science* 5:16 (June 1923), 145–6.

22  Evans, 'Tackling the "Hideous Scourge"'.

23  Royal College of Physicians of Ireland (RCPI), TPCK/3/5/1–2. The former contains eighty-eight pieces of dated correspondence, while the latter comprise thirty-two undated letters. Due to the uncatalogued nature of the correspondence, the entire contents of these files are subject to the one-hundred year rule and thus restricted until 2047. As a result (and in light of the stigmatising nature of the conditions under discussion in these letters), the names of all patients and their relatives have been redacted and replaced with initials. Titles such as 'Mrs' and 'Dr' have been preserved where they offer a clear indication of marital status or qualification. In line with this collection's commitment to patient voice and in light of the relative inaccessibility

of the materials my chapter handles, letters will be quoted at length where relevant. Errors of spelling and grammar will be preserved as an index of the correspondents' levels of literacy, though punctuation will occasionally be introduced parenthetically to aid intelligibility. For a discussion of the difficulties that arise when balancing sensitivity to the privacy of patients and their loved ones with a commitment to bearing historiographical witness to the lived experiences of vulnerable and marginalised individuals, see Jessica Meyer and Alexia Mocrieff's chapter in this collection.
24 I am grateful to Harriet Wheelock, the RCPI archivist, for her opinion on this matter.
25 An example of such criticism is discussed in detail below. 'Mrs B. to T.P.C. Kirkpatrick' (8 May 1935), TPCK/3/5: Kirkpatrick Collection, Patient Letters (1 of 2), RCPI (henceforth TPCK/3/5: Kirkpatrick Collection); 'Anonymous to T.P.C. Kirkpatrick' (August 1945), TPCK/3/5: Kirkpatrick Collection.
26 Riordan, '"A Probable Source of Infection"', 206.
27 Ibid.
28 Finola Kennedy and James M. Smith associate the Criminal Law Amendment Act and the suppressed 1931 Carrigan Report from which it derived with a 'sexual containment culture' and an increasingly stringent policing of female sexuality in the Free State. However, this characterisation has been challenged by Diarmaid Ferriter and Susannah Riordan. See Kennedy, 'The Suppression of the Carrigan Report'; Smith, 'The Politics of Sexual Knowledge'; Ferriter, *Occasions of Sin*, 136–48; Susannah Riordan, '"A Reasonable Cause": The Age of Consent and the Debate on Gender and Justice in the Irish Free State, 1922–35', *Irish Historical Studies* 37:147 (2011), 427–46.
29 For an overview of Ireland's economic performance in the period and its ramifications for living standards, see Cormac Ó Gráda, *Ireland: A New Economic History, 1780–1939* (Oxford: Clarendon Press, 1994), chapter 16; Mary E. Daly, 'Women in the Irish Free State, 1922–39: The Interaction Between Economics and Ideology', *Journal of Women's History* 7:1 (Winter 1995), 99–116; Mary E. Daly, 'The Irish Free State and the Great Depression of the 1930s: The Interaction of the Global and the Local', *Irish Economic and Social History* 38 (2011), 19–36; Gerard McCann, 'Protectionism and the "Economic War" in Interwar Ireland', *The Journal of European Economic History* 43:3 (2014), 39–68.
30 Martin, 'Bodies of Knowledge', 88.
31 Kirkpatrick, 'The Work of a Venereal Disease Treatment Centre', 147. The structure of the clinics at Steevens' mirrored similar patterns of

provision in England and Wales, where demobilisation and the slow acceptance of women and children as 'innocent victims' of venereal diseases conspired to make men the focal-point of medical intervention in the early interwar period. They also reflected a problematic cycle whereby women's objections to being examined and treated by men at male-run clinics and the lower attendance rates to which they gave rise resulted in fewer women's services being established. For a fuller discussion of this dynamic, see Hanley, '"Sex Prejudice" and Professional Identity'.

32 Kirkpatrick, 'The Work of a Venereal Disease Treatment Centre', 147. For an account of the operation of a comparable (albeit entirely female-staffed) women and children's VD ward at the Edinburgh Women and Children's Hospital, see Thomson, 'Between Separate Spheres', 115–17.

33 This policy had been adopted following a series of scandals within the hospital, but also reflected a widely held belief that male sufferers did not deserve treatment on the grounds of their apparent moral culpability. While attitudes on this matter shifted in the intervening century, the hospital's admissions policies did not and it remained a women-only institution until its dissolution in 1950 (most likely due to consistently straitened financial circumstances and administrative neglect). Maria Luddy, *Prostitution and Irish Society, 1800–1940* (Cambridge: Cambridge University Press, 2007), 130; Gary A. Boyd, *Dublin, 1745–1922: Hospitals, Spectacle and Vice* (Dublin: Four Courts, 2006), 167–73; Susannah Riordan, 'In Search of a Broadminded Saint: The Westmorland Lock Hospital in the Twentieth Century', *Irish Economic and Social History* 39:1 (2012), 73–93.

34 'Mr R. to T.P.C. Kirkpatrick' (October 1924), TPCK/3/5: Kirkpatrick Collection.

35 For accounts of drinking cultures in twentieth-century Ireland and Britain, see Diarmaid Ferriter, 'Drink and Society in Twentieth-Century Ireland', *Proceedings of the Royal Irish Academy. Section C: Archaeology, Celtic Studies, History, Linguistics, Literature* 115C (2015), 349–69, 349; Ryosuke Yokoe, 'Alcohol and Politics in Twentieth-Century Britain', *The Historical Journal* 62:1 (2019), 267–87.

36 A belief in the capacity for alcohol to stimulate digestion and aid in gastric health was common in early twentieth-century medical and popular discourse. For a discussion of cultural attitudes to the medicinal use of alcohol in early twentieth-century Britain, see Thora Hands, *Drinking in Victorian and Edwardian Britain* (New York: Springer Berlin Heidelberg, 2018), chapters 9 and 10.

37 'J.D. to T.P.C. Kirkpatrick' (28 December 1935), TPCK/3/5: Kirkpatrick Collection, original emphasis.

38  For an account of syphilophobia and its cultural manifestations, see Ida Macalpine, 'Syphilophobia: A Psychiatric Study', *British Journal of Venereal Diseases* 33 (1957), 92–9; Igor J. Polianski, 'Melancholia Syphilidophobica: Zur Kulturgeschichte der Venerologie', *Der Urologe* 52:11 (2013), 1582–9.
39  'J.D. to T.P.C. Kirkpatrick' (28 December 1935), emphasis added.
40  The venereologist's low opinion of public-health provision may have reflected the increasingly straitened financial circumstances in which Canadian sexual-health services found themselves following cuts to federal funding between 1926 and 1932, when state subsidy ceased entirely. Hamish MacDougall, 'Sexually Transmitted Diseases in Canada, 1800–1992', *Genitourinary Medicine* 70 (1 February 1994), 56–63, 59.
41  '"Noleen's Mammy" to T.P.C. Kirkpatrick' (26 December 1933), TPCK/3/5: Kirkpatrick Collection; '"Noleen's Mammy" to T.P.C. Kirkpatrick' (13 September 1935), TPCK/3/5: Kirkpatrick Collection; '"Noleen's Mammy" to T.P.C. Kirkpatrick' (undated [c. Christmas]), TPCK/3/5: Kirkpatrick Collection.
42  '"Noleen's Mammy" to T.P.C. Kirkpatrick' (13 September 1935).
43  Ibid.
44  For a contemporary description of the Marie Curie Hospital and the treatment 'Noleen's Mammy' was likely to have received there, see Anon., 'The Marie Curie Hospital', *British Journal of Nursing* 78 (September 1930), 242.
45  '"Noleen's Mammy" to T.P.C. Kirkpatrick' (13 September 1935).
46  Ibid.
47  For examples of the project's output, see Michael Brown, 'Surgery and Emotion: The Era Before Anaesthesia', in Thomas Schlich (ed.), *The Palgrave Handbook of the History of Surgery* (Basingstoke: Palgrave, 2018), 327–48; Michael Brown, 'Surgery, Identity and Embodied Emotion: John Bell, James Gregory and the Edinburgh "Medical War"', *History* 104:359 (January 2019), 19–41.
48  'Noleen' herself does not appear to feature among the correspondents in the collection.
49  'E.M. to T.P.C. Kirkpatrick' (3 August 1925), TPCK/3/5: Kirkpatrick Collection, original emphasis.
50  'M.R. to T.P.C. Kirkpatrick' (2 November 1926), TPCK/3/5: Kirkpatrick Collection.
51  While beyond the scope of the present chapter, the ways in which the Irish diaspora navigated networks of healthcare provision such as the VD Service merits further study.
52  'K.C. to T.P.C. Kirkpatrick' (12 March 1927), TPCK/3/5: Kirkpatrick Collection.

53 Ibid.
54 Ibid.
55 For a discussion of the increasing importance of cleanliness and hygiene to working-class British conceptions of sex and sexuality and the practical considerations that informed them, see Szreter and Fisher, *Sex Before the Sexual Revolution*, 298–311.
56 'K.C. to T.P.C. Kirkpatrick' (12 March 1927); 'K.C. to T.P.C. Kirkpatrick' (20 March 1927), TPCK/3/5: Kirkpatrick Collection, original emphasis.
57 'K.C. to T.P.C. Kirkpatrick' (20 March 1927).
58 'T.C. to T.P.C. Kirkpatrick' (undated [c. 20 March 1927]), TPCK/3/5: Kirkpatrick Collection.
59 Szreter and Fisher, *Sex Before the Sexual Revolution*, 100.
60 Ibid.
61 'K.C. to T.P.C. Kirkpatrick' (20 March 1927).
62 'T.C. to T.P.C. Kirkpatrick' (24 April 1927).
63 Ibid., original emphasis.
64 For a fuller discussion of this dynamic, see Anne Hanley's chapter in this collection.
65 'K.C. to T.P.C. Kirkpatrick' (20 March 1927).
66 Hanley, *Medicine, Knowledge and Venereal Diseases*, 53.
67 Riordan, 'Venereal Disease in the Irish Free State', 347; Riordan, 'In Search of a Broadminded Saint'.
68 Ferriter, *Occasions of Sin*, 159.
69 K.C. explains to Kirkpatrick: 'if I should have a course injections [sic], if you'd send them on to Dr Dooley here he'd use them'. 'K.C. to T.P.C. Kirkpatrick' (20 March 1927).
70 Ibid., emphasis added.
71 'B.D. to T.P.C. Kirkpatrick' (26 August 1925), TPCK/3/5: Kirkpatrick Collection.
72 Ibid.
73 This conviction was publicly expressed by both the Medical Women's Federation and the British Social Hygiene Council and was widely held by women VD Medical Officers. For a fuller discussion of this dynamic and its role in facilitating the entry of female medical practitioners into Britain's VD Service in the interwar period, see Hanley, '"Sex Prejudice" and Professional Identity'; Thomson, 'Between Separate Spheres', 115–17.
74 Department of Industry and Commerce, *Census of Population, 1936*, Vol. III: Religions and Birthplaces (Dublin: Stationery Office, 1939), 4.
75 Michel Foucault, *The History of Sexuality* Vol. I: The Will to Knowledge (New York: Pantheon Books, 1978).

76 David Barnard, 'The Physician as Priest, Revisited', *Journal of Religion and Health* 24:4 (1985), 272–86, 284.
77 'B.D. to T.P.C. Kirkpatrick' (21 October 1925), TPCK/3/5: Kirkpatrick Collection.
78 Ibid.
79 Ibid.
80 Ibid.
81 Inglis, 'Foucault, Bourdieu and the Field of Irish Sexuality', 12.
82 In her second letter, B.D. notes that her 'little Baby [sic] would have been a cripple' if not for Kirkpatrick's intervention, suggesting that he complied with her request and granted her daughter admission to Steevens'. 'B.D. to T.P.C. Kirkpatrick' (21 October 1925).
83 'Mrs A.B. to T.P.C. Kirkpatrick' (7 May 1924), TPCK/3/5: Kirkpatrick Collection.
84 Ibid.
85 David Fitzpatrick, 'Divorce and Separation in Modern Irish History', *Past and Present* 114:1 (1987), 172–96; Hug, *The Politics of Sexual Morality in Ireland*; Diane L. Urquhart, '"Divorce Irish Style": Marriage Dissolution in Ireland, 1850–1950', in Niamh Howlin and Kevin Costello (eds), *Law and the Family in Ireland, 1800–1950* (Basingstoke: Palgrave, 2017), 107–24.
86 Fitzpatrick, 'Divorce and Separation in Modern Irish History', 173–4.
87 Hug, *The Politics of Sexual Morality in Ireland*, 12–15.
88 Fitzpatrick, 'Divorce and Separation in Modern Irish History', 174.
89 I am grateful to Diane Urquhart for her opinion on this matter. While not concerned with the transmission of venereal diseases, her study of Irish women's efforts to secure legal separations in cases of domestic violence offers a useful account of the process Mrs A.B. was undertaking. Diane Urquhart, 'Irish Divorce and Domestic Violence, 1857–1922', *Women's History Review* 22:5 (2013), 820–37.
90 For an account of these debates and their implications for the British medical profession, see Ferguson, *Should a Doctor Tell?*, chapter 4.
91 Ibid., 61–3.
92 Inglis, 'Foucault, Bourdieu and the Field of Irish Sexuality', 12.
93 'J.M. to T.P.C. Kirkpatrick' (25 November 1924), TPCK/3/5: Kirkpatrick Collection.
94 'J.M. to T.P.C. Kirkpatrick' (1 January 1925), TPCK/3/5: Kirkpatrick Collection.
95 For studies of welfare provision and its attendant debates in this period (none of which discuss the impact of the RCVD and its recommendations), see Geoffrey B.A.M. Finlayson, *Citizen, State and Social Welfare in Britain 1830–1990* (Oxford: Oxford University Press, 1994), chapter 3; Sophia Carey, *Social Security in Ireland, 1939–1952: The*

*Limits to Solidarity* (Dublin: Irish Academic Press, 2007); Lucey and Crossman, *Healthcare in Ireland and Britain from 1850*; Fred Powell, *The Political Economy of the Irish Welfare State: Church, State and Capital* (Bristol: Policy Press, 2017), chapters 3, 5 and 7; Anthony McCashin, *Continuity and Change in the Welfare State* (Basingstoke: Palgrave, 2018), chapter 3.

96 'M.G. to T.P.C. Kirkpatrick' (29 July 1924), TPCK/3/5: Kirkpatrick Collection, original emphasis.
97 All calculations of inflation in this chapter are made using the Bank of England's online inflation resource: 'Inflation Calculator', Bank of England (22 January 2019), www.bankofengland.co.uk/monetary-policy/inflation/inflation-calculator (accessed 7 August 2019).
98 'F.W.K. to T.P.C. Kirkpatrick' (27 April 1925) TPCK/3/5: Kirkpatrick Collection.
99 'F.W.K. to T.P.C. Kirkpatrick' (15 May 1925), TPCK/3/5: Kirkpatrick Collection.
100 'Mrs B. to T.P.C. Kirkpatrick' (8 May 1935).
101 Ibid.
102 'Mrs B. to T.P.C. Kirkpatrick' (8 May 1935); William Murphy, 'Solomons, Bethel Albert Herbert', in James McGuire and James Quinn (eds), *Dictionary of Irish Biography* (Cambridge: Cambridge University Press, 2009), http://dib.cambridge.org/viewReadPage.do?articleId=a8187 (accessed 25 February 2021).
103 'Mrs B. to T.P.C. Kirkpatrick' (8 May 1935).
104 Terence Denman, '"The Red Livery of Shame": The Campaign Against Army Recruitment in Ireland, 1899–1914', *Irish Historical Studies* 29:114 (1994), 217–18.
105 Oliver St John Gogarty, 'Ugly England (I)', *Sinn Féin* (15 September 1906), 3.
106 Kathleen Lynn and Richard Hayes, *Public Health Circulars, No. 1* (Dublin: Sinn Féin Public Health Department, Dublin, 1918), 1.
107 Ibid.
108 Royal Commission on Venereal Diseases, PP 1913–16 Cd 7475 (Appendix to First Report of the Commissioners, Minutes of Evidence), q. 8, 208. For a discussion of O'Brien's contribution, see Luddy, *Prostitution and Irish Society, 1800–1940*, 184–90.
109 'P. McK. to T.P.C. Kirkpatrick' (18 November 1926), TPCK/3/5: Kirkpatrick Collection.
110 Ibid.
111 For an overview of sexual crime and the discourses surrounding it in Ireland in this period, see William Carrigan (Chairman), *Report of the Committee on the Criminal Law Amendment Acts (1880–85), and Juvenile Prostitution* (Dublin: Stationery Office, 1931); Kennedy,

'The Suppression of the Carrigan Report'; Finnane, 'The Carrigan Committee of 1930–31 and the "Moral Condition of the Saorstát"'; Smith, 'The Politics of Sexual Knowledge'; Maria Luddy, 'Sex and the Single Girl in 1920s and 1930s Ireland', *The Irish Review* 35 (2007), 79–91; Sandra McAvoy, 'Sexual Crime and Irish Women's Campaign for a Criminal Law Amendment Act, 1912–35', in Maryann Gialanella Valiulis (eds), *Gender and Power in Irish History* (Dublin: Irish Academic Press, 2009), 84–100; Cliona Rattigan, '"Crimes of Passion of the Worst Character": Abortion Cases and Gender in Ireland, 1925–50', in Maryann Gialanella Valiulis (eds) *Gender and Power in Irish History* (Dublin: Irish Academic Press, 2009), 115–40; Ferriter, *Occasions of Sin*, 110–45.

112 Population figures are derived from 1911 census data. None of the towns listed are large enough to register in the 1926 published census report. The complete data and records of the 1926 census are held by the National Archives of Ireland but are restricted until 2027. 'M.G. to T.P.C. Kirkpatrick' (2 January 1925), TPCK/3/5: Kirkpatrick Collection; 'F.W.K. to T.P.C. Kirkpatrick' (27 April 1925); 'B.D. to T.P.C. Kirkpatrick' (21 October 1925); 'Census of Ireland, 1911', National Archives of Ireland (August 2009), www.census.nationalarchives.ie (accessed 7 August 2019); Department of Industry and Commerce, *Census of Population, 1926* Vol. I: Population, Area and Valuation of each DED and each larger Unit of Area, 10 vols (Dublin: Stationery Office, 1928).

113 Committee on Venereal Disease, *Report of the Committee on Venereal Disease* (Dublin: Stationery Office, 1926), 3–4.

114 Ireland introduced its first national sexual-health strategy in 2015, inaugurating a five-year programme of research, review and reform intended to address long-standing deficiencies in the nation's sexual-health services. In response to the troubling findings of the 2019 Health and Social Care Committee Report on Sexual Health, the UK Department of Health and Social Care has committed itself to the development of a new national sexual-health strategy 'in partnership with Public Health England (PHE), NHS England and Improvement (NHS E&I), local government and other partners', though, as yet, no timetable has been specified for its delivery or implementation. Department of Health, *National Sexual Health Strategy, 2015–2020* (Department of Health, October 2015), www.gov.ie/en/policy-information/8feae9-national-sexual-health-strategy/ (accessed 25 February 2021); Department of Health and Social Care, *Government Response to the Health and Social Care Committee Report on Sexual Health* (London: Department of Health and Social Care, 24 October 2019), 7.

115 Matthew Peter Hibbert, Aedan Wolton, Harri Weeks, Michelle Ross, Caroline E. Brett, Lorna A. Porcellato, Vivian D. Hope, 'Psychosocial and Sexual Factors Associated with Recent Sexual Health Clinic Attendance and HIV Testing among Trans People in the UK', *BMJ Sexual & Reproductive Health* 46:2 (April 2020), 116–25; Sexual Health and Crisis Pregnancy Programme, *Sexual Health in Ireland: What Do We Know?* (Dublin: Health Service Executive, June 2018), 46–7.

# 9

## 'I caught it and yours truly was very sorry for himself': mapping the emotional worlds of British VD patients*

### Anne Hanley

In 1942, at the height of the Second World War, Mass Observation (MO) surveyed residents in several London boroughs about a public-health advertisement that had recently appeared in the *Daily Mirror*.[1] The advert, titled 'Ten Plain Facts about VD', outlined the dangers of syphilis and gonorrhoea, the tell-tale signs of infection and the necessity of immediate medical treatment. It was part of the Ministry of Health's largest-ever sexual-health propaganda campaign. Alarmed by the wartime spike in infection rates, the Ministry was endeavouring to counteract the 'hush hush' culture that it believed was undermining efforts to protect civilian health.[2] By conducting its survey, MO hoped to understand better how ordinary men and women felt about the very public airing of a subject that, despite heavy campaigning by the Ministry and the British Social Hygiene Council (BSHC), was still very much taboo. MO's interviewers had been warned to expect a spectrum of impassioned responses – from dismay that more was not being done to combat venereal diseases (VD), to indignation that such a distasteful subject was being made acceptable for public consumption. As one outraged middle-aged man from Wandsworth fumed, 'A bloody fine game – syphilis on your breakfast table!'[3] Similarly, a woman from Chelsea, whom the MO interviewer described as coldly antagonistic, insisted that no one would answer such '*impertinent* and [...] insulting' questions: 'You can't deal with a difficult subject in this ham-handed way [...] The point is that you'll get no change out of a person who has *got* VD, they'll only feel what the hell, it's no business of yours and the ones that haven't will only be angry at your bringing up an unpleasant subject they manage to shut their eyes to.'[4]

It therefore seemed unlikely that anyone expected respondents to be as candid as 'M65A' from Notting Hill Gate:

> As a young man, I caught it and yours truly was very sorry for himself. Of course, I read many good books during that time – Macaulay and so on. But I was fleeced by doctors. They had every penny I had! Took two months but I'm told there's a cure now only takes two weeks. Is that possible? [...] It doesn't sound possible to me.[5]

Or, indeed, 'M30D' from Fulham:

> A good many people I have been told catch this disease through using the same lavatories and towels. How to get over this problem is a puzzle. I had a slight dose once which I got from a typist, the last person you would expect it from, but she was most troubled when I told her to go and get treatment and was inclined to [believe] I had given it to her. Several of my pals have had the same experience and it does make you wonder where the origin starts.[6]

As this edited collection has made clear, accessing historical patient voices is challenging at the best of times. But access is doubly difficult when dealing with sexual health, since it carried additional stigma and shame. As our lady from Chelsea vehemently put it, no respectable, right-minded person would talk publicly about VD, let alone admit to having it. In view of this, the ethical implications of scrutinising the intimate lives and traumas of patients such as 'M65A' and 'M30D' are more fraught than normal. But laying bare these stories is also problematic because there is a dearth of surviving material. Individuals afflicted by VD were reluctant to leave records of their infection. As another woman from Chelsea said somewhat contemptuously when approached by MO, 'it's no good asking questions [...] Girls wouldn't talk about it to strangers, only to a doctor or to someone they thought might help them. They certainly wouldn't answer a list of questions from an inquisitive stranger.'[7] Likewise, families, often aided by doctors, suppressed the fact that a relative was suffering from (or had died from) VD.[8]

Recent large-scale digitisation projects, such as that conducted by the Royal London Hospital for the Whitechapel VD Clinic, have been an important step towards making more accessible the few surviving historical records of venereal infection.[9] But these records are primarily institutional. Although they offer up valuable morsels of information about patients' familial and social relationships, they tell us more about how patients were diagnosed and treated. As Claire Brock observes, such mediated accounts are problematic for understanding patient experiences of the clinical encounter.[10] Far more historiographical attention has therefore been given to the health and economic costs of VD. Very little has been written about the emotional and psychological burden of a suspected or diagnosed infection.[11]

In her seminal study of fear, Joanna Bourke articulates the historian's dilemma. Often, 'the reluctance of many historians to analyse emotions stems from problems of nomenclature. Was what people in the 1970s called "fear" the same thing as it was in the 1870s? Probably not. Or, more accurately, many historians feel that they have no way of knowing. Looked at historically, subjective feelings are invisible.'[12] We have records of clinical encounters, but how do we know what men, women and children actually *felt* about these encounters? For the most part, historical patients' emotional worlds seem frustratingly elusive. Today, a diagnosis of syphilis or gonorrhoea might be inconvenient, embarrassing and even stigmatising; certainly, the rise of antibiotic resistant gonorrhoea has created a new urgency for maintaining good sexual-health practices. But for the most part, the profound fear that accompanied such diagnoses in the past is alien to us. The idea that these diseases could lead to death or social ruin seems almost unintelligible.

As Monika Pietrzak-Franger observes, 'the crucial reason behind the socio-political and cultural potency of syphilis [...] lay in the tensions between visibility and invisibility that it produced'.[13] This paradox shaped attitudes to sexual health across the late nineteenth and early twentieth centuries. 'Syphilis was a disease and a metaphor for disease', argues Andrew Smith. 'Both a medical problem and a trope for social and cultural degeneration. In other words, there was the reality of this disease and a cultural fear of it.'[14] As we shall see, these two faces of VD – disease and metaphor – became inextricable. They consumed the public imagination through a flurry of high-profile medical literature and fiction produced from the end of the nineteenth century. Fears about VD became conflated with, and exacerbated by, a variety of national and imperial crises, most notably the Second Boer War (and the resulting 1904 Interdepartmental Committee on Physical Deterioration).[15] These crises directly linked venereal infection to a perceived decline in racial health, challenging heroic ideals of imperial masculinity.[16] As Joanne Townsend puts it, 'in light of the recruiting crisis, a link was drawn from the substandard diseased recruit back to the unhealthy child he had been, thence to his sickly infancy, and finally to his mother, never quite well since marriage'.[17]

Yet at the same time, public discussion of these problems was aggressively suppressed, even into the interwar years when VD was being brought increasingly within the remit of preventative medicine. These tensions between fear and suppression on the one hand, and fascination and scrutiny on the other, fundamentally shaped patient experiences, creating the perfect conditions for the emergence of widespread fears about venereal infection and the threat of infection. This culture of fascination and suppression gave rise to a disorder known as syphilophobia – the 'insane dread of syphilis' or the irrational fear that one has contracted syphilis.[18] Such dread stimulated what Don James McLaughlin describes as 'a psychosomatic generation of symptoms'.[19] Syphilophobia, like other phobias emerging in nineteenth-century medical discourse, derived its phenomenology from a variety of interconnected feelings of shame and fear, producing its own distinct pathologies.[20]

This is where non-traditional sources, especially works of fiction, become so valuable to the historian; they lay bare the emotional and psychological costs of living with VD. With the possible exception of consumption, no other disease category preyed so extensively on the Victorian's literary imagination.[21] Although scholars have drawn heavily on fiction in their study of sexual health, these have been primarily literary critiques or cultural histories.[22] This chapter makes the case for using fiction as a legitimate source for patient-centred social histories of medicine, presenting a methodological model that combines fictional and factual sources in a nuanced and sensitive study of patient experiences. Indeed, fiction should not be a last resort, turned to only when traditional archival materials are unavailable. Rather, fiction's creative reconstructions of real-life struggles and emotional worlds makes it an important source to be considered *alongside* traditional sources. When used thoughtfully, fiction enables historians to access complex and colourful lives otherwise obscured by the clinical nature of patient case notes.

Writing about the ethics of archival research, the political scientist Jelena Subotić insists that 'scholars must avoid visualizing experiences of our subjects by making interpretive leaps and engaging in evocative imagined scenarios that the personal testimonies only hint at but do not fully convey'.[23] Such avoidance is certainly essential for ethically reflexive scholarship. But, as Subotić acknowledges, this cannot be a one-size-fits-all approach. In seeking to understand ordinary lived experiences of VD, we become what Subotić describes as 'a curator of pain', tempted always to seek out extreme instances of emotional, physical or psychological distress.[24] We must avoid that temptation. It is a constant, fine balance, comparing fictional representations – often embellished for literary effect – against what we know of real-life experiences.

In the absence of autobiographical narratives, fiction becomes one of the key collections of material through which historians might access the lives of ordinary VD sufferers.[25] First is the Victorian fiction that used VD as a central plot device to critique the familial and social power structures that endangered health and allowed vice to go unchecked. Victorian writers commonly blurred the boundaries between medicine and literature, playing with popular plot devices like hereditary degeneration and disease transmission.[26] In her work on tuberculosis, Katherine Byrne identifies a 'complex and symbiotic relationship' between medical literature and fiction.[27] As we see in this chapter, these genres drew on each in the creation of venereal stereotypes as well as the socio-cultural conditions in which conditions like syphilophobia thrived. Classic examples include Arthur Conan Doyle's short story 'Third Generation', Henrik Ibsen's sensational play *Ghosts* and Sarah Grand and Emma Brooke's 'New Woman' novels *The Heavenly Twins* and *A Superfluous Woman*.[28]

The diseases depicted in these stories were at the margins of respectable society, but the novelists and playwrights who authored them were not. Doyle (himself a qualified doctor), Grand and Ibsen were among the literary giants of their day. The 'New Woman' – a term coined by Grand in *The Heavenly Twins* – came to define an entire generation of female activism, much of it directed against the sexual double standard that made women vulnerable to infected, reprobate husbands. Likewise, Ibsen's plays became notorious on the London stage and *Ghosts* was no exception. These writers fundamentally reshaped how late Victorian and Edwardian readers and theatre-goers thought about VD and its sufferers.[29]

Each story deals with the hypocrisies of marital respectability; characters must come reluctantly to terms with the degradation that has been concealed behind a façade of morality and respectability. Mental fragility, bodily corruption, despair, familial disorder and social decay define these stories, which are littered with characters desperately trying to keep up appearances while their private lives fall apart. These works gave a public face to a very private problem. If we look past the melodrama, we see in these stories the same pathos, anxieties and fraught personal relationships that real-world doctors recognised in their patients.

The second collection of sources to which we should therefore turn is the extensive corpus of medical literature, especially literature dealing with syphilophobia. Records of syphilophobia, more so than most other medical discussions of VD, prioritised the 'pre-patient' experiences of illness and suspected illness.[30] Such experiences were fundamental to understanding the complex web of social, emotional and psychological factors that fed a patient's phobic state – the stress and fear of exposure and social ruin, the risk of infecting others and acute feelings of isolation, grief and betrayal.

Other records are also of great value, such as those of Britain's VD Service and its accompanying propaganda campaigns, which allow historians to contextualise experiences of infection within the significant shifts in public attitudes towards sexual health across the early twentieth century. Capitalising on the interwar craze for films, voluntary health organisations like the BSHC (formerly the National Council for Combatting Venereal Diseases – NCCVD) released dozens of theatrical health education films.[31] Like the Victorian fiction that preceded them, these films were melodramatic and unsubtle in their messages about personal and collective moral hygiene. But also like their Victorian predecessors, these films drew on real-world dilemmas and therefore offer historians excellent insight into the interwar experiences of living with VD and the *fear* of infection. As we shall see, these films had a significant impact on the numbers of people seeking care and reassurance from the VD Service. The very public presence of syphilis and gonorrhoea on the silver screen began to open up public discussion of sexual health and, by extension, alter people's experiences of illness. But as MO's wartime survey reveals, these diseases continued to carry profound stigma. In many ways, the consequences of infection remained as terrifying in the twentieth century as they had been in the nineteenth, continuing to shape pervasive fears bound up with the spectre of VD.

## 'It is not only the "penny dreadful" novelist, but medical authors who should know better'[32]

Authors and playwrights used VD to critique the real-world problems of middle-class marriage and the sexual double standard. Critics may have decried their work as offensive to public decency and good taste, but it was nonetheless opening up public discussion of the personal costs of infection. Normally, weddings constituted a neat, satisfying plot device for concluding a narrative.[33] But marriage and parenthood are no panacea in these stories. Grand's heroines – Evadne Colquhoun *née* Frayling and Edith Menteith *née* Beale – made socially advantageous but morally compromising marriages. Brooke's heroine, Jessamine Halliday *née* Heriot, similarly found herself tied to a syphilitic reprobate. Both novels are a painful dissection of the ensuing chaos.[34] Likewise, Doyle and Ibsen's tragic protagonists – Sir Francis Norton and Oswald Alving – survived into adulthood only to find themselves blighted by the same disease that killed their fathers.[35] As the New Woman periodical *Shafts* observed in 1893, 'Ibsen's *Ghosts* depicts the "hereditary" question in the most ghastly colours, as rising up like a giant to destroy the young man's life who has been carefully kept in ignorance of the "skeleton in the family closet".'[36] Drawing on the same eugenic themes several decades later in his scandalous interwar novel *The Green Hat*, Michael Arlen used his character Boy Fenwick to explore the destructive potency of the *fear* of infection. Believing himself to be infected, this ill-fated golden boy kills himself on his wedding night. Overcome by despair, he dies 'for purity' – for the fear that he might expose his bride to the ravages of acquired syphilis.[37] Fenwick's tragic end is a common trope of the genre. After much anguish and recrimination, the outcome for such benighted characters is almost always death, either by their own hand or from the insidious consequences of disease.

Throughout their novels, Brooke and Grand remain reticent about the physical impact of VD on the human body. Likewise, neither Doyle nor Ibsen offers much description of characters' corporeal suffering. Arlen went even further – although he coded syphilis into his novel, he never explicitly discussed the disease. For reasons of public decency (and to avoid the ire of the censors), these authors focused on their characters' emotional, psychological and spiritual torment. To find accounts of patients' bodily experiences, we must return to the medical literature and its myriad case histories, many of which have clear fictional parallels.

The case of 'Mrs T. – ', written up in the *Lancet* in 1882 by Frederick W. Lowndes (surgeon to the Liverpool Lock Hospital), was particularly tragic. As a young woman, Mrs T. married a naval officer and soon after developed primary-stage syphilis. She was confined for an extended period to a London hospital, but was eventually discharged without tangible improvement. The couple had only one child, who died in infancy. For several years, Mrs T. continued to be treated unsuccessfully by various doctors. As is the common progression from secondary- to tertiary-stage syphilis, her symptoms disappeared only to manifest aggressively many years later. When Lowndes first encountered her, she was close to death. Recounting his house call, he struggled to convey 'the shocking condition' in which he found her: 'The greater portion of her face was gone, her sight was gone; it was with the greatest difficulty that she was fed, and the stench which filled the room was the most sickening I ever encountered.'[38]

Equally disturbing was the case of the syphilitic and heavily pregnant woman attended by Dr Arabella Kenealy. In 1895 Kenealy wrote to the editor of the *British Medical Journal* about this 'wreck of a young woman', who presented a typical pattern of venereal infertility: three miscarriages in rapid succession, the birth of a child who demonstrated clear symptoms of congenital syphilis and then another two miscarriages. She was again pregnant but bleeding heavily and on the verge of another miscarriage. But more shocking to Kenealy was the woman's congenitally syphilitic child: 'On a low stool with its head supported heavily on long, lean-fingered hands, a child of some four or five years was sitting, watching me out of mournful eyes […] It stretched an elfish hand up and clutching the corner of the chair, made a laborious effort to rise.'[39]

Eventually, the sickly child dragged itself to Kenealy, who claimed that 'you could read the ache of bones in the way it set its feet down; you could hear the patience of hopelessness in its laboured breath'.[40] Kenealy fancied that the child had been deprived of love and 'human companionship' for much of its short life – something she attributed to it being 'so monstrous a "degenerate"'. Fearing that its companion might be about to leave, the child, according to Kenealy, 'looked into [her] eyes with the lonely desolateness of a clouded mind', caught hold of her dress and began to cry.[41] Although probably based on a genuine case of antepartum complication and congenital syphilis, Kenealy's melodrama of wrecked womanhood and hereditary degeneration also drew heavily on the literary style of novelists like Grand and Brooke.[42] As a eugenicist, Kenealy's distasteful descriptions of the child's 'sunken nose, overhung by prominent brows and the dull joyless eyes' were no doubt an attempt to give credence to, and garner support for, her eugenic principles.

Yet when we look beyond Kenealy's eugenic propaganda, we find – as in the New Woman fiction that undoubtedly inspired her – a terrible family tragedy. Such lurid accounts are indeed awful. We do not need to hear these patients' voices directly to know that their suffering was acute. When considered alongside Grand and Brooke's writings (which were themselves laced with eugenic rhetoric), a fuller picture emerges of the personal relationships and social structures that led ordinary women into such misery. The experiences of Mrs T. and Kenealy's unnamed mother and child map on to those of Edith Menteith, Jessamine Halliday and Helen Alving – all were infected by their husbands and gave birth to ill-fated children.

As evidenced in such medical and fictional accounts, VD carried very gender-specific implications that, heavily embedded within a patriarchal social order and its institutions, defined men and women's different experiences of infection. Women came up against what Marilyn Bonnell has described as 'a critical superstructure that was attempting to define and dictate reality according to masculine epistemology'.[43] The long-standing assumption that sexual innocence was predicated on sexual ignorance meant that many women were probably unaware that their ill-health was the result of a venereal infection. We see this double standard especially among the affluent classes. Doctors, whose fees were paid by husbands and fathers, aided these men in controlling the information to which their wives and daughters had access. They cited a man's legal right to medical confidentiality, since informing a woman that she suffered from VD would almost certainly reveal that her husband had infected her. Doctors conspired to keep women in ignorance on the grounds that doing otherwise would lead to familial conflict and undermine paterfamilial authority.[44]

Although many nineteenth-century doctors wrote about the dangers of disease transmission within marriage, none recounted such cases with the same flourish as the French venereologist Alfred Fournier, who warned his fellow doctors that they would have to 'scheme and dissimulate constantly':[45]

> In the vast majority of cases [...] the woman is ignorant of the disease which affects her, and it is your moral duty to deceive her in this matter by hiding from her the name and nature of her malady. And why? [...] A young husband who has infected his wife will come to you, for instance, in the greatest anxiety, and will commence the conversation thus: 'Doctor, a great misfortune has happened to me. I have had syphilis. I have been wrong enough to marry without being thoroughly cured, and I have given the disease to my wife. I have come to ask you to treat my poor wife; but [...] keep her completely ignorant of the name and nature of her disease, for if she knew, I should be lost. There would be an end to her affection and to her esteem; and if she should tell her family, imagine the scene!'[46]

A man might have felt compelled to make such demands by genuine love and concern for a wife whose life had been irrevocably altered by his behaviour. But as we see in Doyle's depiction of Norton, he might also be driven by shame, fear of familial conflict and, by extension, exposure and social ruin. Men such as Sir Mosley Menteith and Captain Alving (Oswald's father) had the wealth and influence to offset their shame and fear by asserting subtle (and not-so-subtle) control over the length, direction and nature of their care and the care of their families. Such control often undermined the wellbeing of their wives and children, who were excluded from conversations and decisions about their own treatment. The following exchange between Dr Frederick Mott (pathologist to the London County Council Asylums) and Dr Armand Routh (consulting obstetric physician to Charing Cross Hospital) during the latter's appearance in 1914 before the Royal Commission on Venereal Diseases beautifully captures the heavy-handed paternalism with which women had to contend:

> If a married woman came to you and you discovered she had syphilis, would you tell her the nature of her disease if she asked you? – No.
> You would not? – I never have.
> You do not think she has a right to know? – She has a right to be treated for it.
> But she has not the right to know the nature of the disease? – I think the doctor is bound to secrecy.
> [...]
> If she asked herself? – No, I do not think I would.
> Why not? – She could be treated probably just as well without knowing. Of course, such a revelation would necessarily lead to divorce or what not if you did.
> [...]
> Supposing you had a syphilitic child to deal with, and there were other younger children born, what would you do in such a case? Say you discovered a late form of syphilis in the child, and the mother is pregnant? – I should speak to the father.
> You would then? – Yes, but I should not tell the mother.
> But you would have to treat the mother? – Yes, and the husband would probably arrange that that could be done.[47]

But women, unfortunately, did not always have conscientious husbands to arrange for their careful, ongoing treatment. The respected British venereologist Jonathan Hutchinson lamented that he and his colleagues frequently encountered men who would allow their wives to go untreated or terminate treatment once the more obvious symptoms had disappeared.[48]

To appreciate properly these patients' experiences, we must understand not only the physical ravages of VD, but also the dynamics of the clinical encounter and the nature and limitations of available treatments. Until the interwar development of sulphonamides, common treatments for gonorrhoea included urethral irrigations and dangerous surgical procedures. The treatment *par excellence* for syphilis was mercury, which might be swallowed as pills or tonics, absorbed through the skin via ointments or vapours, or injected intramuscularly. Each of these methods was dangerous and painful, exposing the patient to the risk of heavy-metal poisoning.[49] But even if women were kept ignorant about the exact nature of their illness, it would not escape their notice that they were being subjected to embarrassing and painful medical interventions for which their husbands and doctors offered little explanation. Indeed, Grand makes pointed use of this exact scenario:

> 'The doctor again!' Edith groaned. 'It has been nothing but the doctor and "tonics" ever since I have been married.'
> 'What does he say is the matter exactly?' Mrs Beale asked.
> All his endeavour seems to be not to say what is the matter exactly', Edith replied.[50]

Although we can bring our historical imagination to bear on the woeful predicament of women in such situations, we can do little more than speculate on how they must have actually *felt*. In doing so, we risk anachronistically imposing our twenty-first-century sensibilities on our historical actors. But in cases such as those outlined above, we may say with relative certainty that patients shared a common set of emotional experiences. As we have seen, a woman's respectability hinged on her ignorance of sexual matters, including sexually transmitted diseases. Pietrzak-Franger even claims that knowledge of syphilis was considered to be pornographic.[51] Having developed one or more symptoms – perhaps a profuse and foul-smelling vaginal discharge, an angry rash across her body or acute abdominal pain and swelling – for which she had no explanation, she would most likely be confused and fearful. She might even have been alerted to the fact that she was unwell by an inability to conceive or carry a pregnancy to full term – traumatic enough without the added burden of a venereal infection. Or she might be left with a generalised anxiety after a few deliberately ambiguous words from her doctor.

Even when women did know themselves to be suffering from VD, their emotional responses were mediated through male doctors' expectations of appropriate womanly behaviour. Fournier, for example, admired what he saw as the self-sacrificing stoicism of a patient who maintained an appearance of ignorance for the sake of the husband who had infected her.[52] This is precisely why fiction is so important. Whereas Fournier and Routh ironed out the complexities of female experience, Grand gave voice and nuance to women's 'mental torture'. Far from preserving her innocence, Edith's sexual ignorance leaves her vulnerable to a dissipated husband. It made her 'a lovely specimen of a well-bred English girl' but condemned her to a miserable marriage, disease, insanity and early death. In Edith, Grand provides what so much of the medical literature cannot – an articulate female-oriented perspective on the day-to-day emotional and psychological impact of living with syphilis. It is rendered all the more moving and confronting because society's rigid morality – its 'conspiracy of silence' – denied Edith legal recourse or, indeed, any mechanisms for articulating her anger and betrayal.

> Edith had been robbed of all means of self-defence by the teaching which insisted that her only duty as a wife consisted in silent submission to her husband's will. Her intellectual life, such as it was, had stopped short [and] only her senses had been nourished, and these were now being rendered morbidly active by disease [...] The mental torture was extreme; but she fought for her reason with the fearful malady valiantly; and all the time presented outwardly only the same dull apathy, giving no sign and speaking no word which could betray the fury of the rage within.[53]

The same long-standing assumption that innocence was predicated on ignorance meant that, although women in Edith's predicament might have suspected that something was gravely wrong, they lacked the sexual knowledge and vocabulary to articulate their concerns. And by deliberately not naming the disease that afflicts her protagonist, Grand's novel becomes what Livia Arndal Woods describes as 'a particularly pointed *fin-de-siècle* attack on the threats that unsaying and unknowing pose'.[54] Central to these medical and fictional accounts were the power dynamics of knowledge, specifically who was entitled to knowledge. The assumption that the possession of sexual knowledge was immoral persisted well into the twentieth century, as evidenced by the middle-aged woman from Wandsworth who felt that the Ministry of Health's war-time propaganda campaign created 'the wrong way of thinking in our younger people, who become curious [...] find out what it all means and become debased through the knowledge'.[55] Indeed, as we shall see, a chief criticism across the nineteenth *and* twentieth centuries was that the sexual knowledge imparted through fictional representations of VD would lead to greater promiscuity.[56]

However, knowledge was not always a guarantee of health or happiness. Syphilophobia, for example, was thought to be exacerbated by misinformation or information conveyed inappropriately.

As we see in Evadne's troubled marriage, knowledge could not guard against the expectations of a family whose principle concern was not the moral or physical health of their son-in-law, but the material gains of a socially advantageous marriage.[57] Her spiral into hysteria, which causes her to fixate on the dangers of congenital syphilis, is heavily infused with the language of syphilophobia. Rather than protecting her, Evadne's wide reading of medical texts gave her the knowledge to fixate on syphilis's morbid qualities and to imagine herself to be infected. Dr Galbraith – her second, untainted husband – observes of Evadne that 'it was always what she imagined that made her morbid'.[58] Even though she did not consummate her marriage to Colquhoun, she became convinced that his sexual vices had imprinted themselves on to her and the unborn child she conceived with Galbraith.[59]

The mercenary self-interest that forced women like Evadne into such predicaments was aggressively criticised by New Woman writers, such as Nora Brownlow in her scathing 1892 *Shafts* article, 'The Modern Slave Market'. What do a bride's parents demand from 'the purchaser'? According to Brownlow, '*money*, that's the chief thing, good houses for the slave to live in, fine clothes for the slave to wear, servants to wait upon her, and a place in Society [...] The moral character of those who buy [...] is not considered.'[60] As various writers to *Shafts* lamented, young women had been conditioned to accept this status quo:

> Talking one day of Evadne's treatment of her husband [...] to a girl to whom I had recommended the book, I heard with sorrow arguments against it which seemed to me terrible from one who may someday be a wife and mother [...] There are girls who know so little of the existence of this evil that they have no power of selecting a fit husband; and there are those who, from various sources outside the home, have learnt of, and become blunted to, the immorality surrounding them.[61]

To understand the historical experiences of women living with VD, we must first recognise these larger inequalities and the patriarchal structures that buttressed them.[62] When we think about how men and women might have exercised agency, we must consider not only the therapeutic limitations of their care, but also the social and political obstacles they faced – obstacles that would have seemed especially insurmountable for persons with stigmatising conditions like syphilis or gonorrhoea. Evadne understood the medical dangers of consummating her marriage, but social convention denied her the freedom to act on that knowledge and break from her husband.[63] Women's agency was conditional, defined within strict moral boundaries. As Lynn Thomas encourages us to do, we must think of their agency as a process of 'just getting by'.[64] Infected men and women were not overthrowing an unjust system. Rather, they were trying to navigate that system to achieve the least-worse outcome for themselves and their families. As historians, we should read conditions like syphilophobia as one particular manifestation of such navigations.

## 'I am polluted to the marrow, soaked in abomination!'[65]

Before the establishment in 1917 of Britain's VD Service, which guaranteed universal care that was free at the point of use, men and women who believed themselves to be infected with syphilis or gonorrhoea had limited options.[66] One option was to seek mainstream medical care. Those who could afford doctors' fees, might – as Sir Francis Norton did – visit private consulting rooms. Those who could not afford such fees were at the mercy of the Poor Law and the few voluntary hospitals willing to treat VD patients.[67] Alternatively, infected men and women, driven by shame, fear or a lack of financial resources, might turn to irregular or 'quack' remedies.[68] Or they might forgo treatment entirely. Regardless of their choice, a chronic lack of information characterised many patients' experiences. In a society that looked ambivalently on discussion of VD, reliable public-health information was scarce. In its place existed a web of misinformation and charlatanism. Caught in this web, the patient or 'non-patient' faced lengthy periods in which they were left to speculate and fret. Doctors before the First World War insisted that syphilophobia was brought on and exacerbated by this dearth of reliable and responsible information. When asked whether boys should be taught about the dangers of syphilis, Dr Arthur Powell (London School of Hygiene and Tropical Medicine) insisted that:

> a great deal of tact would be required lest an undue syphilophobia should be produced. The dangers of syphilophobia are by no means small. I have held autopsies on eleven cases of suicide due to

syphilophobia, and I know many cases of lunacy due to the same cause. I am not sure that some of the suicides which came under my official notice might not be more appropriately termed homicide caused by ignorant friends and medical advisers giving an unjustifiably lurid prognosis. I am sorry to say it is not only the 'penny dreadful' novelist, but medical authors who should know better, who have painted such monstrous pictures of the bogey syphilis. Most of us have met the type of syphilitic who, primed with such old wives' fables, carefully shakes his socks each night to see if any of his toes have been left behind.[69]

Although hyperbole, Powell's description of patients anxiously shaking their socks to check for missing digits reflected wider patterns of behavioural change witnessed in those with syphilis and syphilophobia.

That more men than women presented with syphilophobia was attributed to 'the double standard of morality, with its extra-marital sexual exposures and subsequent conflicts and repressions'.[70] Large numbers of men, fearing the worst, attended VD clinics during the early interwar years. Having had sexual liaisons while on active service during the First World War, they became anxious about their health and the health of their families. 'As a young man in Mesopotamia', one syphilophobe had 'been frequently exposed to infection, and nothing would remove his belief that he had got syphilis; he claimed it was incurable and that an unkind fate awaited him, and he refused to consult anyone else.'[71] Likewise, a syphilophobic 'ex-naval man' had convinced his son that the latter was congenitally syphilitic. But both men's Wassermann blood tests were negative.[72] In keeping with its pre-war emphasis on hygiene, the British armed forces employed a variety of punitive methods and scare tactics to discourage servicemen from illicit sexual liaisons. During the latter years of the First World War, these included 'moral prophylaxis' lectures organised by army chaplains, members of the Royal Army Medical Corps and the NCCVD. As Mark Harrison has shown, these efforts, which prioritised the necessity of clean living and focused in visceral detail on the physical and moral dangers of sexual immorality, fed men's morbid preoccupations as well as an ingrained sense of guilt.[73] Our phobic ex-servicemen probably picked up fragments of information from such lectures and from conversations with comrades, which in turn fuelled their fears in civilian life.

The breakdown of these double standards in sexual knowledge and medical care – which had begun in the 1890s and accelerated during the Great War and interwar years – was part of a wider shift in attitudes towards sex.[74] As Lloyd (Meadhbh) Houston demonstrates in Chapter 8 through close readings of correspondence from Dr Kirkpatrick's female patients, despite the strategic projection of a self-conscious image of sexual innocence, many women were nonetheless speaking with increasing awareness and openness about their sexual health.[75] This breakdown of gendered knowledge barriers was also due to the establishment of the VD Service and the accompanying propaganda campaign orchestrated by the BSHC. Health-education films, for example, were destabilising both the gendered and class-based boundaries of sexual-health knowledge. Case notes from the Whitechapel VD Clinic exemplify this trend. Alongside a patient's symptoms and other personal information, medical officers listed the motivating cause for attendance. Many patients had been sent by their GP or were transferred from a hospital. But the commonest motivating factor for attendance was advertisements. For example, 590 of the 2,310 male patients seen in 1930 attributed their attendance to flyers, posters, public lectures and films.[76] 'Adverts' became so common a reason for attendance that it was eventually given its own column on the confidential registers.

Interwar VD health-education films, many of which were commissioned by the BSHC, had very different plots and tropes from the fatalistic Victorian novels and plays that had dealt with similar subjects. In Grand, Ibsen and Doyle's writing, innocent virgins married degenerate reprobates and lived only long enough to watch their children succumb to the ravages of congenital syphilis. Wholesome young men were felled in their prime by the emergence of a previously dormant congenital taint. And the outcome was inevitably the same: misery, heartbreak and death. Although interwar films continued to promote eugenic ideas about the dangers posed to racial health by illicit sex, they were much more upbeat than their Victorian and Edwardian predecessors.

Such a step change was due in large part to the diagnostic and therapeutic innovations that were heralding a more optimistic era of care in the 1920s and 1930s. The spirochete had been identified in 1905. The diagnostic Wassermann blood test for syphilis had been developed in 1906. Salvarsan and its derivates were developed from 1909 and marked a major improvement on older mercury treatments.[77] Interwar health authorities had a new-found confidence that, with timely and thorough treatment, they could achieve a complete cure. And health-education films were an essential means of ensuring the public also knew this. As Kirsten Ostherr has observed, health-education films were often scripted deliberately to transcend the specificities of class, gender and locale – the aim being to reach the largest possible audiences.[78] Their popularity with the huge cinema-going audiences of the interwar years offered health authorities an unprecedented opportunity to reshape public behaviour, assuage anxieties and manage expectations about medical interventions.[79] And these large audiences did indeed translate into large attendance numbers at clinics.[80]

VD health-education films packaged up uncompromising morality tales as light entertainment, intending that audiences – men and women, working- and middle-class alike – would identify with one of the protagonists and realise how close they themselves might have come to danger. Some films, such as *Test for Love* (1937), were produced for female audiences.[81] Others, such as *Trial for Marriage* (1936), were intended for men.[82] The plots of both films were typical of the genre: a foolish young person falls in with a 'fast' crowd, commits a sexual transgression and subsequently discovers that they have been infected with syphilis or gonorrhoea. This would be followed by a period of acute suffering and self-recrimination. But, importantly, the films also promised eventual atonement.[83] Such sexual transgressions would have been morally unforgivable *and* medically untreatable only a few decades earlier. Although still a grievous social misstep, it was now nothing that a prompt visit to the local VD clinic could not fix.

John, the flawed protagonist in *Trial for Marriage*, is corrupted by Hermione Strange – 'the bad girl of Chelsea'. Bored, lonely and missing his fiancée, he declares that he would 'like to be wild again for once'. Hermione obliges, inviting him to a party where, having plied him with absinthe, she seduces him. Fearing the worst, John's cousin Henry (who is, incidentally, a venereologist) takes John to visit his hospital's VD wards. As Henry explains to the senior surgeon, John is 'really a jolly good chap. But he's got in with a fast gang [...] I want to open his eyes a bit. I feel this is the only way to do it.' At this point, the plot descends into pointed, unsubtle dialogues on the dangers of VD and the exceptionalism of the new VD Service.

> *Henry*: You wouldn't get sights like this if people were compelled to come early for VD treatment.
> *Surgeon*: It's a mistake to use force. Here in England, we pin our faith to persuasion and to educating public opinion.[84]

In contrast to the controls on sexual health in the United States and other parts of Europe, Britain's VD Service was designed around a principle of utilitarian non-coercion.[85] *Trial for Marriage* was not alone in emphasising that the new scheme was a deliberate move away from older systems like the Contagious Diseases Acts. The intention was to normalise the clinics and to make approachable the health professionals who staffed them. In these films, we see reflections on contemporary attitudes as well as carefully choreographed attempts to change those attitudes.

They captured the internal conflicts besetting persons suffering from, or fearing that they suffered from, VD, presenting these conflicts as the by-product of a society that was itself conflicted in its attitudes to sex and the possession of sexual knowledge.[86] As such, these films tell us a great deal about the emotional and mental state in which interwar men and women might find themselves when confronting the possibility they were infected and infectious. While awaiting his test results, John is tormented by the possibility that he might be endangering his future wife. His guilt and anxiety play out in a surreal dream sequence in which he is on trial for criminally reckless conduct. Although warned about the dangers of VD and the wrongness of society's sexual double standard, he insists that his 'bad habits' were an unavoidable consequence of inadequate sex education:

> I had been brought up to believe that a man was entitled to sow his wild oats before marriage. I was aware that as a result of my past indiscretions since coming to London I had to undergo treatment and although I know that that treatment was not completed, I considered myself sufficiently cured. I did not realise that by marrying my wife I had committed any offence against the laws of this court of public opinion.

But the judge (and 'right-minded' people everywhere) remained unconvinced. Just in case the audience harboured any lingering doubts, his closing monologue – the most hard-hitting in the film – made it abundantly clear that the consequences of sexual transgression were a matter for individual *and* collective concern:

> The prisoner has sought to justify what he has done by referring to the principles of sowing wild oats. Now, I am sure that no right-minded person would accept this for a single moment as an excuse. As regards falsely making the declaration of good health, the prisoner admits that he is to blame for studying his own convenience instead of acting on advice of skilled medical opinion [...] Had you been ignorant, the fact that you did not realise what the results of your act would be might have been an argument in your favour. But you had the knowledge, were warned by friends and medical advisors and was [sic] trusted by your wife. Your act is an unpardonable offense against the community.

As evidenced in these films, experiences of venereal infection were becoming bound up with a complex web of external pressures and competing gendered assumptions about acceptable behaviour and an individual's responsibility to the community. As *Trial for Marriage* demonstrates, the culture of concealment and secrecy that had shaped Victorian and Edward experiences of VD had begun to break down. Society was making space to discuss sexual health. The sexual double standard and patriarchal medical high-handedness were becoming increasingly unsustainable.

Awaking, John receives a letter confirming that he will need lengthy treatment and that, consequently, the wedding must be postponed. Although the film ends without his much-anticipated marriage, it is not fatalistic. Throughout the film, the message is clear: despite John's transgressions, he can be cured and happily married provided that he commits to the necessary treatment. John will not meet the same fate as Ibsen and Doyle's protagonists because modern medicine is on his side.

While such films were generally well-received, not everyone was thrilled by their subject matter. Reflecting on the problem in 1942, a young woman from Balham told her MO interviewer that 'if people saw us going to a film on the subject, they would think we have got dirty minds. So many people would not go for fear they might be seen by their friends.'[87] Although VD health-education films were trying to reshape what Julian Carter describes as 'the epistemological environment' in which people experienced sex and sexual ill-health, they could not entirely overcome the common assumption that sexual knowledge was intrinsically corrupting.[88] A young woman from Poplar articulated a similar reluctance to engage with public-health information about VD:

> It's a thing we know about but don't [like] to talk about it. We British [...] are snobs and don't have any truck with dirt of that kind. I saw a film at work, but it made everybody so embarrassed and shocked that they could make pictures like that. And there were a lot of men in the canteen. It was uncomfortable. We don't want to think of our chaps in Egypt (husband two years in the Middle East) doing indecent things. We just couldn't. We think of them as brave and fighting.[89]

For these women, the government's public-health messages were neither informative nor reassuring, but distasteful and demoralising. Moreover, they revealed a problematic disconnect between medical and lay attitudes. With support from the state, the medical profession was trying to reshape the discourse around sexual health by playing down persistent associations with shame, transgression and moral pollution. But public opinion remained firmly rooted in these older paradigms. Indeed, lingering stigma, combined with the proliferation of sexual-health information, meant that VD propaganda was thought to be inadvertently facilitating the spread of syphilophobia. Certainly, by the late 1930s, health authorities worried that excessive use of shock and fear to bring home the dangers of VD was having adverse effects:

> Following educational campaigns on this subject, people were sometimes found to go to VD clinics under the belief, based on what they had heard in lectures, that they had syphilis. This occasionally caused medical officers of clinics to be a little caustic about these propaganda efforts [which] might not always be carried out as wisely as it should be.[90]

Interwar and war-time VD propaganda might have begun to open up discussion on sexual health, but it also triggered anxiety and (in some cases) compulsive, paranoid behaviours that we would classify as syphilophobia. As one woman admitted to her MO interviewer, 'I keep thinking I've got it, every pain I have – I wipe the lavatory seat and use the old douche can.'[91]

However, health authorities believed that such risks to individual wellbeing were necessary for the protection of communal health.[92] This was a view shared by some MO survey participants, like the twenty-eight-year-old Scottish engineering foreman who was interviewed in a pub in Hammersmith. 'I know some of my workers have venereal disease. They deny it and won't go to a doctor [...] What you want to do is to show by films how bad it is. People hate it. If they know how bad it is, they'd go to a doctor, but they're scared to show it up.'[93]

Certainly, admission registers from the larger clinics reveal that increasing numbers of men *and* women from across classes were attending without referral because they feared that an unidentified rash or discharge might be venereal. For example, in 1939, Adela, a middle-class housewife, presented with her twenty-year-old daughter for examination at Westminster Hospital's VD Department. Both were diagnosed as 'N.V.D.' (no VD or non-VD). Around that same time, Florence brought her sixteen-year-old daughter, Peggy, to the clinic. But they were not so lucky; Florence was diagnosed with acquired syphilis and her daughter with congenital syphilis.[94] Infants as young as two weeks were brought for precautionary examination and treatment, as in the case of baby Ronald, whose 'occupation' was humorously listed by the medical officer as 'feeder and sleeper'. Ronald was diagnosed as 'N.V.D.'[95] We can only speculate on the troubled marital relationships that might have lead Adela, Florence and Ronald's mother to suspect that they and their children were infected. But we can assume that their clinic visits – like those of countless other men, women and children during the 1920s and 1930s – were prompted by the film and poster campaigns spearheaded by the BSHC.

But just as attendances were dramatically increasing, so too were rates of defaulting. Given the stigma surrounding VD, it is unsurprising that many people resisted mainstream medical interventions. Their reliance on quack remedies or their reluctance to continue treatment was motived by fear of exposure and social ruin. As the interwar health films demonstrate, stigma and shame continued to shape experiences of infection, even if health authorities were pushing for more open discussion. High rates of defaulting were also indicative of a fundamental distrust of medical authority, especially when that authority was sanctioned by the state. As 'M65A' from Notting Hill Gate complained, 'I was fleeced by doctors. They had every penny I had!'[96] Patients' uneasy relationships with medical authority also reveal much about their experiences of living with

VD. The decision to default suggests that many lacked, or believed themselves to lack, control over the direction of their treatment. They may have baulked at dangerous and invasive treatments, but as we have seen, very few were actually consulted about their own care.[97] That so many decided to discontinue their treatment once their symptoms began to disappear also suggests that their expectations and understanding of their own wellbeing differed from the clinical metrics used by their doctors. Aside from the important social factors that influenced a person's decision to discontinue treatment, some patients probably saw the disappearance of symptoms as equal to cure, regardless of the assertions and entreaties of their doctors.[98] As Christopher Crenner observes in his study of general practice, radically divergent expectations of the diagnostic and therapeutic process were not unique to the twentieth century. But these divergences became increasingly conspicuous as wider and wider gaps opened up between the technological practice of medicine and patients' understanding of that practice.[99]

## 'The influence of the bloody Church'

Until the mid-twentieth century, syphilophobia was assumed to have a specific set of familial and social triggers, among the commonest being religiously inspired guilt. VD was long understood in terms of divine punishment or a father's 'sins' visited on his children. We see this clearly in many cases of syphilophobia, such as the 'young fellow' who 'had led a reasonable life, but during his somewhat long engagement, rather than befoul his approaching matrimony, satisfied himself sexually elsewhere'. Although the man was symptomless and had negative Wassermann results, he was consumed by the fear that he had infected his wife – a fear that his doctor attributed to a profound sense of guilt. His doctor therefore encouraged him 'to tell all' to his wife, whose blood was also tested and found to be negative. This confession may have had its intended cathartic effect because within two years the couple had a healthy child and the husband was seemingly free from his phobia.[100]

Illness, argues David Barnard, is never simply a 'biophysical event', but an 'existential crisis' that carries psychological, social and spiritual significance in its contraction and cure. This was especially so in suspected and diagnosed cases of syphilis and gonorrhoea, especially among patients who had strict religious upbringings.[101] These patients not only imbued their doctors with priestly qualities, but also viewed their own illnesses as personal and familial crises that transcended mere medical concerns. VD was as much a spiritual crisis as a biophysical one. As such, the act of unburdening oneself to a doctor in the confessional space of the consulting room – transposing a ritual for spiritual healing into the realm of the physiological – was thought to have a powerful health benefit.[102] In their distress, patients pinned 'intense existential hopes' on their doctors and invested considerable faith in their therapeutic powers.[103] This faith was as critical to a successful cure as mercury pills, salvarsan injections or urethral irrigations. Faith and placebos are not enough to combat aggressive microbial infections like syphilis or gonorrhoea, but as David Harley puts it, 'the immune system of a *despairing* patient will be hard pressed to cope with the therapeutic assault'.[104] Houston argues in Chapter 8 that the *process* of confessing an illness or the fear of illness to one's doctor and family came to be seen as a form of emotional and psychological therapy – something that deviated markedly from Victorian and Edwardian practices of concealment. In Britain, this shift was due in large part to the VD Service, which, along with the BSHC's propaganda, began to break down gendered boundaries of secrecy and divisions in sexual knowledge.

Doctors saw genuine therapeutic value in these secular confessions because they believed syphilophobia often to be the product of a zealous religious worldview, in which sin and divine punishment were very real. For example, the delusions of one young man, who attributed a collection of undiagnosed psychological symptoms to neurosyphilis, 'soon became firmly fixed in his mind and grew progressively worse until, at last, he was fearful that his brain was "rotting away"'. The attending doctor deemed it noteworthy that the man had been raised by a family 'who were almost puritanistic [sic] in their religious beliefs' and had therefore been imbued at an impressionable age with 'deeply fixed conceptions of right and wrong'. This, along with numerous pre-marital sexual encounters, created the psychological conditions for his syphilophobia, which was finally triggered by 'the shock' of being diagnosed with syphilis. The young man became convinced that his infection was 'just retribution for marital infidelity. A primary conflict was initiated, resulting in repression, mental fatigue and depression, and subsequent phobic tendencies.'[105]

For the most part, women diagnosed with syphilophobia had – or feared they had – been infected by their husbands; Evadne's fixation with her supposedly compromised health and that of her baby are good examples. As we see over eighty years later in Dorothy Baldwin's 1974 report to the Albany Trust on conditions in a major metropolitan VD clinic, such emotional turmoil was universal:

> The most painful factor about having VD is that your partner, your beloved, has probably/certainly been unfaithful to you. This knowledge, on its own, without the added stress of VD can and does cause intense misery. The sort of misery that brings out the worst behaviour in all of us.[106]

But some women were also consumed by the shame of pre-marital sexual encounters and the fear of a lingering 'taint'. One woman, who had been discharged 'cured' long before her wedding, returned to her local VD clinic after five years of marriage and the birth of a healthy child. She was convinced that she was still infected and infectious: 'I have come back. I shall soon have a nervous breakdown. I am nearly insane. I have gonorrhoea.' Doctors believed that such women – like men – were tormented by 'an old fear or sense of guilt'.[107] Indeed, it is in such cases that we see the beginnings of syphilophobia's pathologisation as a form of mental degeneration. When elaborating on the above case, J.A. Hadfield speculated that the woman's:

> sense of guilt might have originated from some earlier experience; if she was guilty of masturbating when she was a small child and she was told that if she continued she would go mad, that fear would become impressed upon her mind, and now took the form that if she was sexual she would go mad; and if later she got syphilis she would regard it as punishment for the earlier guilt.[108]

While a puritanical upbringing might produce a morbid preoccupation within the individual, religious teachings and institutions were thought to exert a malignant influence on society's sexual attitudes more broadly. Syphilophobia was thought to result from the belief, 'deeply rooted in the minds of the solid, conservative, middle class', that VD was 'a direct consequence of infractions of the Seventh Commandment'.[109] This deeply rooted belief had created the atmosphere of secrecy and shame against which interwar and war-time propaganda campaigns were pushing. And as we see in responses to the MO survey, the perceived influence of religion on matters of sexual health was a growing source of frustration.[110] On hearing that the *Daily Mirror*'s 'Ten Plain Facts about VD' did not actually include any information about medical prophylaxis, one middle-aged man from Chelsea asked indignantly, 'do you mean to say they're going to all the trouble of an advertising campaign and yet aren't telling people what to do to avoid VD? I suppose that that's the influence of the bloody Church.'[111] Another Chelsea resident was equally exasperated, claiming that 'of course, they're infernally hypocritical, with all that about "abstinence is best" or however they put it. I suppose that was to placate the Church. As if it would make a difference to people's behaviour.'[112]

However, as we see in case after case of syphilophobia, the continued insistence on abstinence, along with harsh social penalties for those found to have been unchaste, subtly (and not-so-subtly) shaped people's behaviour and attitudes. Syphilophobia was heavily bound up with feelings of guilt and fears of reputational damage for having transgressed moral boundaries. As such, it became something that health authorities viewed as a uniquely middle- and upper-class condition:[113]

> Syphilophobia is almost unknown in the lower strata of society. It is largely a disease of respectability [...] The eminently respectable person [...] has sharply defined values of right and wrong. Viewed in this light, syphilis is regarded as a punishment for wrong doing, a branding or stigmatization, or at times, the scourge of a vengeful deity. Basic conflicts are thus established by the *fait accomplait* [sic] of a sin against the Lord and may have a grave bearing on the outcome of the phobic state.[114]

Medical professionals assumed that the better-educated classes also had greater access to pseudo-medical literature as well as the mental acumen and imagination to ruminate on the information contained therein. They were thought to be more sensitive to the dangers of infecting others and more likely to fret over that danger. Likewise, these patients were thought to have more social and reputational capital to lose – something that supposedly caused the spectre of VD to loom more largely for them than the working classes.[115] This was certainly the stereotype perpetuated in fictional representations;

with the exception of the interwar health-education films, writers focused exclusively on the mental, spiritual and emotional suffering of the middle and upper classes.

F.J. Lambkin (lecturer in syphilology at the Royal Army Medical College) insisted that syphilophobia was 'one of the greatest difficulties met with in treating syphilitic patients, *especially among the educated and well-to-do classes*'.[116] In his opinion, 'the first thing to be done in such cases is to endeavour to divert the mind from the exciting cause'.[117] One syphilophobe – 'a generally healthy, single man of 36 years' – had, through a 'morbid interest in syphilo-literature', acquired considerable pseudo-knowledge of the 'minutiae of diagnosis', which he used to interpret and fret over every ache, pain or blemish.[118] But doctors also believed that patients' fixation with 'syphilo-literature' and accompanying oppressive thoughts could be gotten over through mental application – something that they also believed to be beyond the working classes.[119]

Although syphilophobia offers historians a rich picture of patient experiences, these experiences were nonetheless mediated through the writings of health professionals. It is entirely possible that, when characterising syphilophobia as a middle-class phenomenon, doctors were simply not 'seeing' syphilophobia among the working classes – instead mistaking it for another condition. Moreover, these medical accounts increasingly shifted away from the social causes of syphilophobia towards neurological explanations. The twentieth-century syphilophobe was increasingly diagnosed as 'psycho-neurotic'.[120] Speaking in the late 1930s, one doctor doubted that 'the present-day comparative laxity of morals made much difference, as it was not a question of whether the moral standard was high or low, but whether there was a conflict in the mind'.[121] Whereas syphilophobia was initially thought to be brought on by 'an old fear or sense of guilt' (and exacerbated by the rigid morality that shaped British society in the late nineteenth and early twentieth centuries), later diagnostic practices drew heavily on psychiatric explanations. Doctors increasingly believed that 'the shock of the syphilitic infection' was only a precipitating cause of insanity among highly strung or maladjusted individuals. Regardless of their gender, the syphilophobe was characterised using traditionally feminine tropes – emotional, melancholic, hysterical and fragile – which reinforced the view slowly crystallising among medical professionals that syphilophobia was simply one of many 'personality defects' common to patients already predisposed to mental instability.[122] Such psychiatric readings marginalised the social and familial factors that fed syphilophobes' fears, shame and guilt.

## Conclusions

As with every other chapter in this collection, the aim has been twofold: to bring to the fore patients' experiences of illness and to use this historical research to reflect on current healthcare debates or challenges. In this case, the focus has been on the provision of sexual-health services as well as the social inequalities and moral sensibilities that impeded people's access those services. Britain's historical VD Service was established to combat diseases about which the state had done nothing for thirty years and for which treatments were experimental. But its establishment also began to shift the discourse around sex and dismantle the Victorian socio-moral order that, as we have seen, trigged feelings of shame, fear and isolation in so many men and women.

As this chapter has demonstrated, these keen feelings of shame, along with the stigma surrounding matters of sex, present historians with a variety of methodological and ethical challenges. When patients' interactions with health professionals were motivated as much by feelings of shame and fear as a desire for wellness, how can historians discern when those patients were obfuscating or lying? How can historians negotiate the fact that surviving records of people's sexual ill-health are mere slivers of richer, more complex lives? How can we excavate personal stories from impersonal records? And, given the traumatic and historically taboo nature of these patients' sexual-health conditions, should we even try?

The short answer is yes. Although historians must grapple with a variety of ethical issues surrounding the access and use of records containing information about intimate, sexual relationships – information about women and men at some of the most vulnerable, embarrassing and traumatic moments in their lives – there is great potential to make a positive impact with our research.[123] As Jessica Meyer and Alexia Moncrieff have shown in Chapter 2, sensitive historical analysis of records that contain intensely personal information has the potential to nuance and change our understanding of stigma. Historians can read quite successfully (and ethically) against the grain of historical medical records to build up a picture of patient experiences. Moreover, understanding how ordinary people experienced sexual ill-health in the past is important for responding effectively to sexual-health challenges today. It has, for example, important policy implications for issues around the inequalities in access to contemporary services.

As the House of Commons Health and Social Care Committee's 2019 Report on Sexual Health made abundantly clear, Britain urgently needs a new national strategy for designing effective awareness campaigns, managing the provision of clinical services and tackling persistent inequalities in health outcomes and access to those services. Falling overall sexually transmitted infection (STI) rates, though welcome, mask 'a number of seriously concerning underlying trends and inequalities'.[124] Today, with STI diagnoses at record levels and multi-drug-resistant strains of infection rising, Britain's sexual-health services are as essential as ever. But their availability is being eroded by funding cuts to local authorities. This perfect storm of public-health pressures is not so much a 'turning-point' for sexual health as a troubling re-emergence of long-standing challenges. While surveying twentieth-century British sexuality and sexual health, I was unsurprised to find that the challenges of disease prevalence, misinformation and inequalities in access to services are much the same in 2020 as they were in 1920. As we confront these challenges in the twenty-first century, our historic struggles against these diseases hold invaluable lessons.

For example, by today's ethical standards, which prioritise a patient's right to be able to make *informed* decisions about their own care, the historical exclusion of women from decision-making processes seems shocking. Such inequalities are difficult to sustain in a nationalised health service, where doctors are not subject to market pressures or coercion from patients' fee-paying families. With a mandate to provide care that was universal and free at the point of use, Britain's socialised sexual-health services – delivered first via the interwar VD Service and later through the National Health Service – have broken down the economic power imbalances that shaped the types of medical neglect and patriarchal doctor–patient relationships to which women like Edith and Evadne would have been subjected.

Only by understanding how health systems in the past were (mis) used to sustain a variety of social inequalities can we hope to avoid similar failings going forward. Only by understanding how health systems developed to serve population needs can we hope to design successful responses to new biomedical, infrastructural and financial challenges. If historians are to open up meaningful dialogue with health professionals and policy-makers, it is important that we also build up – as far as possible – a picture of ordinary men and women's experiences as they navigated evolving health systems in the past.

For this picture to be nuanced, historians must draw on more than just medical records. A patient's experience of VD did not begin with their first visit to the doctor. It began weeks, months or even years earlier. As Michael Worboys urges in Chapter 1, historians of medicine therefore need radically to revise how they think about the medical encounter. So much of the care, concern, anxiety, self-diagnosing and self-treating that preceded the act of seeking professional medical intervention all too often slips below the historian's radar. This was especially evident in the realm of sexual health, where many afflicted persons would exhaust irregular or 'quack' remedies before reluctantly turning to mainstream medicine.[125] To understand the complex lives and emotional worlds of these people, historians must look to sources that offer up information about patient experiences beyond the narrow confines of the consulting room.

## Notes

  * Many thanks to Lesley Hall for her guidance on archival searches and for the time she generously gave to talking over the ideas for this chapter. Rebecka Klette offered invaluable advice on syphilophobia. Thanks also to Jessica Meyer for her comments on an earlier draft and to Lloyd Davies for his diligent editing.

  1 For more on Mass Observation as a social-research organisation, including its establishment in 1937, see James Hinton, *The Mass Observers: A History, 1937–1949* (Oxford: Oxford University Press, 2013); Peter Gurney, '"Intersex" and "Dirty Girls": Mass-Observation and Working-Class Sexuality in England in the 1930s', *Journal of the History of Sexuality* 8:2 (1997), 256–90.

  2 For more on the Ministry of Health's wartime campaign, see Adrian Bingham, 'The British Popular Press and Venereal Disease during the

Second World War', *The Historical Journal* 48:4 (2005), 1055–76; University of Sussex Special Collections, Mass Observation Archive, Instructions to Investigators (24 February 1943) SxMOA1/2/12/1/C/1.

3 University of Sussex Special Collections, Mass Observation Archive, Second Venereal-Disease Survey (February–March 1943) SxMOA1/2/12/1/D (henceforth Second Venereal-Disease Survey, SxMOA1/2/12/1/D).

4 Second Venereal-Disease Survey, SxMOA1/2/12/1/D, original emphasis.

5 University of Sussex Special Collections, Mass Observation Archive, First Venereal-Disease Survey (November–December 1942) SxMOA1/2/12/1/B (henceforth First Venereal-Disease Survey, SxMOA1/2/12/1/B).

6 First Venereal-Disease Survey, SxMOA1/2/12/1/B.

7 Second Venereal-Disease Survey, SxMOA1/2/12/1/D.

8 For more discussion of this, see Anne R. Hanley, *Medicine, Knowledge and Venereal Diseases in England, 1886–1916* (Basingstoke: Palgrave, 2017), 152–4; Royal Commission on Venereal Diseases, PP 1913–16 Cd 7475 (Appendix to First Report of the Commissioners, Minutes of Evidence), qq. 16–36 (henceforth, Royal Commission on Venereal Diseases, Appendix to First Report, Cd 7475); Select Committee on Death Certification (First and Second Reports, Proceedings, Evidence, Appendix, Index), PP 1893–94 XI (373) (402), qq. 1624–7.

9 See, for example, Royal London Hospital Archives and Museum, The Ambrose King Centre (formerly the Whitechapel Clinic), Female Confidential Registers (1930–2000) RLHAK/1/2/1–43; Male Confidential Registers (1930–2000) RLHAK/1/3/1–77.

10 Claire Brock, *British Women Surgeons and their Patients, 1860–1918* (Cambridge: Cambridge University Press, 2017), 70.

11 Important exceptions include Joan Sherwood, *Infection of the Innocents: Wet Nurses, Infants, and Syphilis in France* (Montreal: McGill-Queen's University Press, 2010); Lindsay R. Watson, 'Tom Tiddler's Ground: Irregular Medical Practitioners and Male Sexual Problems in New Zealand', *Medical History* 57:4 (2013), 537–58.

12 Joanna Bourke, *Fear: A Cultural History* (London: Virago Press, 2005), 6.

13 Monika Pietrzak-Franger, *Syphilis in Victorian Literature and Culture: Medicine, Knowledge and the Spectacle of Victorian Invisibility* (Basingstoke: Palgrave, 2018), 1.

14 Andrew Smith, *Victorian Demons: Medicine, Masculinity and the Gothic at the Fin-de-Siècle* (Manchester: Manchester University Press, 2004), 95.

15 For more on the Physical Deterioration Committee (PDC), see Simon Szreter, *Fertility, Class and Gender in Britain, 1860–1940* (Cambridge: Cambridge University Press, 1996), 207–18.

16  For more on these crises and anxieties, see Joanne Townsend, 'Marriage, Motherhood and the Future of the Race: Syphilis in Late-Victorian and Edwardian Britain', in Kari Nixon and Lorenzo Servitje (eds), *Syphilis and Subjectivity: From the Victorians to the Present* (Basingstoke: Palgrave, 2018), 67–89.
17  For more on these crises and anxieties, see Townsend, 'Marriage, Motherhood and the Future of the Race', 69.
18  Henry Morris, Norman Moore, D'Arcy Power and F.W. Mott, *Syphilis: From the Proceedings of the Royal Society of Medicine* (Longmans, Green and Co., 1912), 139, 143, 187. Some doctors also referred to a condition that they termed 'syphilomania' – the 'insane obsession as to the results of an attack of syphilis'. For the most part, however, doctors used 'syphilophobia' to describe both the fear of contracting venereal diseases and the fear of its ravages on the body. Although not a common usage, syphilophobia was also used by some doctors (writing before the codification of knowledge around neurosyphilis) to describe the effects of tertiary-stage infection on a patient's brain and behaviour. See, for example, Frank E. Cormia, 'Syphilophobia and Allied Anxiety States', *The Canadian Medical Association Journal* (October 1938), 361–6.
19  For more on the emergence of phobias, see Don James McLaughlin, 'Hydrophobia's Doppelgänger: Toward a Literary History of Emotions in Early American Rabies Narratives', *Literature and Medicine* 37:1 (2019), 116–17.
20  For philosophical reflections on the experiences of illness, see Havi Carel, *Phenomenology of Illness* (Oxford: Oxford University Press, 2016).
21  For more on how diseases functioned as metaphors for wider social anxieties, see Katherine Byrne, *Tuberculosis and the Victorian Literary Imagination* (Cambridge: Cambridge University Press, 2011).
22  See, for example, Kari Nixon and Lorenzo Servitje (eds), *Syphilis and Subjectivity: From the Victorians to the Present* (Basingstoke: Palgrave, 2018); Pietrzak-Franger, *Syphilis in Victorian Literature and Culture*.
23  Jelena Subotić, 'Ethics of Archival Research on Political Violence', *Journal of Peace Studies* (2020), 1–13, 7.
24  Ibid., 7.
25  An important exception is Alphonse Daudet's nineteenth-century autobiographical account of living with neurosyphilis. See Alphonse Daudet, *In the Land of Pain*, translated by Julian Barnes (London: Penguin, 2018). Although not a patient-authored account, Freud's *A Case of Hysteria* also engages with the phenomenon of syphilophobia. See Sigmund Freud, *A Case of Hysteria (Dora)*, A New Translation by Anthea Bell (Oxford: Oxford University Press, 2013).

26 Laurence Talairach-Vielmas, *Wilkie Collins, Medicine and the Gothic* (Cardiff: University of Wales Press, 2009), 1, 7.
27 Katherine Byrne, *Tuberculosis and the Victorian Literary Imagination* (Cambridge: Cambridge University Press, 2011), 4.
28 There is also a large collection of novels, plays and short stories that use VD as a literary device. See, for example, Norah Hoult, *There Are No Windows* (1944); James Hanley, *Boy* (1931); Michael Arlen, *The Green Hat* (1924); Eugène Brieux, *Les Avariés* (1913) and its subsequent English film and novel adaptations as *Damaged Goods*; Wilkie Collins, *Armadale* (1866). Arguments have also been made for the syphilitic subtext of the degenerative portrait in Oscar Wilde's *The Picture of Dorian Gray* (1890) and Robert Louis Stevenson's *The Strange Case of Dr Jekyll and Mr Hyde* (1886). See Lesley A. Hall, '"Sons of Belial": Contaminated/Contaminating Victorian Male Bodies', in Andrew Mangham and Daniel Lea (eds), *The Male Body in Medicine and Literature* (Liverpool: Liverpool University Press, 2018), 159–76.
29 For further discussion of the Victorians' reception of these works, see Anon., 'The Question of "Ghosts"', *Pall Mall Gazette* (14 March 1891), 1; Anon., 'The Question of "Ghosts"', *Pall Mall Gazette* (16 March 1891), 3; William Archer, 'Ghosts and Gibberings', *Pall Mall Gazette* (8 April 1891), 3; Sally Ledger, 'Ibsen, the New Woman and the Actress', in Angelique Richardson and Chris Willis (eds), *The New Woman in Fiction and in Fact: Fin-de-siècle Feminisms* (Basingstoke: Palgrave, 2001), 79–93; Elaine Showalter, 'Syphilis, Sexuality and the Fiction of the Fin-de-Siècle', in Ruth Bernard Yeazell (ed.), *Sex, Politics and Science in the Nineteenth-Century Novel* (Baltimore: John Hopkins University Press, 1986), 88–115.
30 For further discussion of the 'non-patient' and 'pre-patient', see Michael Worboys's chapter in this collection.
31 The BSHC/NCCVD was established in 1913 following the appointment of the Royal Commission on Venereal Diseases and was tasked with overseeing programmes of sexual-health education and propaganda following the recommendations laid out in the Royal Commission's final report in 1916. For more on the work of the interwar activities of the BSHC/NCCVD, see S.M. Tomkins, 'Palmitate or Permanganate: The Venereal Prophylaxis Debate in Britain, 1916–1926', *Medical History* 37:4 (1993), 382–98. The term 'theatrical' is used to denote films using fictional plots, as opposed to documentary-style films. For further discussion of this distinction, see Christian Bonah, David Cantor and Anja Laukötter, *Health Education Films in the Twentieth Century* (Rochester: University of Rochester Press, 2018).
32 Morris et al., *Syphilis*, 187.

33 Gail Cunningham, *The New Woman and the Victorian Novel* (London: Macmillan, 1978), 11; Chris Willis, '"Heaven Defend Me from Political or Highly-Educated Women!": Packaging the New Woman for Mass Consumption', in Angelique Richardson and Chris Willis (eds), *The New Woman in Fiction and in Fact: Fin-de-Siècle Feminisms* (Basingstoke: Palgrave, 2001), 53–65, 56.

34 Martha Vicinus, Teresa Mangum and Judith Walkowitz have identified the appeal of melodrama to female authors because it emphasised gendered power relations and highlighted the role of the heroine. See Martha Vicinus, '"Helpless and Unfriended": Nineteenth-Century Domestic Melodrama', *New Literary History* 13:1 (1981), 132–4; Teresa Mangum, *Married, Middlebrow and Militant: Sarah Grand and the New Woman Novel* (Michigan: University of Michigan Press, 1998), 91–4; Judith Walkowitz, *City of Dreadful Delight: Narratives Of Sexual Danger In Late-Victorian London* (Chicago: University of Chicago Press, 1992), 85–8; Marilyn Bonnell, 'The Legacy of Sarah Grand's *The Heavenly Twins*: A Review Essay', *English Literature in Transition* 36:4 (1993), 467–78, 470.

35 Arthur Conan Doyle, 'Third Generation', *Round the Red Lamp: Being Facts and Fancies of Medical Life* (London: John Murray, 1894). For more short stories about venereal diseases, see from the same collection 'The Surgeon Talks' and 'The Doctors of Hoyland'.

36 E.E. Abney-Walker, 'Heredity', *Shafts* (March 1893), 4.

37 Michael Arlen, *The Green Hat* (Robin Clark, 1991), 72–3.

38 Frederick W. Lowndes, 'Syphilis and Marriage', *Lancet* (8 July 1882), 7–9.

39 Arabella Kenealy, 'A Question of Conscience', *British Medical Journal* (14 September 1895), 682.

40 Kenealy, 'A Question of Conscience', 682; For further discussion of this case, see Anne Hanley, '"The Great Foe to the Reproduction of the Race": Diagnosing and Treating Venereal Diseases-Induced Infertility, 1880–1914', in Tracey Loughran and Gayle Davis (eds), *Infertility in History: Approaches, Contexts and Perspectives* (Basingstoke: Palgrave, 2017), 335–58.

41 Kenealy, 'A Question of Conscience', 682.

42 Sarah Grand, *The Heavenly Twins* (London: William Heinemann, 1893); Emma Frances Brooke, *A Superfluous Woman* (London, 1894). See also Teresa Mangum, *Married, Middlebrow, and Militant: Sarah Grand and the New Woman Novel* (Michigan: University of Michigan Press, 1998).

43 Bonnell, 'The Legacy of Sarah Grand's *The Heavenly Twins*', 473. See also, Mary Spongberg, *Feminizing Venereal Disease: The Body of*

the Prostitute in Nineteenth-Century Medical Discourse (New York: New York University Press, 1997).
44 Jill Harsin discusses at length the cultural and legal structures that maintained women's ignorance within a late nineteenth-century French context. See Jill Harsin, 'Syphilis, Wives, and Physicians: Medical Ethics and the Family in Late-Nineteenth-Century France', *French Historical Studies* 16:1 (1989), 72–95.
45 Alfred Fournier, *Syphilis and Marriage. Translated by Alfred Lingard, with prefatory remarks by Jonathan Hutchinson* (London: David Bogue, 1881), 170–1.
46 Ibid., 169–70.
47 Royal Commission on Venereal Diseases, Appendix to First Report, Cd 7475, qq. 9573–83.
48 Jonathan Hutchinson, *Syphilis* (London: Cassell, 1887), 496.
49 For more discussion of the different methods of administration as well as the dangers of mercury treatment, see Hanley, *Medicine, Knowledge and Venereal Diseases*, 93–6. For more on the treatments for gonorrhoea, see Hanley, '"The Great Foe to the Reproduction of the Race"', 335–58.
50 Grand, *The Heavenly Twins*, vol. 2, 58.
51 Pietrzak-Franger, *Syphilis in Victorian Literature and Culture*, 20.
52 Fournier, *Syphilis and Marriage*, 172.
53 Grand, *The Heavenly Twins*, vol. 2, 51.
54 Livia Arndal Woods, 'Not-So-Great Expectations: Pregnancy and Syphilis in Sarah Grand's *The Heavenly Twins*', in Kari Nixon and Lorenzo Servitje (eds), *Syphilis and Subjectivity: From the Victorians to the Present* (Basingstoke: Palgrave, 2018), 115–36, 115–16.
55 Second Venereal-Disease Survey, SxMOA1/2/12/1/D.
56 For further discussion of these concerns, see Julian B. Carter, 'Birds, Bees, and Venereal Disease: Toward an Intellectual History of Sex Education', *Journal of the History of Sexuality* 10:2 (2001), 213–49; Alison Bashford and Carolyn Strange, 'Public Pedagogy: Sex Education and Mass Communication in the Mid-Twentieth Century', *Journal of the History of Sexuality* 13:1 (2004), 71–99.
57 Anna Maria Jones, '"A Track to the Water's Edge": Learning to Suffer in Sarah Grand's *The Heavenly Twins*', *Tulsa Studies in Women's Literature* 26:2 (2007), 217–41, 235; Bonnell, 'The Legacy of Sarah Grand's *The Heavenly Twins*', 470.
58 Grand, *The Heavenly Twins*, vol. 3, 267.
59 Woods, 'Not-So-Great Expectations', 124–9.
60 Nora Brownlow, 'The Modern Slave Market', *Shafts* (December 1892), 87.

61 Mary Fordham, 'Knowledge Is Power', *Shafts* (September 1893), 137.
62 For an extended critique of these structures, see Christabel Pankhurst, *The Great Scourge and How to End It* (London: E. Pankhurst, 1913).
63 Bonnell, 'The Legacy of Sarah Grand's *The Heavenly Twins*', 468.
64 For more on the conceptual challenges of understanding historical agency, see Lynn M. Thomas, 'Historicising Agency', *Gender & History* 28:2 (2016), 324–39.
65 Doyle, *Round the Red Lamp*.
66 For more on the interwar VD Service, see Anne Hanley, '"Sex Prejudice" and Professional Identity: Women Doctors and their Patients in Britain's Interwar VD Service', *Journal of Social History*, 54:2 (2020), 569–98; Samantha Caslin, 'Transience, Class and Gender in Interwar Sexual Health Policy: The Case of the Liverpool VD Scheme', *Social History of Medicine* 32:3 (2019), 1–21; Roger Davidson, 'Venereal Disease, Sexual Morality and Public Health in Interwar Scotland', *Journal of the History of Sexuality* 5:2 (1994), 267–94.
67 For more on these health inequalities, see Hanley, *Medicine, Knowledge and Venereal Diseases*.
68 Venereal Disease: A Bill Intituled an Act to Prevent the Treatment of Venereal Disease Otherwise than by Duly Qualified Medical Practitioners, and to Control the Supply of Remedies therefore; and for other Matters Connected therewith, PP 1917–18 (17); Report from Standing Committee A on the Venereal Disease Bill (Lords) with the Proceedings of the Committee, PP 1917–18 (77). For further discussion of quack medicine, see Roy Porter, *Health for Sale: Quackery in England, 1660–1850* (Manchester: Manchester University Press, 1989); Takahiro Ueyama, *Health in the Marketplace: Professionalism, Therapeutic Desires and Medical Commodification in Late-Victorian London* (Society for the Promotion of Science and Scholarship, 2010), 59–111; Watson, 'Tom Tiddler's Ground', 537–58.
69 Morris et al., *Syphilis*, 187.
70 Cormia, 'Syphilophobia and Allied Anxiety States', 364.
71 J.A. Hadfield, 'The Nature and Cause of Phobias, with Special Reference to Syphilophobia. Discussion', *British Journal of Venereal Disease* (April 1938), 128–9.
72 Ibid., 133.
73 For more on the hygiene lectures delivered to servicemen during the First World War, see Mark Harrison, 'The British Army and the Problem of Venereal Disease in France and Egypt during the First World War', *Medical History* 39:2 (1995), 133–58; Royal Commission on Venereal Diseases, Appendix to First Report, Cd 7475, qq. 316–21, 392–3, 396, 527–33, 535–41, 3618–23, 3720–3, 3960–5.

74 For further discussion of these generational shifts, see Lucinda McCray Beier, '"We Were Green as Grass": Learning about Sex and Reproduction in Three Working-Class Lancashire Communities, 1900–1970', *Social History of Medicine* 16:3 (2003), 461–80.
75 For further discussion of the tensions between the projection of sexual innocence and the possession of sexual knowledge, see Simon Szreter and Kate Fisher, *Sex Before the Sexual Revolution: Intimate Life in England, 1918–1963* (Cambridge: Cambridge University Press, 2010).
76 Royal London Hospital Archives and Museum, The Ambrose King Centre (formerly the Whitechapel Clinic), Male Confidential Register (1930) RLHAK/1/3/1.
77 For more on these developments, see Hanley, *Medicine, Knowledge and Venereal Diseases*, 117–34.
78 Kirsten Ostherr, *Medical Visions: Producing the Patient through Film, Television and Imaging Technologies* (Oxford: Oxford University Press, 2013), 45.
79 Bonah, Cantor and Laukötter, *Health Education Films in the Twentieth Century*, 1.
80 University of Sheffield Special Collections, Records of Lydia Henry: VD Medical Officer, Blackburn, Lancashire, Audio Recording MS110/1/3A.
81 British Film Institute, Vernon Sewell (dir.), *Test for Love* (Central Council for Health Education Film Unit, UK, 1937).
82 British Film Institute, *Trial for Marriage* (Central Council for Health Education Film Unit, UK, 1936).
83 Timothy Boon, 'Health Education Films in Britain, 1919–39: Production, Audiences and Genres', in Graeme Harper and Andrew Moor (eds), *Signs of Life: Cinema and Medicine* (London: Wallflower Press, 2005), 45–57, 46; Timothy Boon, 'Films and the Contestation of Public Health in Interwar Britain' (unpublished PhD Thesis, University of London, 1999), 133–75.
84 British Film Institute, *Trial for Marriage* (1936).
85 Prevention and Treatment of Venereal Diseases. Recommendations of the Royal Commission; Action Taken by the Local Government Board; Progress Made with Schemes of Treatment; and Particulars of Certain Schemes, PP 1917–18 Cd 8509. For more on the different sexual-health controls enacted across Europe, see Roger Davidson and Lesley Hall (eds), *Sex, Sin and Suffering: Venereal Disease and European Society since 1870* (London: Routledge, 2001).
86 For more on these conflicts, see Carter, 'Birds, Bees, and Venereal Disease': 213–49.
87 First Venereal-Disease Survey, SxMOA1/2/12/1/B.
88 Carter, 'Birds, Bees, and Venereal Disease', 215.

89 First Venereal-Disease Survey, SxMOA1/2/12/1/B.
90 Hadfield, 'The Nature and Cause of Phobias', 129.
91 First Venereal-Disease Survey, SxMOA1/2/12/1/B.
92 For more on the long history of tension between individual and communal sexual-health interests, see Anne Hanley, 'Syphilisation and its Discontents: Experimental Inoculation Against Syphilis at the London Lock Hospital', *Bulletin of the History of Medicine* 91:1 (2017), 1–32.
93 First Venereal-Disease Survey, SxMOA1/2/12/1/B.
94 London Metropolitan Archives, Venereal Disease Department Registers of the Westminster Hospital H02/WH/B/14/025.
95 Ibid.
96 First Venereal-Disease Survey, SxMOA1/2/12/1/B.
97 Claire Brock found similar patterns of resistance among gynaecological patients at the Royal Free Hospital, London. See Brock, *British Women Surgeons and their Patients*, 108.
98 For more on defaulting, see Hanley, '"Sex Prejudice" and Professional Identity'.
99 Christopher Crenner, *Private Practice: In the Early Twentieth-Century Medical Office of Dr Richard Cabot* (Baltimore: Johns Hopkins University Press, 2005), 71–2. For more on this disconnect in relation to VD treatment, see Simon Szreter, 'The Prevalence of Syphilis in England and Wales on the Eve of the Great War: Revisiting the Estimates of the Royal Commission on Venereal Diseases 1913–1916', *Social History of Medicine* 27:3 (2014), 508–29.
100 Hadfield, 'The Nature and Cause of Phobias', 130.
101 David Barnard, 'The Physician as Priest, Revisited', *Journal of Religion and Health* 24:4 (1985), 272–86, 278.
102 For further discussion of the placebo effect in history, see, for example, Anne Harrington, *The Cure Within: A History of Mind–Body Medicine* (New York: W.W. Norton Company, 2008); Anne Harrington (ed.), *The Placebo Effect: An Interdisciplinary Exploration* (Harvard: Harvard University Press, 1999).
103 Barnard, 'The Physician as Priest, Revisited', 272.
104 David Harley, 'Rhetoric and the Social Construction of Sickness and Healing', *Social History of Medicine* 12:3 (1999), 407–35, 426, emphasis added.
105 Cormia, 'Syphilophobia and Allied Anxiety States', 363.
106 London School of Economics Special Collections, Grey Papers, VD Correspondence, Dorothy Baldwin's account of her visit to a VD clinic (c.1974), HCA/Grey/4/22.
107 Hadfield, 'The Nature and Cause of Phobias', 127–8.
108 Ibid.

109 Cormia, 'Syphilophobia and Allied Anxiety States', 362.
110 Second Venereal-Disease Survey, SxMOA1/2/12/1/D.
111 Ibid.
112 Ibid.
113 Cormia, 'Syphilophobia and Allied Anxiety States', 362.
114 Hadfield, 'The Nature and Cause of Phobias', 129.
115 Ibid., 127–8.
116 F.J. Lambkin, *Syphilis: Its Diagnosis and Treatment* (New York: William Wood and Company, 1911), 147–8, emphasis added.
117 Ibid., 147–8.
118 Cormia, 'Syphilophobia and Allied Anxiety States', 361.
119 Lambkin, *Syphilis*, 147–8.
120 Cormia, 'Syphilophobia and Allied Anxiety States', 364–5.
121 Hadfield, 'The Nature and Cause of Phobias', 130.
122 Cormia, 'Syphilophobia and Allied Anxiety States', 364–5; Lambkin, *Syphilis*, 147–8. See also Ida Macalpine, 'Syphilophobia: A Psychiatric Study', *British Journal of Venereal Disease* 33:2 (1957), 92–9.
123 For further discussion of the ethical challenges accompanying the 'mass digitised turn', see Julia Laite, 'The Emmet's Inch: Small History in a Digital Age', *Journal of Social History*, 53:4 (2020), 963–89. For further reflections on the ethical implications of archival research and the researcher's ethical obligations to their dead subjects, see Subotić, 'Ethics of Archival Research on Political Violence'.
124 For more on current challenges facing sexual-health services, see House of Commons, Health and Social Care Committee, 'Sexual Health: Fourteenth Report of Session 2017–19. Report, Together with Formal Minutes Relating to the Report', HC 1419 (House of Commons, 2019).
125 Royal Commission on Venereal Diseases, Appendix to First Report, Cd 7475, q. 9794–800. Such attempts at self-medication existed even into the latter half of the twentieth century. See, Kevin Anderson, 'Self-Medication by Patients Attending a Venereal Diseases Clinic', *British Journal of Venereal Disease* 42 (1966), 44–5.

# Index

Literary works can be found under authors' names. Footnotes are indicated by 'n.' after a page reference. Captions are indicated by italics.

'3 Before GP' 52

ableist 211
abortion 199
activism 3, 14, 91–5, 102, 107, 113, 303
agency 2, 5, 7–8, 13, 14–15, 21, 26n.29, 62, 65, 66, 79–80, 127, 139, 140, 148, 158, 161, 163, 173, 174, 189, 223–5, 234–5, 256–7, 282, 312–13
Alleged Lunatics' Friend Society 92, 114n.6
anonymisation 62, 71, 72, 81
archives 62, 64–5, 68, 70, 72, 79, 81–2, 158, 160, 215n.43
    Friends of the National Archives 72
    National Archives (TNA) 61, 63, 65, 67, 68, 73, 160
    Discovery 64, 72
    National Archives of Australia 73
    National Archives of Ireland 297n.112
Arlen, Michael 305–6
Army Medical Officers (MOs) 227, 230, 235, 237
aspirin 43, 48, 50
Association of British Insurers 75
asylum 73, 92, 93–100, 102–3, 105–6, 108–13, 125, 127–8, 130–1, 132–3, 135, 137, 138, 140–4, 147–8, 150n.32
    Carlton Hayes Asylum (Leicestershire and Rutland) 136–41, 145
    East Riding Asylum (Beverley) 146
    farm 14, 20, 125–39, 141–5, 146–8, 150n.32
    patients 132, 133, 134, 136–42, 145–6, 147
    residence 143–4
    Graylingwell Asylum (West Sussex County Asylum) 133
    Hull Borough Asylum 133
    Lancaster County Lunatic Asylum 133
    Lincoln County Asylum 135
    Menston Asylum (West Riding of Yorkshire) 144

## Index

Northampton Asylum 134
Parkside Asylum (Cheshire) 144
rule books 133
Wexford County Lunatic Asylum / St Senan's Psychiatric Hospital 280
Asylums Act (1808) 130

biomedicine 5, 43, 223–5, 228, 236–8, 241–2
biopower 2
boots 232, 235, 237, 238, 239, 241
Both, Edward T. 188
  Both iron lung 188
  Both respirator 192, 195, 197, 199
Bourke, Joanna 40, 227–8, 231, 234–5, 301
Bragg-Paul Pulsator 184, 185, 187, 189–92, 195, 107, *198*, 213n.14, 215n.40, 216n.46, 217n.76
Bragg, William H. 183, 185, 189–90, 194, 212n.1, 215n.36, 215n.38
breathing 3, 22, *103*, 105, 183–9, 191–5, 197, 199–203, 205, 215n.33, 216n.47
  breath 34, 39, 166, 186, 189, 197, 201, 307
  breathe 183, 186, 189, 195, 200, 203
  breathlessness 187, 199, 207–8
  dyspnoea 199, 207
  machine 183–9, 192–5, 197, 200–1, 203, 217n.66, 217n.69, 217n.71
*British Medical Journal (BMJ)* 206, 306
British Oxygen Company (BOC) 203–4, 206, 211
British Social Hygiene Council (BSHC) 294n.73, 299, 304, 315, 320, 322, 331n.31
  see also National Council for Combatting Venereal Diseases
Brooke, Emma 303–4
  Jessamine Halliday *née* Heriot 305, 307
Bund für Irrenrechts–Reform und Irrenfürsorge 103
bureaucracy 64, 75–80, 226

Chance, Arthur 259
charity 262, 279
Chronic Obstructive Pulmonary Disease (COPD) 203, 205, 207, 210
clinical reality 229, 231
Code on Genetic Testing and Insurance (2018) 75
Committee of Inquiry Regarding Venereal Disease (ICVD) 261, 284
Concordat and Moratorium on Genetics and Insurance (2014) 75
Conolly, John 97, 131–2, 134
conscientious objection 78
conspiracy of silence 311
  see also sexual double standard
Constitution of the International Committee of Historical Sciences (2005) 81
Contagious Diseases Acts 101, 259, 137
COVID-19 6, 17, 19, 26n.25, 36, 52, 53, 186, 199, 202, 212, 225, 242, 251n.142
Creative Commons 68, 70
Criminal Law Amendment Act (1935, Ireland) 262, 291n.28

*Daily Mirror* 299, 324
Davies, J.N.P. 47–8, 59n.65

defining illness 34
degeneration *see* eugenics
diaries 6, 40, 49–50, 61, 224, 227, 230, 231
dietary remedies 50
digitisation 21, 62, 64–5, 68, 81–2, 300
  digital humanities 66
disability 68, 71, 72, 80, 165, 173, 183, 186–7, 201–2, 205, 214n.20
  Disability Living Allowance / Universal Credit 168
  disability paradox 201
  disabled innovation 202
  disabled users 187, 201, 212
  history 93
  respiratory disability 185
  studies 108
disease 3, 7, 8, 22, 37, 38, 40, 43–6, 53, 54, 80, 105, 106, 168, 202–4, 210, 216n.47, 224, 229, 232, 234, 239, 270, 283, 286, 292n.31, 300–1, 303, 305–6, 308–11, 324, 326, 327
  ignorance 33, 48, 256, 271, 276, 305, 307–8, 310–11, 333n.44
  metaphor 301, 330n.21
  prevalence 48, 286, 327
  prognosis 314
disgust 231–2, 234
divorce 276–9, 309
  Constitution or Ireland 277
  Divorce and Matrimonial Causes Act 277
  divorce *a vinculo matrimonii* 277
  *divortium a mensa et thoro* 277
  doctor-patient confidentiality 279
doctor 1, 2, 6, 7, 11, 19, 33, 34–6, 38, 39, 43, 46, 47, 49, 52–4, 55n.6, 65, 67, 97, 99–102, 104–6, 108–9, 112, 154–9, 164, 166, 168, 170–1, 195, 197, 201–2, 212, 215n.38, 224, 226–7, 229–30, 238, 257, 265, 273–4, 276, 284, 289n.8, 300, 306, 315, 320–1, 323, 325, 328, 330n.18
  doctor-patient relationship 5, 8, 18, 22, 256, 304, 320–2
    confession 41, 272, 274–5, 321, 322
    trust / distrust / mistrust 156, 168, 256, 264, 266, 272–4, 276, 285, 320
    fees 7, 279, 307, 313, 327
    paternalism 307–10
Doyle, Arthur Conan 303
  Francis Norton 305, 308, 313
Dr Steevens' Hospital, Dublin 257–9, 274–7, 280–2, 291n.31
Drinker, Phillip 188
  Drinker–Collins respirator 192, *196*
  Drinker device 188, 190, 192, 197
  Drinker Iron lung 192
  Drinker respirator 188, 190–2, 195–7, *196*, 199–200

economy 112, 128–3, 136, 146, 263
emotion 11–13, 18, 19, 42, 91, 129, 141, 147, 224, 231–6, 241–2, 256, 266–9, 273, 275–6, 279, 281, 285, 301–4, 306, 310–11, 317, 322–3, 325, 328
empowerment / disempowerment 3, 92, 108, 110–11, 147–8

endurance 232, 234–5, 239, 241, 248n.86
environment / environmental 37, 95, 126, 127, 136, 138, 139, 144–5, 204, 217n.70, 224–5, 229, 231–2, 237–42, 243n.13, 246n.51, 318
escape 37, 94, 101, 128, 140–1, 143, 145–7, 225, 310
eugenics 305, 307, 315
  degeneration 301, 304, 307, 323
  eugenicist 307
  hereditarianism 95, 105, 112
  racial health 302, 315
Evans, Reg 70–1
Eve's Motor Rocking Bed 192
ex-patient organisation 93–4, 103, 111, 113
exposure diseases 224

family history 65, 68, 73, 75, 78, 105
fear 13, 18, 98, 109, 148, 166–7, 173, 204, 207, 210, 227, 231–4, 242, 270, 301–2, 304–5, 307–8, 310–11, 313–14, 316–26, 330n.18
femininity 269
First World War / Great War 22, 58n.38, 61–5, 67–8, 70, 74–7, 102, 106, 223–4, 227, 229, 233–4, 241–50, 258, 313–14
folk medicine / folkloric remedies 43–4, 154
footnotes 71–2
four-nations history 256–7, 288n.4
Fournier, Alfred 308, 310
fungal diseases 38

Garner, Clara 278
gas 45, 203, 206, 224, 230, 233–5, 237, 239–40, 251n.128

general practitioner / GP *see* doctor
Germany 21, 92, 95, 106–7, 109, 111, 113
Gillies, Harrold 70
Gogarty, Oliver St John 283
gonorrhoea 283, 299, 301, 304, 309, 313, 316, 322–3
  Pelvic Inflammatory Disease 269
  Sulphonamides 309
  urethral irrigations 309
Grand, Sarah 303, 305–7, 310–11, 315
  *The Heavenly Twins* 303
  Edith Menteith *née* Beale 305, 307, 310–11, 327
  Evadne Colquhoun *née* Frayling 305, 312–13, 323, 327
  Mosley Menteith 308
Guardians / Board of Guardians 158–9, 161, 166–7, 169, 171–3, 280

Habermas, Jürgen 79
healthcare systems 42, 157–8, 225, 242
health consumers / health users 5, 13–14, 17, 154–6, 164, 171, 205
  rejection 195, 210
  survivor 91, 93, 111, 113, 203, 215
  user experience 15–16, 93, 186–7, 191, 195, 201, 206–7, 210
  user involvement 91, 93, 185–6
Heidelberg University Clinic 103–4
Helman, Cecil 43–5
history from below 9, 53, 95, 158, 161
Holloway's Pills 46–7

hospital 2, 5, 6, 7, 41, 71, 107,
    125, 148, 156–7, 164–5,
    176, 185–91, 197,
    199–200, 203–7, 210,
    212, 216n.46, 226–7,
    232–3, 239, 257–60, 264,
    267, 269–70, 272–4, 276,
    278–81, 283, 292n.33,
    315–16
  Liverpool Lock Hospital 306
  Liverpool Royal Infirmary 191
  Marie Curie Hospital for Cancer
    and Allied Diseases 267
  records 65, 148
  Royal London Hospital 300
  scandal 92–4, 112, 156, 165,
    292n.33
  voluntary hospitals 259, 313
  Westminster Hospital 278, 320
  Westmoreland Lock Hospital
    259, 264
House of Commons 99, 191, 204,
    327
House of Lords 100, 206
humour 232, 235–6, 240, 241
Hutchinson, Jonathan 309
hysteria 98, 99, 312
  hysterical 199, 325

Ibsen, Henrik 303, 305–6, 315,
    318
  *Ghosts* 303, 305
    Helen Alving 307
    Oswald Alving 305, 308
illness experience 2, 4–5, 9, 229,
    231, 234, 235, 241
imperial 111, 301–2
  crisis 301
  masculinity 302
institutions 62–3, 66, 68, 73, 79,
    94, 95, 97, 99, 105–8,
    112, 125–47, 155, 256–9,
    264, 279–80, 285,
    292n.33, 307, 323
  authority 8, 140, 276
  care 172, 197, 301

institutionalisation 14, 18, 108,
    102, 130
  psychiatric 21, 95, 125–8,
    131–3, 146
  space 127–9, 133, 140, 142–7
  welfare 262
Interdepartmental Committee on
    Physical Deterioration
    301–2
Iron Lung 187–90, 192, 197,
    200–1, 212, 213n.3,
    217n.76
  *see also* Both, Edward T.,
    Both iron lung

Kandinsky, Saloman 278
Kenealy, Arabella 306–7
Kerridge, Phyllis 190–2
Ketton-Cremer, Robert Wyndham
    69
Kirkpatrick, Thomas Percy Claude
    256–86
  correspondence 256, 260–5,
    272–3, 275
  father–confessor 272–5
  feminine / femininity 266–7,
    269–70, 284
  masculine / masculinity 265–7,
    284
  petitioning 281
  practice 258
  record-keeping 260

Lacks, Henrietta 69
*Lancet* 11, 41, 101, 201, 205,
    207–8, 226, 306
legalism 92, 111
Legion of Mary Catholic Girls'
    Hostel 262
letters 21–2, 49, 67, 96, 98, 104,
    155, 158, 161–9, 166–7,
    172–3, 178n.33, 224,
    239, 255, 258, 260–86,
    261, 290n.23, 318
lice 224, 226, 230, 232, 235–6,
    239–41

# Index

Lin, Maya 70
London School of Hygiene and Tropical Medicine 190, 313
Lowndes, Frederick W. 306
Lunacy Acts
  1845 97, 125, 130
  1890 92, 95, 101, 109, 112
Lunacy Commission 97, 130
  Commissioners 97–100, 109, 128, 144
Lunacy Law Amendment Association (LLAA) 99, 101–2
Lunacy Law Reform Association (LLRA) 99–102, 112
lunatics' rights activism 92, 93, 95, 102, 107

McIndoe, Archibald 70
madhouse literature 113
Mass Observation (MO) 299, 305, 318–19, 324
maternity 281
Max Weber 76
medical care 17–19, 53, 67, 74, 77, 156, 158, 168, 173, 258, 269, 304, 308, 312–13, 315
  physiotherapy 199–200
  placebo 42, 46, 52, 322
  radiotherapy 193, 267
  therapy 106, 129–33, 185, 203–9, 275, 322
  treatment 3, 5, 8, 17, 18, 36, 42–4, 54, 64, 66, 71, 94, 98, 103–5, 108, 109, 113, 125–6, 131, 133–4, 136, 139, 145–7, 161, 168–71, 173, 188, 194–5, 199, 201–2, 205–6, 208–9, 255–60, 264–8, 270–3, 275, 279–81, 283, 285–6, 299–300, 308–9, 313, 316–18, 320–1, 326
medical data 68, 81

medical records / patient records 21, 48, 65, 68–71, 102, 125, 129, 133, 135, 224, 255, 278, 301, 304, 327–8
Medical Research Council (MRC) 47, 185, 187–8, 191, 193–5, 197, 207
  Respirators (Poliomyelitis) Committee 192
*Medicine Without Doctors* 41–2
Men, Women and Care project 63–4, 68, 71, 73
military medicine 8, 16, 226–7, 229–30
Ministry of Health 160, 191–2, 278, 299, 311
Ministry of Pensions 63, 66–8, 77
modernity 65, 76–7, 93, 226
morality 304, 311, 314, 316, 325
moral treatment / moral therapy 127–31, 134, 136, 146
Mott, Frederick 308
mud 224, 232–3, 240–1

National Council for Combatting Venereal Diseases (NCCVD) 304, 315, 331n.31
  *see also* British Social Hygiene Council
National Health Service (NHS) 5–6, 7, 10, 16, 18, 34, 36–7, 47, 48, 52, 53, 55n.8, 68, 102, 157, 148, 157, 160–1, 188, 204, 206, 211–12, 297n.114, 327
  Patient Experience Framework 147
national prayer days 40
National Trust 69
nausea 38
negative pressure 187–8, 191, 193, 201, 217

# 344  Index

New Woman, the 303, 305, 307, 312
noise 186, 190, 194, 205
'Not to call the doctor' 52
nutrition 20, 135, 193

O'Brien, Brian 283–4
occupational identity 134, 137, 141–2
over-the-counter medicines 35, 36, 39, 44, 45–8
oxygen 185–6, 188, 192, 202–13

pain 1, 21, 34, 38, 39–40, 69, 70, 193, 197, 227, 232–3, 267–8, 270, 275, 278, 281, 303, 305, 309–10, 319, 323, 325
Parliamentary and Health Service Ombudsman 148
patent medicines 38, 42, 45–6, 48, 51–2, 57n.37
patient
  case notes / case books 3, 67, 125–6, 128, 133–42, 145–7, 199–200, 212, 230, 302, 315
  clinical encounter 3, 5, 11, 16, 18, 21, 285, 301, 309
  confidentiality 65, 67, 278–9, 308
  co-operation 208, 210
  expert by experience 102, 106, 186, 195, 273
  gender 111, 256, 263–4, 266, 285, 307, 315–16, 318, 325
  groups 9, 92, 165, 174–5
  non-patient 21, 22, 33–5, 36–8, 43–4, 48–50, 52–4, 111, 262, 313
  outpatient 95, 156, 264
  rights 77, 92, 94–5, 102, 107, 110, 111–13, 158, 161, 174

  view 54, 147, 154–5, 161, 173, 224–5, 228
Paul, Robert W. 184
pauper 129, 155, 158, 160–2, 164–6, 173–4
  letter 155, 158, 161, 162–4, 166–9, 172–3
  lunatics 99, 101, 130
pensions 61–8, 71–2, 76–80
personal correspondence 66, 200, 255, 274, 315
phenomenology 302
physiology 47, 229–31, 272
Poliomyelitis / Polio 186, 188, 191–3, 195, 197, 199, 201, 203
Poor Law 8, 15, 21, 87n.54, 155, 157–67, 172, 313
  union 159–69, 171–3, 177n.24
  workhouse 112, 130, 158–9, 161–2, 164–6, 169–71, 173–4
positive pressure 184, 187, 189, 191, 193, 195, 215n.35
Porter, Roy 1–2, 4, 5, 8, 13, 14, 20, 33, 37, 41–2, 55, 93, 95, 113, 132, 154, 223
Powell, Arthur 313–14
power 7, 9, 11, 18, 19, 38, 39, 41, 42, 47–8, 63, 66, 70, 72, 77, 80, 82, 100, 136, 158, 161–2, 171–2, 174, 183, 192–4, 224, 226–8, 230, 234, 236–7, 241–3, 256, 269, 277, 303, 311–12, 322, 327
  coercive 100, 112, 159
  contesting 158, 161, 171, 174
prayer 34, 39–41, 46, 269
pregnant 169, 197, 199, 306, 309
privacy 14, 65–6, 73, 75–80, 184, 210, 279, 291n.23
private madhouse 92, 101
privatisation 211–12
prosthetic 186–7, 194, 200, 202

protest 9, 78, 91, 95, 105, 108, 112, 173, 278
Prudential Insurance, Ltd 262
psychiatry 93–5, 102, 108, 110, 111, 113, 130, 132, 154
  anti-psychiatry 106, 110–11
  criticism of 92–3, 111
public sphere 65, 76, 78–81, 109
public's view 36–7

quack 42, 43, 46, 57n.37, 58n.39, 238, 313, 320, 328
  charlatanism 313
  irregular practice 194, 313, 328
quality of life 201–2, 204, 206–9

rejection 195, 210
relapsing fever 224
religion 39–41, 56n.22, 277, 324
  church 39, 41, 168, 257–8, 276, 321, 324
  faith 39–40, 48, 173, 238, 267, 272–4, 278, 317, 322, 323
  guilt 276, 314, 317, 321, 323–6
  sin 276, 324
*Report on Taking Medicines in War-Time* 50
resistance 9, 14, 15, 18, 21–2, 113, 139–41, 147, 166, 209, 223, 230–1
respiration 183–5, 188, 192, 195, 199, 203
  artificial 183–5, 188, 192, 195, 199
  natural 195
respirator 185, 186–92, 195, 197, 199–200, 203
  Barospirator 192
  Biomotor 192
  breathing machine 183, 185–7, 192, 194–5, 197, 201, 203
  Burstall Jacket respirator 192, 198
  Cuirass respirator 192

Emerson respirator 192
Henderson respirator 192
Laffer Lewis Apparatus 192
mechanical respirator 185–7, 189, 199, 203
Siebe–Gorman 'drinker' respirator 192
respiratory 5, 183, 185, 186–204, 208–10, 216n.47
  disability 185, 201
  illness 204, 209
  paralysis 183, 186, 188, 191, 195, 199
restraint 99, 129, 134, 234
resuscitator 183
Routh, Armand 308
Royal Army Medical College 229, 325
Royal Army Medical Corps 61, 230
Royal College of Physicians of Ireland 258, 260
Royal Commission on Venereal Diseases (RCVD) 255, 259, 278, 283, 308
Royal Historical Society 81

Schramm, Cyril 73, 74
Second Boer War 301
Second World War 67, 197, 299
'Secret Remedies' 46
self-
  advocacy 91–4, 107–11, 113, 156, 168
  care 4, 5, 19, 42, 52–3, 225, 243n.13
  diagnosis 5, 6, 33, 54, 270
  medication 48, 50, 337n.125
  narratives 93
  treatment 6, 36, 42, 53–4
Self Care Forum 36, 53
separation *see* divorce
Serocalcin 50
sexual double standard 272, 303, 305, 307, 314–15, 317, 318

sexual health *see* venereal disease
sexuality 7, 69, 256, 263, 276, 285, 327
  historiography 257
  Irish 257–8, 276
  purity 283–4, 305
  urban–rural divide 283–4
sexual knowledge 271–3, 308, 310–12, 315, 317–19, 322–3
*Shafts* 305, 312
  Nora Brownlow 312
shame 17–18, 22, 69, 74–5, 78, 210, 255, 257, 270, 275, 279, 300, 302, 308, 313, 319–20, 323–4, 326
Sinn Féin 283–4
  Public Health Committee 283
  *Public Health Circular* 283
smoke
  smokers 208
  smoking 207–8, 210
social control 4, 131, 146, 308
social movement 93, 107, 109, 112
Social Welfare Act 1952 (Ireland) 282
soldiers 5, 8, 22, 57n.38, 74, 223–42, 248n.86, 283
Solomons, Bethel 281
speaking out 108–9, 111
spiritualism 97–9
standardisation 76, 95, 187
standardising 17, 194
stigma 8, 17–18, 20, 22–3, 36, 62–3, 70, 98, 105, 108, 206–7, 210, 255, 278–9, 284, 300, 305, 319–20, 326–7
  stigmatising 4, 7, 18, 21, 66, 74, 256–8, 268, 272–4, 276, 301, 312
  stigmatisation 14, 111, 324
  taboo 271, 299, 326
suicide 97, 104, 156, 167, 313–14
'symptom iceberg' 6, 34, 35, 38–9, 52

syphilis 18, 259, 278, 283, 299, 301–16, 319–20, 322–4
  congenital 306–7, 312, 314–15, 320
  mercury 309, 316, 322
  salvarsan 273, 315, 322
  spirochete 315
  syphilophobia 302–4, 311–14, 319, 321–5, 330n.18
  neurological 325
  Wassermann (*blood test*) 271, 273, 314–15, 321

trauma 5, 14, 66, 199, 224, 234–5, 239, 242, 300, 310, 326
travel 6, 158, 169, 211
  distance 156, 168–9, 224, 270
  time 169
trench fever 224, 232, 246n.42
trench foot 224, 229, 232, 234, 235, 237, 238, 246n.42
Tuke, William 131
typhus 168, 224, 230

UNESCO Recommendation Concerning the Status of Higher–Education Teaching Personnel (1997) 81

VD *see* venereal disease
venereal disease 8, 18, 22, 36, 66, 74, 259, 269, 283, 292n.31, 295n.89, 299, 300, 302–4, 306, 308, 310, 320, 330n.18, 331n.31
  class 268–9, 271, 277, 307, 320
  emotional impact 268–9, 279, 302–4, 306, 310, 328
  fiction 302–4, 306–7, 310, 331n.31
  melodrama 304, 307, 332n.34

health-education films 304,
    315–18, 325, 331n.31
  *Test for Love* 316
  *Trial for Marriage* 316–18
infertility 306
knowledge of 271, 310, 318
miscarriage 306
promiscuity 311
propaganda 299, 304, 311,
    315, 319, 322, 324,
    331n.31
psychological impact 301–4,
    306, 311, 321–2
  melancholic 325
VD Service 255, 257, 263, 278,
    294n.73, 304, 313, 315,
    317, 322, 326–7

VD clinics 259–60, 263–4,
    266, 269, 274, 279,
    291–2n.31, 300, 314–17,
    319–20, 323
venereal infection *see* venereal
    disease
vernacular medicine 225, 228,
    236, 238–9, 242
Visiting Committee 133, 146
vomiting 38, 195, 197
  *see also* nausea

Wellcome Library 61
whooping cough 44–5

York Retreat 127, 131

EU authorised representative for GPSR:
Easy Access System Europe, Mustamäe tee 50,
10621 Tallinn, Estonia
gpsr.requests@easproject.com